Understanding Voice Problems

A Physiological Perspective for Diagnosis and Treatment

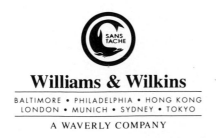

Williams & Wilkins

BALTIMORE • PHILADELPHIA • HONG KONG
LONDON • MUNICH • SYDNEY • TOKYO

A WAVERLY COMPANY

Understanding Voice Problems

A Physiological Perspective for Diagnosis and Treatment

RAYMOND H. COLTON, Ph.D.

Professor of Otolaryngology and Communication Sciences
Department of Otolaryngology and Communication Sciences
SUNY Health Science Center at Syracuse
Syracuse, New York

JANINA K. CASPER, Ph.D.

Associate Professor of Otolaryngology and Communication Sciences
Department of Otolaryngology and Communication Sciences
SUNY Health Science Center at Syracuse
Syracuse, New York

With contributions from
MINORU HIRANO, M.D.

Professor and Chairman
Department of Otolaryngology—Head and Neck Surgery
Kurume University School of Medicine
Kurume, Japan

Color photography by Eijii Yanagisawa, M.D.

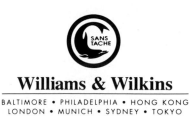

Williams & Wilkins

BALTIMORE • PHILADELPHIA • HONG KONG
LONDON • MUNICH • SYDNEY • TOKYO

A WAVERLY COMPANY

Editor: John P. Butler
Associate Editor: Linda Napora
Project Editor: Rebecca Marnhout
Designer: JoAnne Janowiak
Illustration Planner: Ray Lowman
Production Coordinator: Charles E. Zeller

Copyright © 1990
Williams & Wilkins
428 East Preston Street
Baltimore, Maryland 21202, USA

Printed in the United States of America

Library of Congress Cataloging-in-Publication Data

Colton, Raymond H.
    Understanding voice problems: a physiological perspective for diagnosis and treatment / Raymond H. Colton, Janina K. Casper; with contributions from Minoru Hirano.
        p.   cm.
    Bibliography: p.
    Includes index.
    ISBN 0-683-02058-7
    1. Voice disorders—Pathophysiology.   I. Casper, Janina K.   II. Hirano, Minoru, 1932-   . III. Title.
    [DNLM: 1. Larynx—physiology. 2.Voice Disorders—diagnosis. 3. Voice Disorders—therapy.   WV 500 C725u]
    RF510.C65   1990
    616.2′2—dc20
    DNLM/DLC
    for Library of Congress   89-9170
                                                                                          CIP

94

7   8   9   10

To David W. Brewer, M.D.
our teacher, colleague, friend, and
a fine human being

PREFACE

Ten years ago books on the topic of the voice and its disorders were few and far between. Happily for those of us who have found this a fascinating and rewarding area of work and study, the past decade has witnessed a miniexplosion of interest in, study of, and writing about the voice by clinicians, scientists, and physicians. Specialization in the study and treatment of voice gained even further recognition with the 1987 initiation of the *Journal of Voice*, devoted solely to articles pertinent to the topic. Even further subspecialization is taking place as some practitioners delve into the unique needs and problems of the professional voice user. We are indebted to those who pioneered and pursued an interest in phonation, in how the larynx works, and in how to alter or correct its function, despite the critical attitude of some who found these attempts lacking in scientific stringency. Their persistence, coupled with major technological advances, has resulted in significant enlargement of the scientific knowledge base of the study of laryngeal function. However, even with this growth of interest in the study of the voice, we have been dismayed by its continuing stepchild status in training programs for speech-language pathologists and otolaryngologists. On the other hand, we have been heartened by the growing numbers of practitioners in these fields and, also, of voice coaches of both the singing and speaking voice who attend conferences and courses in search of greater knowledge and understanding about the voice and its disorders.

Why this book? We have been fortunate in being part of a multidisciplinary team that has studied normal and disordered phonation both clinically and experimentally for many years. Through this experience we have evolved a philosophy and framework for the examination of laryngeal function and for clinical management of the voice-disordered patient that we believe differs from others in its emphasis. Over the years we have presented our ideas in many lectures and courses and, if we are to judge by feedback received, have found our approach to be well received and helpful, especially to those who routinely work with the voice. It seemed appropriate, thus, to prepare this book, which we intend to be used by students and practitioners alike in all of the specialty areas involved in the management of the voice, including otolaryngology, speech pathology, and coaching of the singing and dramatic voice. If not used as a text for study, we would hope that this book would be used as a reference text by other medical specialists, such as pediatricians, family practitioners, and internists, who might be the first to come in contact with a voice-disordered patient.

We believe that understanding voice disorders must begin with an understanding of normal phonatory physiology and acoustics. Based on such knowledge, it is then possible to understand the pathophysiology that results from misuse, abuse, pathology, or neurological involvement. Because there is not a one-to-one relationship between physiology and acoustics, it is not possible to predict specific pathology or alterations in physiology on the basis of acoustics or perception alone. Thus, neither acoustic nor perceptual data are sufficient for the diagnosis and treatment of voice disorders. Knowledge of the pathophysiology together with understanding the acoustic and perceptual factors and individual psychodynamics must all be added to the equation in determining diagnosis and planning treatment.

We are firm advocates of the differential diagnosis model and have attempted to emphasize that throughout the text. A differential diagnosis can only be carried out if it is based on knowledge. Indeed, one of the fascinations of the area of voice is the amalgamation of knowledge from various fields that must be brought to bear on the diagnostic process. The team approach is thus an ideal mechanism to support this need. The approach to management has at its core the normalization of physiology, which we believe will bring with it normalized phonation. When normalization is not a realistic goal due to structural or neuromotor constraints, then the approach builds on making the most of what remains functional. The choice of therapy technique is predicated upon a knowledge-based problem-solving approach, rather than on an uninformed gunshot approach. The ''if it works, use it'' approach may be successful occasionally but may be totally inappropriate at other times. It is important to know when to use a technique and to be able to at least speculate about why it works or fails to do so. The clinician must understand the nature of the altered physiology, must take into account the psychological dynamics that may be operative, and must then be able to select an appropriate approach to rehabilitation that will address these issues. The intertwined relationship between the voice and the person is an essential component in both diagnosis and management. However, even in the patient with a psychologically based voice disorder, the deviations in the manner of voice production and voice use must be understood. In writing this book we have presumed that the reader will have been exposed to the study of laryngeal anatomy, physiology, neuroanatomy, and neurophysiology. Therefore, the chapters dealing with these topics appear at the end of the book and are designed to be sources of reference rather than extensive teaching chapters.

There is much written about the voice that has yet to be substantiated by experimental data. We have made note of such gaps in our knowledge base in many parts of the book. We have also chosen to put ourselves out on a limb by raising questions about some long-held beliefs. In doing so, we have brought to bear whatever data are available to support our positions, and where data have been lacking, we have had to rely on theoretical constructs. Although some differences exist in the types of voice problems that occur at various points along the life-span, we have chosen to embed that information wherever appropriate in the text, rather than to devote entire chapters to specific age groupings. Similarly, we have not set aside a chapter specific to the problems of the professional voice user; there is liberal mention made of matters specific to that group throughout the chapters.

We have confined ourselves to those problems having laryngeal integrity and function at their core. Thus, there is little discussion of the difficulties with voice experienced by the deaf and by those with severe hearing impairment. Although we have come to learn that there may be physiological differences in phonation between the hearing and the (congenitally) deaf, the problem usually lies primarily in the absence of acoustic input, not in abnormality of the larynx. For the same reason we have excluded discussion of the resonance problems of hyper- and hyponasality. The velopharyngeal mechanism and the anatomical structures involved in that mechanism are at the core of most resonance problems, rather than the phonatory mechanism. Another problem area that is absent from this book is that of the patient without a larynx. The phonatory demands of that population require the learning of an alternative mode of sound production that can no longer involve the larynx. Such problems are unique to this group and are well and thoroughly covered in other readily available publications.

Chapter 1 introduces the study of the larynx, beginning with its important biological functions. The uniqueness of our human ability to speak is dependent in part on the ability of the larynx to produce the acoustic signal we call voice. The changes in that signal that accompany life-span changes are reviewed, as is voice production. The team approach to the diagnosis and management of voice disorders is introduced. Chapter 2 is key to the philosophy of this book. We have approached the process of differential diagnosis in the manner usually experienced in the real world when the patient presents with certain symptoms. We follow the process through the steps that the practitioner must pursue in narrowing the possibilities until a diagnosis and etiology are assigned. Case studies are presented as an aid to understanding the process. Our scheme rests on eight primary symptoms of disorders of voice and expands from there to the various signs—perceptual, acoustic, physiologic, laryngoscopic, and stroboscopic—that would be consistent with the symptom.

In Chapter 3 Dr. Minoru Hirano discusses the histology of laryngeal structures and the histopathology of laryngeal lesions. Chapter 4 addresses misuse and abuse of the larynx, with a focus on the physiological effects related to specific behaviors. One of the unique aspects of this book is a lengthy section in this chapter devoted to the effects of drugs on the voice. The use of over-the-counter as well as prescription drugs is extensive. Their effects on the laryngeal mucosa have been largely overlooked. There is still a paucity of experimental evidence about these effects. Voice problems associated with nervous system involvement are discussed in Chapter 5. Although voice problems in this population are extensive, the available data on the acoustic parameters of the voice or the physiological parameters of airflow and laryngeal muscle action potentials are exceedingly limited.

Chapter 6 is devoted to a discussion of voice problems associated with organic disease and trauma. These are areas about which the speech pathologist must be knowledgeable, even though voice therapy may only occasionally be an appropriate treatment modality. An extensive section on taking the voice history introduces Chapter 7, and its length emphasizes our concern about the relatively minimal training speech-language pathologists and otolaryngologists usually receive in this critical area of communication between patient and practitioner. The remainder of the chapter is given over to descriptions and discussion of methods of laryngeal examination and testing procedures, both instrumental and noninstrumental. Dr. Hirano's discussion of phonosurgery, the surgical management of voice problems, is the topic of Chapter 8.

The focus of Chapter 9 is vocal rehabilitation, the primary method used to alter phonatory behavior. The chapter begins with a discussion of some general concepts, principles, and guidelines that we feel are critical to the undertaking of a vocal rehabilitation program. The role of voice therapy in the treatment of disorders associated with voice misuse or abuse, pathology, neuromotor involvement, and some unusual problems is discussed. A variety of specific treatment techniques are offered. Each is described, and a rationale for its usefulness is provided. Some controversial areas related to voice therapy and some unresolved issues are discussed, and the final sections of this chapter briefly address the issues of prevention and malpractice.

Chapters 10 to 12 were described earlier as reference chapters. They deal with the anatomy, physiology, and neuroanatomy and neurophysiology of the vocal mechanism, in that order. It is our intent that these chapters be referred to frequently as a differential diagnosis is pursued. Chapter 13, the final reference chapter, provides normative data against which patient data can be compared. By placing this material in a separate chapter, we have made it readily accessible for reference use. And finally, the Appendix offers a variety of forms and protocols that we have found to be useful in our assessment and examination procedures.

As much as possible, we have attempted to construct our sentences so as to avoid the use of sex-specific pronouns. When this attempt resulted in convoluted language structure that became an obstacle to understanding, we have chosen to use gender pronouns (i.e., his or her) interchangeably. The reader should be aware that despite the particular pronoun used, we are speaking of both sexes unless it is clearly stated otherwise. Furthermore, because this book is intended for a broad audience, we have adopted the use of the English alphabet rather than phonetic symbols to describe vowel sounds (such as /ee/ for the sound in ''see'').

We are indebted to Minoru Hirano, M.D., for his valued additions to this book with the chapters on histopathology (Chapter 3) and on surgical intervention (Chapter 8). Dr. Hirano has been a leader and innovator in the study of vocal fold physiology and in many other aspects of the study of the larynx and the voice.

Many others have helped in diverse ways with the preparation of this book. Dr. David W. Brewer has, throughout the years, been a source of constant support and encouragement, and he has been so for this project as well. We thank him for that and for his insightful reading and critique of much of the text. We acknowledge the help of Samuel Mallov, Ph.D., Professor Emeritus of Pharmacology, SUNY Health Science Center at Syracuse, who checked the accuracy of our comments about the effects of drugs on the voice. Martha Hefner, medical illustrator at the SUNY Health Science Center, along with Elinor Griep, Brian Harris, and Craig Palmer, provided splendid illustrative material, and always with a smile. We are grateful for the generosity of Eiji Yanagisawa, M.D., in sharing with us his superb photographic skills. Others have read various sections of the manuscript in preparation and have given us valuable direction. We wish to thank Peak Woo, M.D., Fran Lowry, Carol Friedenberg, Herbert N. Wright, and Joanne Chilton.

We each have families who have been supportive and patient throughout this process. They have been deprived of attention, of our presence, and of the availability of the computer, but not of our gratitude and love.

CONTENTS

PREFACE vii
COLOR PLATES xiii

1   Introduction and Overview 1

2   Differential Diagnosis of Voice Problems 11

3   Laryngeal Histopathology 51

4   Voice Misuse and Abuse: Effects on Laryngeal
    Physiology 73

5   Voice Problems Associated with Nervous System
    Involvement 107

6   Voice Problems Associated with Organic Disease
    and Trauma 151

7   The Voice History, Examination, and Testing 165

8   Surgical and Medical Management of Voice Disorders . . 211

9   Vocal Rehabilitation 235

10   Anatomy of the Vocal Mechanism 271

11   Phonatory Physiology 285

12 Neuroanatomy of the Vocal Mechanism 297

13 Some Normative Data on the Voice 309

    APPENDIX: FORMS USED IN VOICE EVALUATION
    LABORATORY AND COMMUNICATION DISORDER UNIT 317

    REFERENCES 329

    INDEX 347

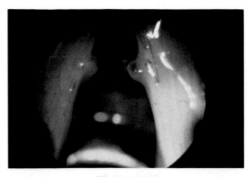

Figure 4.1.

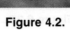

Figure 4.2.

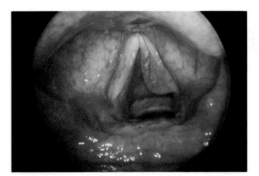

Figure 4.3.

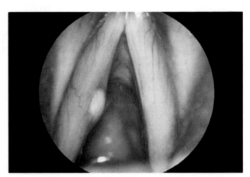

Figure 4.4.

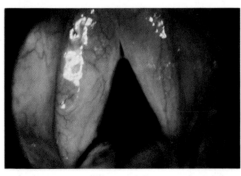

Figure 4.5.

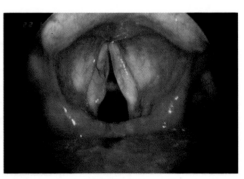

Figure 4.6.

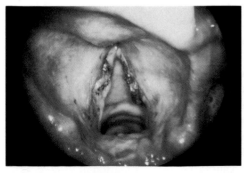

Figure 6.1.

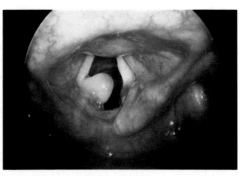

Figure 6.2A.

reflect the unique place of speech in human existence. Clear evidence of this evolution is seen in the multiplicity of the protective laryngeal reflex mechanisms. It is important to recognize that these protective "natural" acts may sometimes be the cause of a voice disorder. For example, excessive coughing, a protective act, can result in trauma to the vocal folds and cause edema, which in turn will interfere with the vibratory characteristics of the vocal folds. By the same token, rapid, random movements of the vocal folds at rest may interfere with normal vibratory motion. Central neurological dysfunction or disruption in a reflex arc may create abnormal motions, which may interfere with phonation or, indeed, threaten life.

The biological function of the larynx can never be ignored. The otolaryngologist who accidently touches the back wall of the pharynx when performing an indirect mirror examination can attest to the rapid reflexive motions of the pharynx and larynx that result from the "gag" reflex. But the reflex or biological functions of the larynx can be subtle in their effects and less apparent to both the untrained and the experienced eye. Many reflex endings are sensitive to small changes of movement or air pressure that serve to inform the central nervous system about the normal operation of the airway. The respiratory cycle itself and the activity of the nerve controlling the diaphragm may be affected by these changes. They also affect the discharge pattern of the intrinsic laryngeal muscles. The effects of these subtle changes are important to consider for an understanding of the physiology of normal voice production.

We are still young in our understanding of the physiology of the human body. Our fascination with modern instrumentation has produced a good deal of information about human voice production (Baken, 1987). Nevertheless,the fundamental mechanisms of bodily function and regulation must not be ignored. Reflexes are primitive neural control subsystems. They operate at a very low level in the hierarchy of neural functioning and control large muscle actions. But these mechanisms are always there, waiting in the wings, so to speak, to alter body function. Our awareness and appreciation of their role should be apparent to us and to our patients if we are truly to understand human voice function.

The Larynx and the Voice

The voice is an integral part of that uniquely human attribute known as speech. The larynx and its capabilities are important in two broad areas: biological function and speech. The larynx houses the major source of sound used during speaking. The vocal folds produce a tone that becomes modified by the pharynx, palate, tongue, and lips to produce the individual sounds of speech. Voice is present for all normally produced vowels and for half of the consonants. The point in time at which the vocal folds begin to vibrate relative to the movement of the other articulators (i.e., lips, tongue, palate, etc.) is critical if the speaker is to produce the intended sound. The larynx must operate in close synchrony with other parts of the speech production apparatus if intelligible speech is to be produced. Although the voice is not visible to the eye during speech production, its absence or malfunction is obvious.

In addition to its role as a carrier of words, the voice is a producer of musicality; it is also an expresser of emotion and acts as a mirror on persons' inner selves. The singer with superb control of the vocal instrument brings immense pleasure to the listener. Although the singer's words may be conveying a message, the phrasing, control of pitch, and dynamic range may communicate even more strongly. In classical singing, for example, it is the rare listener who is not enthralled by the sound of a clear and beautiful high C, sung with ease, power, and majesty. The singing of a choir or the chanting of prayers can lead to a unique religious experience.

The actor's voice, resonant and full of meaning, can add significantly to the message and the intensity of emotion. Indeed, the actor's delivery of the words can sometimes be more engrossing to the listener than the words themselves.

The voice serves as an emotional outlet valve. Laughter and crying are both releasers of emotion and frequently serve important cathartic functions. Shouts of joy and screams of rage or fear convey meanings that are easily recognized.

The voice reveals the inner self. It is a reflection of the personality of the individual. We recognize the stereotypical driving, hard-hitting voice of the salesperson, the nasal singsong of the perpetual whiner, and the monotonous de-energized voice of the depressed. The voice of an outgoing person may be characterized by variety in the pitch, loudness, or quality. On the other hand, a monotone voice, one with little variety, may characterize the withdrawn individual or the loner who wishes not to be disturbed. Markel and his colleagues (1964, 1973) have shown that the pitch, loudness, and tempo of the voice can be used to reflect the personality of the individual and correlate well with other standardized tests of personality measurement.

The speaker's voice is used to attract as well as repel people. The soft, "soothing" voice is more apt to calm an agitated person than a strident and loud voice. On the other hand, a strident, loud voice may be effectively used to repel someone. How many times have we used the loud, "firm" voice to dispense with a pushy salesperson or avert a physically threatening situation?

The voice can reveal a person's physical state, as well as the physical state of the larynx. The weak or tremulous voice identified with illness is easily identified, and the voice altered by laryngeal pathology is identified as abnormal.

Yes, the voice is a powerful tool that not only delivers the message but also adds to its meaning. In learning to understand the voice, it is not enough to understand its mechanical functioning. It is also necessary to recognize the important information the voice conveys about the speaker.

Voice Changes in Life

The voice changes dynamically, minute by minute. But there are long-term changes that are associated with growth and decline in life. At the major stages of life, the uses of the voice are different, as are the demands placed upon it. The reasons for these differences are many and include biological maturation and the emotional and social changes that occur in the individual's life.

The Voice in Infancy and Childhood

In the first few weeks of life, the infant voice is used to express pain, pleasure, displeasure, and hunger. Crying, the major avenue of communication for the infant, is rich in its ability to communicate (Lester, 1985).

Crying reflects the beginning ability of the infant to control his or her voice. It is a gross physical act that can be described as ballistic in nature. In other words, crying, once started, runs its time course and stops. Little can be done to stop the crying once it has begun. As the child grows older, he is more responsive to the environment and also gains more control of the physical apparatus used to produce the cry. Consequently, crying is seen to reflect physical and psychological growth. As the child gains finer and finer motor control, the cry becomes increasingly controllable and much more purposeful in its usage.

The next most obvious voice use change occurs as the child begins to use the voice in the production of speech sounds. Concurrently, the child is learning the sounds of his specific language. Then, the child can use the voice to express ideas and moods. As the child matures, increasingly complex and sophisticated differentiation of acceptable modes of vocal behavior develop. This differentiation begins in infancy. The child's vocal response to a caretaker's familiar voice differs from that to an unfamiliar voice. Generally, the child's vocal response differs based on the familiarity of the voice heard. Children learn that the voice of the playground is not the voice of the classroom. Such differentiation continues through life in many subtle ways.

The voice reflects the physical development of the child. The young infant possesses a larynx that is pliable and has a low level of neuromuscular coordination. It is also small, with short vocal folds. The small structure means that the pitch of the infant's voice will be high. The infant's ability to control the tension of the vocal folds is limited. Moreover, the limited ability of the infant to control the air pressure required for speech results in short bursts of sound, much of which is rather loud. As the child grows, the ability to control vocal pitch and loudness increases (Boone,1987). This development is reflected in the longer cries, which are lower in pitch and vary in loudness depending on the circumstances.

In summary, during infancy and childhood the characteristics of the voice depend on the degree of physical, cognitive, and emotional maturation exhibited by the child. The physical size of the vocal folds is a major determinant of the fundamental frequency of the child's voice. The infant, with a small larynx and short vocal folds, exhibits the highest vocal pitch, whereas the older child, whose larynx has grown, possesses a lower vocal pitch. Adult vocal pitch is not attained until puberty, when the larynx reaches its adult size.

Loudness variation is less affected by these growth changes and more affected by the level of motor control exhibited by the child. Quality variation reflects physical growth changes of the vocal folds, changes in the size and shape of the entire vocal tract, and finer control of the neuromuscular system. Differentiation of appropriate voice use characteristics depends not only on physical abilities but also on cognitive and social growth and awareness.

The Voice of the Adult

By age 18 years or so, the voice reaches its mature or adult stage. The fundamental frequency is about where it will remain for several decades. The individual has full control over the dynamic range (loudness) of the voice and can produce many variations of pitch and voice quality. These vocal abilities reflect the maturation of the anatomical and physiological systems for the support of speech (Kahane, 1982).

Although the adult voice has been attained by age 18 years, there is still much refinement that can occur to expand vocal abilities. Indeed, vocal training for the singer or the actor most appropriately begins when this level of maturation has been reached. Pitch range can be extended, vocal control can be increased, and voice quality can be enriched.

The way the voice is used depends on the demands of the situation. These demands may include the teacher's need to instruct and maintain discipline, the minister's need to deliver a forceful sermon or to be consoling, the salesperson's need to sell a product, and so on.

It is easy to take the voice for granted. Often we abuse it with constant use and frequent misuse. We abuse it with smoke and alcohol and expect it to be unaffected. It is only when we experience difficulty talking that we cease taking it for granted and seek help. Often we have difficulty recognizing abusive habits and making the necessary changes, even when our lives are threatened.

The Aged Voice

After 65 years of age or so, the voice begins its decline, much the same way other body functions begin their decline (Beasley and Davis, 1981; Kahane, 1981). The voice, however, does not always mirror the extreme or rapid changes that may occur in the physical functioning of the body. Aged individuals in good physical condition possess voices that are similar in their characteristics to the voices of those of younger persons (Ramig and Ringel,1983). Some singers can maintain their voices well into the 70s. The voice may retain the essential elements of beauty, although it may not exhibit the range or degree of vocal control that was present in younger years.

But for others, the voice readily betrays the effects of aging. Voices that show a decline or increase of vocal pitch, decreased control of loudness, or changes of voice quality may be showing signs of diminished physical status. Acoustic changes such as upward or downward frequency shifts, poorly controlled loudness, and quality changes reflect to some degree the physiological changes that occur in the larynx with increasing age.

The vocal demands of the aged adult are different from those of the younger adult. After retirement, the salesperson no longer must use that voice to sell a product. The retired minister no longer has to deliver that forceful Sunday sermon. The decline of bodily function is usually accompanied by reduced demand on the system. That is not to say that the voice is no longer important to the elderly. On the contrary, the voice is important, but in a different way. It retains its importance in the communication process. It is used to maintain contact with friends and relatives. For some individuals, verbal communication is the only way to maintain human contact and control the environment.

Production of the Voice

To most laypeople, the way in which the voice is produced is a mystery. The term "voice box" is commonly used to refer to the larynx, the voice-generating mechanism. Most people know they have one and that it is somewhere in the throat below the chin. From experience they know that when they have laryngitis, they cannot talk, or their voices sound "funny," but few understand why those changes occur. Some people may be aware that after strenuous voice use, such as yelling at a sports event, their voices may sound hoarse. They surmise that the hoarseness has to do with "straining" the voice. Some people may even realize they can manipulate their voices in many ways, for example, raise or lower pitch, increase or decrease loudness, and change their voice quality. This is such common knowledge that it is taken for granted without thought about the workings of the mechanism that is capable of producing such changes.

Understanding phonatory physiology goes beyond knowing laryngeal anatomy and recognizing various laryngeal pathologies (Kahane, 1982; Aronson, 1985). Treatment of the voice-disordered patient demands such a knowledge base. Disturbed physiology may be a by-product of pathology and may persist after the pathological condition is resolved. On the other hand, disturbed physiology may be the cause of tissue changes. Whatever the treatment modality, restoration of normal function, or the closest possible approximation of it, is the goal.

The basic concepts of phonatory physiology have been understood for many years (van den Berg, 1958; Lieberman, 1968). Recent technological advances have, however, significantly increased our knowledge base (Kahane, 1981; Hirano, 1981b). The inaccessibility of the larynx, especially during the phonatory act, has hindered our ability to understand its functioning more fully. In 1855 Garcia developed the laryngeal mirror (Garcia,

1855; Moore, 1937) and made it possible to visualize the larynx with the naked eye. Since then, greatly improved techniques of laryngeal visualization as well as sophisticated analyses of laryngeal acoustics and improved methods of measuring physiological events related to phonation have resulted in a greater understanding of phonatory physiology (Fritzell and Fant, 1986).

Understanding of the physiology of phonation is intimately bound up with an understanding of laryngeal anatomy and neuroanatomy, as well as respiratory function. Changes in the structures, in the tissues, or in motor control, whether the result of neurological insult, trauma, congenital anomaly, lesion, or disease process, will distort normal physiology in some fairly predictable ways. This disturbed physiology will, in turn, have an effect on the acoustic characteristics of the voice. Physiology can also be altered by changes in muscular and skeletal tensions, with concomitant changes in the acoustics. Therefore, there is an interdependence and interaction among anatomy, physiology, neurology, and acoustics. It is necessary to understand this interaction in order to treat the voice problem effectively. It is imperative that teachers of the professional voice increase their working knowledge of the complex phonatory process.

All users of voice, as well as those who treat or train it, can benefit from an understanding of how the voice works. Simple knowledge of the effects of vocal abuse and the need for good vocal hygiene could be potent preventive measures for reducing the incidence of vocal nodules and certain polyps. There are some people who, without the benefit of specific voice training, are able to use their voices in strenuous ways without encountering any vocal problems. They are the exceptions. Most people who use the voice in strenuous ways will develop vocal difficulty.

Most professional voice users have had vocal training, although it is rare for such training to include more than a cursory understanding of phonatory physiology. Typically, voice coaches have been taught by other voice coaches, and techniques are passed on that are believed to produce the desired results. There is little objective evidence that these techniques do what they are purported to do. Although some techniques appear to be spectacularly successful, others have done unwitting damage to voices.

Professional voice users need to understand the workings of their instrument in order to use it most effectively and maintain its health. In addition to professional singers and actors, the category of professional voice users should be expanded to include teachers, coaches, ministers, salespersons, cheerleaders, and others who use their voices extensively and strenuously.

The Voice Team

There are many professionals representing numerous disciplines or fields of study who are concerned with the voice. Some are concerned with basic studies of laryngeal function, others are concerned with medical problems affecting the voice, and others are concerned with the treatment of voice problems. Still other disciplines are focused on developing the voice to its pinnacle for performance purposes. Each discipline brings its particular focus and area of expertise to bear on diagnosis, treatment, or teaching.

The internist, the family practitioner, or the pediatrician may be the first specialist to come in contact with a patient with a voice problem. These primary care physicians must be aware of the voice as a sign of health or illness. For example, persistent hoarseness is recognized among medical personnel and the public as one of the early warning signs of cancer. There are other vocal symptoms that if recognized can be helpful in the early diagnosis of certain disease processes. Recognition and identification of the existence of a problem is only the first step. This must be followed by appropriate treatment or referral for further evaluation and/or treatment.

Medically, the otolaryngologist is the most appropriate specialist for the diagnosis and treatment of laryngeal problems. Although relatively few otolaryngologists specialize in the treatment of voice problems, most will be expected to treat a variety of laryngeal problems. Laryngitis, vocal fold nodules, polyps, loss of voice, or hoarseness of undetermined etiology are among the problems that affect the voice and are typically seen by otolaryngologists.

As is true for otolaryngologists, there are many speech pathologists who are engaged in working with the voice disordered patient, but relatively few have made this an area of specialization. The mode of treatment offered by speech pathologists focuses on the modification of phonatory behavior. Indeed, the speech pathologist's broad-based understanding of behavior, whether it be the result of inappropriate voice usage, disturbed physiology, or a manifestation of underlying psychological problems, uniquely qualifies this professional to aid in the diagnostic process, as well as to provide a primary resource for nonmedical treatment.

Voice scientists have added immeasurably to our understanding of phonatory physiology and acoustics through experimental verification of hypotheses. They are not usually directly involved in either treating or teaching the voice user. However, the information available from laboratory studies of the voice can be helpful in establishing a diagnosis and in documenting change in vocal function as a result of treatment. Furthermore, much can be learned about phonatory physiology from the study of abnormal function.

Neurolaryngology, the specialized neurological approach to laryngeal function, is a fairly new and developing area of knowledge, with far-reaching clinical implications. Many movement disorders have laryngeal components that have not been well documented and are not well understood. Indeed, it is not unusual for a phonatory problem to be the first symptom of a motor disorder. A neurolaryngologist could be a valuable member of any team concerned with voice disorders.

Imaging techniques are powerful tools assisting in the diagnosis of pathologic conditions. Radiologists whose special area of expertise focuses on head and neck problems are frequently involved in initial and subsequent assessments of laryngeal function. The information relative to the size, location, and extent of a lesion, which can be obtained through a variety of imaging techniques, is frequently critical to diagnostic and management decisions, especially those that involve surgery. Videofluoroscopic imaging of the larynx during the act of speaking or singing can provide helpful information relative to the level of the vocal folds and their movement.

Patients whose voice problems are an expression of deep-rooted emotional problems may require psychotherapy (Diehl, 1960; Aronson, Peterson, and Litin, 1966). Referral to a psychotherapist is indicated when it has been determined that the vocal problem exhibited by the patient may be an expression or symptom of significant psychiatric disability. Our understanding of the bond between voice and personality has been enhanced by the contributions of the fields of psychiatry and psychology.

Teachers and coaches of the singing and the speaking voice are interested in maximizing the individual potential of each of their students while maintaining the health and structural integrity of the vocal mechanism. Their unique knowledge of the professional voice and their deep interest in its correct use necessitates a good knowledge of vocal anatomy and physiology. This is especially true because the vocal demands on singers and actors are frequently much greater than for the average speaker. Furthermore, even subtle changes in vocal production may be critical to a performance.

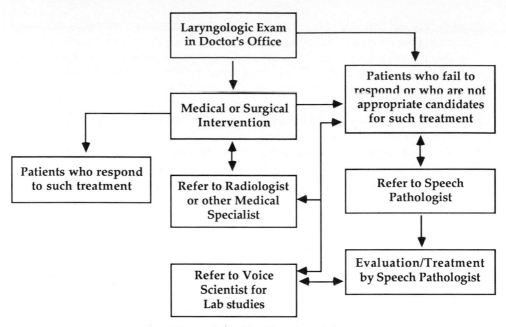

Figure 1.1.   Traditional model.

The number and variety of disciplines involved in the understanding and management of the voice give testimony to the complexity of the process of phonation. Our experience in the "team approach" to understanding the voice and its disorders has led us to an appreciation of the value of active involvement of a variety of disciplines working together in the assessment process. The benefits of the team approach accrue not only to the patient but also to the professionals involved. In the traditional model (Fig. 1.1), patients may have to be seen by three or more specialists for individual assessments. This model results in greater costs to the patient both in money and in time. The time spent with each specialist, the elapsed time between appointments, and the time required for coordination of findings may add up to produce a significant delay between presentation of symptoms and beginning treatment. Furthermore, because patient vocal behavior may vary from day to day, each professional may be presented with different vocal behavior for evaluation.

In the team approach, schematized in Figure 1.2, the patient is seen simultaneously by a number of specialists. In our experience, the team most frequently includes the otolaryngologist, the voice scientist, and the speech pathologist, who jointly examine the patient through a variety of techniques. All test results are then reviewed and discussed by the team. Because the patient is seen simultaneously by all team members, the same vocal behavior is evaluated by each.

Summary

The larynx serves essential reflexive biological functions that protect the airway and maintain life. These basic functions determine the limits of voice and may occasionally affect its function. The larynx also provides the acoustic signal for speech, that uniquely human capability. Singing, dramatic exposition, laughing, and crying fulfill additional human needs through the voice. The voice reflects individual identity, personality, and life stage. An understanding of phonatory physiology, as well as of those factors that may disturb it, is necessary for all professionals involved in the care of the voice and for all

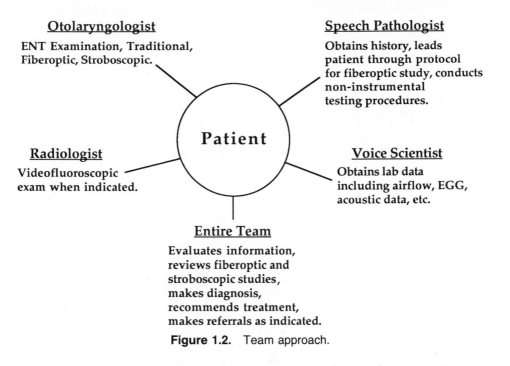

Otolaryngologist

ENT Examination, Traditional, Fiberoptic, Stroboscopic.

Speech Pathologist

Obtains history, leads patient through protocol for fiberoptic study, conducts non-instrumental testing procedures.

Patient

Radiologist

Videofluoroscopic exam when indicated.

Voice Scientist

Obtains lab data including airflow, EGG, acoustic data, etc.

Entire Team

Evaluates information, reviews fiberoptic and stroboscopic studies, makes diagnosis, recommends treatment, makes referrals as indicated.

Figure 1.2. Team approach.

professional voice users. Assessment of the voice-disordered patient is enhanced by input from various disciplines through a team approach.

2

Differential Diagnosis of Voice Problems

In this chapter, and throughout this book, we will be using the term "diagnosis" in two distinct ways. In the first sense, it will refer to the process involved when attempting to determine the nature of a problem. That process involves examination and observation, a problem-solving approach. However, in the second sense, the word "diagnosis" refers to the decision that is the end product of the diagnostic process.

The diagnostic process can be likened to solving a puzzle. Each piece of the puzzle must be examined from many perspectives. Each piece is only a part of the global picture. As a piece is found, it is placed into the puzzle, until the picture is complete. As often happens, one or more pieces may be missing. In those instances, more time is required to search for the missing pieces. In the process of diagnosis of voice disorders, there may also be missing pieces. The solution may not be apparent, and ongoing examination of all relevant information must continue.

Analysis of voice problems involves the examination of many individual components. These components include the statement of the problem, the symptoms, and the history or related information, as well as a set of signs observed or measured by the examiners. The examination of these components may involve a variety of procedures, including the following: interview; examination of medical records; rating of auditory perceptual characteristics; measurement of acoustic, aerodynamic, vibratory, and muscle action events; examination of the laryngeal structures and their function; and experimental therapy in which attempts are made to manipulate the patient's vocal behavior.

The successful completion of the diagnostic process requires a solid base of information. Diagnosis of voice disorders requires a thorough understanding of laryngeal anatomy and physiology. A fundamental understanding of phonatory physiology is essential so that rational hypotheses can be formulated about the voice problem and the conditions accompanying it.

Moreover, the clinician must be able to formulate hypotheses concerning the expected changes in physiology based on analysis of perceptual and acoustic information. The clinician must be aware of and sensitive to the relationship between personality and voice. Knowledge about the various pathologies and how they affect phonation is, of course, essential.

The diagnostic process is differential. That is, it is necessary to consider all the possible causes of a problem and to proceed through them all as if each is the real cause until proven otherwise. The differential aspect of the diagnostic process involves consideration of the basic question, what specific problem might demonstrate all these component parts? The available information relative to the patient is then matched against each of these hypotheses in the search for a match, a good fit.

The process of differential diagnosis begins anew with each patient. In the clinical setting, patients present themselves with a complaint. The challenge for the diagnostician is to track down all the pieces of data essential to an understanding of the physiology, to the making of a diagnosis, and perhaps to knowledge about etiology.

What Is an Etiology?

Etiology is defined as ''a science or doctrine of causation or of the demonstration of causes'' (*Webster's Third New International Dictionary*). Symptoms and signs describe various components of the problem, providing part of the raw data necessary for determination of an etiology. The first step in the treatment of any medical problem is determination of its cause, its etiology. Recognition of the correct etiology is essential for proper treatment. It is not only unwise but also potentially dangerous to treat a problem for which a well-considered etiology has not been established. An incorrect etiology may result in improper treatment, lack of needed treatment, or, at the very worst, may compromise a patient's life. For example, laryngitis is a common cause of hoarseness and is treated not only by otolaryngologists but also by pediatricians, family physicians, and internists. In many cases, laryngitis is caused by an upper respiratory infection and is appropriately treated with medication. However, hoarseness may be a sign of many other laryngeal pathologies, including malignant lesions, and as such should be evaluated with all possible etiologies in mind. In our experience, some patients have followed a protracted and unsuccessful course of medical treatment only to have subsequent examination reveal the presence of a vocal fold lesion as the etiology of the hoarseness.

Assigning an etiology is not always easy to accomplish. It is possible for a condition to be unobservable and to escape careful and thorough examination. It is also possible for a condition to persist when the original cause of the problem is no longer present. An untrained singer may have developed vocal nodules while engaged in strenuous voice use and abuse for a period of several months. That abusive behavior may no longer be present, but the resultant tissue changes persist. It is important to be aware of antecedent conditions that may be responsible for the present problem.

Symptoms and Signs

The words ''signs and symptoms'' are used frequently in medical literature. What do they mean, and how can the distinction between them help the diagnostic process?

What Is a Symptom?

A symptom is a complaint. It is what the patient reports about the problem and its characteristics. Symptoms may be described in various ways. The patient may complain of sensations associated with phonation, such as pain along the side of the neck, or soreness in the throat region after prolonged conversation. Other complaints may refer to perceptual characteristics of the voice, such as hoarseness, scratchiness, or perhaps a wobbly voice. Some symptoms can be verified; some cannot. For example, you cannot "feel" the patient's pain or record it. However, the report of pain is a very important symptom and can be a potent factor in directing the clinician's thinking about a problem. Other feelings (e.g., dry throat, scratchy throat, etc.) may also be difficult to verify. Symptoms, verifiable or not, have reality for the patient and must be given serious consideration by the speech pathologist and the otolaryngologist.

What Is a Sign?

Signs are characteristics of the voice that can be observed or tested. For example, hoarseness may be the patient's complaint, but it is also a sign that can be observed and measured independently. Signs represent an inventory of vocal characteristics based upon examination, observation, and measurement.

Signs Versus Symptoms: Why the Distinction?

Despite the fact that patients' symptoms have reality for them, they do not tell the full story. Sometimes they can be misleading, they are frequently underreported, and they may not be the most salient and significant vocal characteristics present in the voice. Thus, symptoms may provide only part of the picture of the patient's vocal difficulty.

Signs provide more objective information. Because each sign is not unique, there may be redundancy in the data. For example, hoarseness may include the following acoustic signs: low fundamental frequency, less variability of fundamental frequency, increased frequency perturbation, increased spectral noise, and large s/z ratio (see pp. 19–27, this chapter, for a more complete discussion on these acoustic signs). Which of these component signs are significant is sometimes difficult to determine, and it is not always possible to record all of them in a single patient. However, knowing how one relates to another and to the underlying pathophysiology will assist the speech pathologist or otolaryngologist in properly interpreting the sign and evaluating its significance.

Major Symptoms and Signs of Voice Problems

In this section, the major symptoms and signs of voice problems will be presented. In the next three sections, we will discuss perceptual, acoustic, and physiological signs. Finally, each of the symptoms discussed in this section will be presented in greater detail, with listing of the major perceptual, acoustic, and physiological signs, as well as potential etiologies that might produce the symptoms and signs. The emphasis throughout this chapter will be on the process of discovering and interrelating the perceptual, acoustic, and physiological signs to the underlying pathology or pathophysiology and eventually to the etiology of the problem.

In our experience, patients with voice problems tend to present eight major symptoms. Not included in this list are symptoms reflective of a problem with resonance, which have been traditionally considered voice problems but are not phonatory problems. There may be some other minor symptoms or different classification schemes, but we believe that these eight primary symptoms are basic. It is important to recognize that symptoms do not usually occur singly but more often appear in combination with others.

The eight symptoms shown in Table 2.1 are as follows:

Table 2.1.
Eight Primary Symptoms of Voice Problems

Hoarseness
Vocal fatigue
Breathiness
Reduced phonational range
Aphonia
Pitch breaks or inappropriately high pitch
Strain/struggle voice
Tremor

1. Hoarseness: This symptom reflects aperiodic vibration of the vocal folds. Some patients will use the term ''hoarse'' to refer to this symptom, whereas others might use terms such as ''raspy voice'' or ''rough voice.''

2. Vocal fatigue: Patients complain of feeling tired after prolonged talking and often state that continued talking requires a great deal of effort. Moreover, they may report occasional raspiness or hoarseness, which tends to be most apparent at the end of a working day.

3. Breathy voice: Patients sometimes complain that they are unable to say complete sentences without running out of air and needing to replenish the air supply in order to continue talking. They further report having difficulty being heard, especially in noisy situations. We usually label the voice as breathy, although patients will not always use this term.

4. Reduced phonational range: This symptom is usually associated with singers who complain that they are experiencing difficulty producing notes that had previously presented no problem. Typically these are the notes that occur at the upper end of their singing range. They may also complain of tiredness and soreness in the throat area.

5. Aphonia: Aphonia means absence of voice. The patient speaks in a whisper and may sometimes complain of a variety of symptoms, including dryness in the throat, soreness, and a great deal of effort in attempting to speak.

6. Pitch breaks/inappropriately high pitch: A patient may complain of periodic squeakiness and of voice cracks. The voice seems out of control, and the patient reports never knowing what sound will come out. Therefore, we have labeled this symptom as pitch breaks, although it is also possible to describe it as the inappropriate use of falsetto or puberphonia. Often this symptom is reported by a male adolescent who uses an inappropriately high pitch as the habitual voice rather than the more typical lower pitched male voice.

7. Strain/struggle voice: These patients report that it is difficult to talk. This may include inability to get voicing started or to maintain voice. They report that it is a strain to talk; they experience a great deal of tension while speaking and become fatigued due to the effort involved. For these reasons, we have labeled this symptom as strain/struggle voice.

8. Tremor: Patients may complain that the voice is wobbly or shaky. They are unable to voluntarily produce a steady sustained sound. We use the word ''tremor'' to refer to this voice characteristic.

These eight symptoms are the most common in our experience, and the terms used are those patients have used themselves in discussing their problem. Some patients may use slightly different terms, but the meaning is similar. Patients also may not report just a single symptom. Rather, they may report several of these symptoms, but usually the symptom mentioned first or emphasized should be considered the primary symptom and probably will relate most directly to the eventual etiology of the vocal problem.

Perceptual Signs

Perceptual signs of voice problems are the characteristics of an individual's voice that are perceived by the listener/observer. Although they are often considered subjective, they have psychological reality and may be assessed objectively and compared across listeners (see Chapter 7 for methods of scaling perceptions). Clinically, the perceptual signs—the clinician's perception of voice characteristics—paired with the history serve as initial guideposts in the process of differential diagnosis.

Many adjectives have been used to describe voice qualities (Perkins, 1971; Colton and Estill, 1981; Aronson, 1985). The list of perceptual signs to be presented in this chapter encompasses a variety of perceptual characteristics that serve to focus our attention on clinically useful voice characteristics. Some of these characteristics have reasonably clear acoustic correlates that can be measured. Others do not have clear or well-defined acoustic correlates. For example, we are not able to differentiate hoarseness and roughness acoustically. Both hoarseness and roughness have increased perturbation and a noisy spectrum. As another example, tension can be observed by a clinician, but its measurement becomes problematic. Indeed, we would be hard put to specify the exact loci of vocal tension, its acoustic parameters, and how to measure it.

Perceptions by their very nature are hard to describe verbally. They are subjective and individual, being influenced by personal preference, experience, and culture. In the following discussion of perceptual signs of voice (see Table 2.2), we have grouped them within the broad areas of pitch, loudness, quality, nonphonatory behavior, and aphonia (absence of phonation). The definitions of the terms are worded so as to provide meaningful guidelines without undue restriction on individual experience.

Pitch

Pitch is the perceptual correlate of fundamental frequency.

Monopitch.   This term refers to a voice that lacks variation of pitch during speech. There is a marked absence of inflectional variation and in some instances an inability to voluntarily vary pitch. The fundamental frequency curve of a speaking voice can be displayed by various instruments, such as the PM Intonation Unit (Voice Identification) or the Visi-Pitch (Kay Elemetrics). These instruments make it possible for the clinician's perception to be verified and for the voice-disordered patient to receive valuable visual feedback. Monopitch can be one of many signs characteristic of neurological impairments that may affect the voice. It may also simply be a reflection of an individual's personality or, more significantly, of psychiatric disability.

Inappropriate Pitch.   This refers to the voice that is judged to exceed the range of acceptable pitch for age and/or sex, being either too low or too high. Norms for fundamental frequency (the acoustic correlate of pitch) are available for age and sex (see below under "Acoustic Signs"). The high pitched voice of a young child is perceived to be inappropriate when produced by an adult, and vice versa. Similarly, the pitch range for an adult female voice does not generally extend as low as might be acceptable in an adult male. The perception of voice pitch and the subsequent judgment of the acceptability of that pitch, based solely on perception, can be fraught with danger. Research has shown (Plomp, 1976, pp. 111–142; Wolfe and Ratusnik, 1988) that other characteristics of voice quality can affect our perception of pitch. Thus, although the hoarse voice of a person with a vocal lesion may be perceived to be lower than acceptable, actual measurement of the fundamental frequency may fail to corroborate that perception (Shipp and Huntington, 1965). The pitch of a voice is related to the size of the larynx and its structures. A vocal pitch higher than expected may reflect underdevelopment or immaturity of the larynx

Table 2.2.
Perceptual Signs of Voice Problems

Pitch
   monopitch
   inappropriate pitch
   pitch breaks
Loudness
   monoloudness
   loudness variations (soft, loud, or uncontrolled)
Quality
   hoarseness/roughness
   breathiness
   tension
   tremor
   strain/struggle
   sudden interruption of voicing
   diplophonia
Nonphonatory behavior
   stridor
   excessive throat clearing
Aphonia
   consistent
   episodic

based on endocrinological factors or perhaps a congenital anomaly. Vocal pitch may also be excessively low due to endocrinological factors such as hypothyroidism or the use of male hormone by women. It is also possible for vocal pitch to be too high or too low based on individual preferences or habit.

Pitch Breaks. These are characterized by unexpected and uncontrolled sudden shifts of pitch in either an upward or downward direction. These are readily perceived even by the untrained and unsophisticated listener. They are frequently associated with the changing voice of the adolescent male and are usually a temporary stage that resolves with time. Occasionally pitch breaks persist beyond the expected laryngeal growth period. Pitch breaks, however, may also occur as a result of laryngeal pathology or as an accompaniment to conditions that involve some loss of neural control of phonation.

Loudness

Loudness is the perceptual correlate of intensity.

Monoloudness. This refers to voice that lacks variation in loudness level. The use of increased loudness for emphasis is absent, and there may be an inability to voluntarily vary loudness. As with monopitch, the loudness curve of a voice may be displayed by the PM Intonation Unit (Voice Identification), or the Visi-Pitch (Kay Elemetrics), in order to provide visual feedback and verification of the perception. In this category, the perception does not attend to the actual level of loudness being used but rather to the variability of the level during speaking. Monoloudness may be an indication of neurological impairment in which the ability to voluntarily control and vary loudness may be lost, it may be a reflection of psychiatric disability, or it may reflect habit associated with personality.

Loudness Variations. When these are at the extremes of the loudness continuum, either too soft to be heard easily in average conversational settings or excessively loud for the setting, they are perceived as a sign of a problem. Although norms are available for dynamic range (the softest to the loudest sound a person is able to produce; see "Acoustic Signs," below), appropriate loudness levels are dependent upon the specific speaking situation. Unpredictable and uncontrolled variation of loudness level, explosive to fading, constitutes another sign of loudness variability that is beyond accepted norms. Voices that are too soft or too loud may often be a reflection of personality and habit. A habitually loud speaker may have grown up in a large and noisy family in which excessive loudness was the norm, or she may have had to speak loudly in order to be heard by a hearing-impaired relative. The inability to control vocal loudness may also be due to the loss of neural control of the phonatory mechanism or to problems affecting the respiratory mechanism. It is also possible that variations in vocal loudness, from explosive to almost aphonic, may be a reflection of psychological problems.

Quality

Hoarseness and Roughness.   These words are descriptors of a voice quality that is noticeably aberrant in its lack of clarity, its increased noisiness, and its discordance. Although hoarseness/roughness may be the primary perceptual characteristic of an abnormal voice, its perception may be paired with other characteristics such as breathiness, tension, or strain. The degree of hoarseness/roughness in the voice is related to the amount of perturbation (see below under "Perturbation") and to the noisiness of the spectrum (see below under "Spectral Noise"). Pathologies that affect the vibratory behavior of the vocal folds will usually result in some degree of perceived hoarseness/roughness.

Breathiness.   This designation refers to the perception of audible air escape during phonation. The voice lacks clarity of tone and is usually reduced in loudness. A breathy voice quality is related to the amount of airflow produced. Norms for airflow measures are available (see Chapter 13), and its measurement can verify the perception of breathiness. Excessive airflow through the glottis is usually a reflection of inadequate glottal closure. Inability to fully adduct the vocal folds during phonation may be the result of peripheral neurological problems, of central neurological impairment, of the presence of a lesion that interferes with closure, or of improper use.

Tension.   Tension in the voice suggests to the listener a "hard edge" to the voice, combined with hard glottal attacks and sometimes observable muscular tension in the external neck. Tension is a perception that is difficult to verify through measurement. Assumptions can be made about the dynamics of vocal tension, such as increased tension of certain muscle groups, but we do not have adequate data to determine the most salient muscle groups nor the amount of tension that is acceptable in the normal voice. In many instances tension seems to be related to "hyperfunctional" usage patterns. However, it may also be a reflection of compensatory behavior in the presence of some laryngeal pathology or neurological disability.

Tremor.   This sign may be described as regularly rhythmic variations in pitch and loudness of the voice that are not under voluntary control. The voice is perceived as unsteady, "wobbly," quavering. Tremor is a perception that can be verified through measurement. Indeed, the rate of the tremor can be an important factor in determining the underlying pathology (see pp. 25–27). Tremor of any type is usually a reflection of a central nervous system dysfunction that results in some loss of control of the phonatory mechanism.

Strain/Struggle Behavior.   The voice perceived to reflect strain/struggle behavior suggests difficulty in initiating phonation and struggle to maintain phonation. As speech is produced, there is the perception of inability to control voicing as it fades in and out. Actual voice stoppages may occur. Physical correlates of these perceptions, such as voice onset time, silence, and variations of fundamental frequency and sound pressure level, are accessible to objective measurement. However, the perception of the strain and struggle behavior is qualitatively unique and is not well expressed by the various measurements. There continues to be considerable controversy (Dedo, Townsend, and Izdebski, 1978; Aronson, 1985) regarding the etiology of this type of vocal behavior. However, it would probably be fair to say that neurological dysfunction of some sort is implicated in most cases. Some experts continue to believe that in a certain percentage of these patients, the etiology is psychological.

Sudden Interruption of Voicing.   A sudden unexpected drop in loudness and an equally unexpected change in voice quality to breathy voice is a quite noticeable sign. The breathy voice may last only a fraction of a second and may occur repeatedly within an utterance, alternating with essentially normal voicing. This perceptual sign of an abnormal voice may be the result of sudden, unexpected, and involuntary abduction of the vocal folds, the etiology of which is usually neurological dysfunction. Again, these perceived voice characteristics (e.g., loudness variability, airflow changes) are accessible to objective measurement.

Diplophonia.   This word literally means double voice. It is said to be present when two distinct pitches are perceived simultaneously during phonation. Theoretically this occurs when the vocal folds are under differing degrees of tension and each vibrates at a different frequency. Although it is a fairly frequently used term, we have found its occurrence to be relatively infrequent. There does not seem to be a consistent pattern of the perception of diplophonia as a consequence of a given pathology.

Nonphonatory Behaviors

Stridor.   The term refers to noisy breathing, involuntary sound that accompanies inspiration, expiration, or both and is indicative of a narrowing of the airway at a certain point. Although the pitch or quality of the stridorous sound is taken by some to be diagnostic (Cotton and Richardson, 1981), the judgments of these factors appear to be based entirely on perception. Although the frequency and intensity of stridor could be measured, we know of no such measurements. The presence of stridor is always an abnormal finding and one with potentially serious implications since it is a reflection of blockage of the airway.

Excessive Throat Clearing.   A frequent accompaniment to a variety of voice disorders, excessive throat clearing probably represents an attempt by the patient to clear excess mucus from the vocal folds, or it may be a response to the sensation of "something in the throat." It is a natural behavior but is considered a perceptual sign of disordered voice when it occurs with excessive frequency and consistency.

Aphonia

Consistent Aphonia.   This is an absence of voicing, usually perceived as whispering, that is constantly present. Aphonia may be the result of bilateral vocal fold paralysis in which the vocal folds are unable to adduct or a result of central nervous system dysfunction, or it may be a psychogenic problem.

Episodic Aphonia.   This may take a number of forms. A patient may exhibit unpredictable, involuntary aphonic breaks in voice production that last for only a fraction of a second. Another patient may experience aphonic periods lasting minutes, hours, or even days. Yet another patient may experience a gradual fading of voice to the aphonic state, particularly with increased physical fatigue. Momentary involuntary aphonic breaks are not uncommon during the speech of patients with laryngeal pathology. Episodic aphonia may be observed in patients with central neurological dysfunction of the flaccid type, as noted in myasthenia gravis. However, it is possible that episodic aphonia may be psychologically based.

Acoustic Signs

Voice is produced by movements of the vocal folds interrupting the egressive airstream. The movements of the folds are controlled by the biomechanical characteristics of

Table 2.3.
Acoustic Signs of Voice Problems

Fundamental frequency
  mean or average speaking fundamental frequency
  frequency variability
  phonational range
  perturbation
Amplitude
  average overall sound pressure level
  amplitude variability
  dynamic range
  perturbation
Spectral noise
Vocal rise or fall time
Voice tremor
Phonation time
Voice stoppages
Frequency breaks
Normal acoustics

the folds themselves, the magnitude of the air pressure beneath the folds, and their neural control. Pathology may affect these movements by interfering with any of these variables.

Vocal fold movement results in periodic interruption of the airstream at rates appropriate for the perception of sound. Acoustics is the study of sound, and voice acoustics can provide important information about vocal fold movement. But acoustics is one stage removed from the movements of the vocal folds. Although acoustic signs are, at best, imperfect mirrors of the underlying vocal fold physiology, there is a great deal of correspondence between the physiology and acoustics, and much can be inferred about the physiology based on acoustic analysis. Moreover, acoustic parameters are probably the easiest to record and to analyze objectively.

There are many acoustic signs that may be associated with any given pathology (see Table 2.3). Some are unique and others redundant. For example, jitter (variations of period from one pitch period to the next, also known as frequency perturbation) and noise spectrum may reflect the basic aperiodicity of the vibrating vocal folds. Jitter may be easier to measure and therefore have greater clinical utility. But all acoustic signs reflect some aspect of the underlying pathology of interest.

Fundamental Frequency

The vibrating frequency of the vocal folds is referred to as fundamental frequency. This acoustic characteristic is usually defined as average fundamental frequency or, in the instance of spontaneous speech or reading, speaking fundamental frequency. Also of interest is the variability of fundamental frequency usually expressed as the standard deviation of frequency and sometimes labeled the pitch sigma. The range of frequencies that can be produced by the voice may also be of interest and is called phonational range. Finally, there is considerable interest in the short-term stability of the vocal folds. This stability (or lack thereof) is reflected in the measure termed frequency perturbation.

Mean Fundamental Frequency.   There are considerable normative data on fundamental frequency for males and females of all ages (Baken, 1987). Males should produce fundamental frequencies between 100 and 150 Hz, whereas females should produce fundamental frequencies between 180 and 250 Hz (Hollien, Dew, and Philips, 1971). Figure 2.1 presents an example of fundamental frequency as a function of time for a sentence pro-

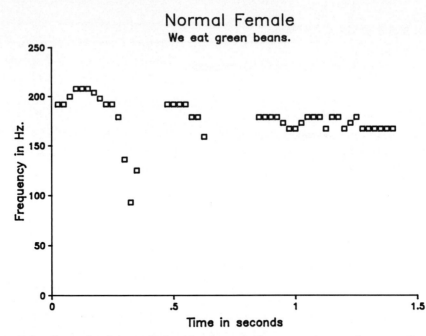

Figure 2.1. Example of an analysis of fundamental frequency in a sentence produced by a normal female speaker. Each square plots the fundamental frequency measured over a 20-msec time period. Note the gaps in the plot, indicating places where there was no measurable fundamental frequency. These gaps correspond to the voiceless sounds in the sentence.

duced by a normal female speaker. The speaking fundamental frequency was 189.4 Hz. Pathology may affect the vibrating frequency, with the result that males or females will produce either too high a frequency or too low a frequency. By too high or too low, we mean frequencies that lie outside these approximate limits.

One should not confuse pitch with frequency. Pitch is the psychological feature of the voice, whereas frequency is the physical feature. It is possible to perceive a voice as having excessively low pitch without an excessively low fundamental frequency (Wolfe and Ratusnik, 1988).

Frequency Variability. The standard deviation of fundamental frequency (or pitch sigma) reflects frequency variability for a reasonably large time segment or passage. During speech, both fundamental frequency and intensity vary depending on the sounds, the words uttered, and the intent of the message. Computing the standard deviation of frequency during a sentence or paragraph will provide an estimate of this longer-term variability. In Figure 2.1 the standard deviation of fundamental frequency for the sentence of the normal speaker was 20.98 Hz. In the literature the standard deviation of fundamental frequency is usually expressed in semitones and labeled the pitch sigma. Converting frequency to semitones yields a pitch sigma of 4.32 for this speaker. As a general guideline, one should expect normal speakers to exhibit frequency standard deviations between 2 and 4 for both males and females (Mysak, 1959; Stoicheff,1981; Linville and Fisher,1985; Baken, 1987). Patients are sometimes unable to produce normal variability. This acoustic measure would presumably be related to the perceptual features of monopitch, although little research has been done on these relationships.

Phonational Range. Phonational range refers to the range of frequencies that a person can produce. Normal young adults should be able to produce a phonational range of

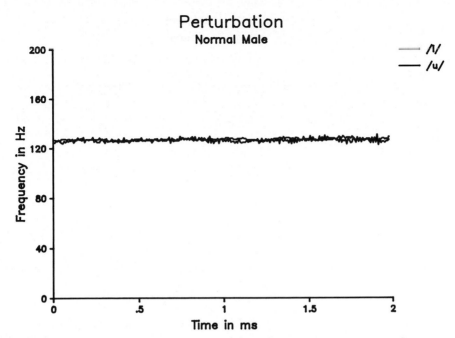

Figure 2.2. Example of an analysis of fundamental frequency during sustained vowels. Unlike Figure 2.1, fundamental frequency was measured for each glottal cycle. Note the small changes of fundamental frequency, although the speaker was attempting to produce a steady phonation.

about three octaves, with singers slightly higher than nonsingers (Colton, 1972; Baken, 1987). Phonational range decreases with age.

Perturbation. Perturbation refers to the irregularity of vibration of the vocal folds that is sometimes called vocal jitter. Such irregularity may be manifested either by irregularities in the time of vibration or in the amplitude of vibration. Variation of glottal period or frequency perturbation refers to the change of frequency from one successive period to the next (Horii, 1979, 1980, 1982; Casper, 1983). Normal speakers have a small amount of perturbation, which may represent variation in vocal fold mass, tension, muscle activity, or neural activity (Baer, 1979). An example of perturbation in a normal speaker's sustained vowel production is shown in Figure 2.2. Chapter 13 summarizes some of the data on normal perturbation.

Perturbation or jitter may be expressed in a variety of ways. One way is to report the average differences of period for all of the periods analyzed, in microseconds or milliseconds. Another way is to create a ratio of the average period differences divided by the average period for the utterance. If the result is multiplied by 100, the result is the jitter factor (Hollien, Michel, and Doherty, 1973). If the result is multiplied by 1000, the result is the jitter ratio (Horii, 1979). Another measure of perturbation involves subtracting the current cycle from the mean of adjacent cycles, averaging over all periods to be analyzed and dividing by the mean period. The result is called relative average perturbation, or RAP for short (Davis, 1981). There are several other variants of this basic procedure. Baken (1987) discusses the technique for the collection and calculation of frequency perturbation very completely.

When pathologies affect the vocal folds, their vibrations will show increased aperiodicity (Lieberman, 1963; Koike, 1967b; Hecker and Kreul, 1971). There are many possible pathologies that can affect vibration, including but not limited to growths on the vocal folds, changes in the mucosa, variations in the composition of the vocal folds, variations

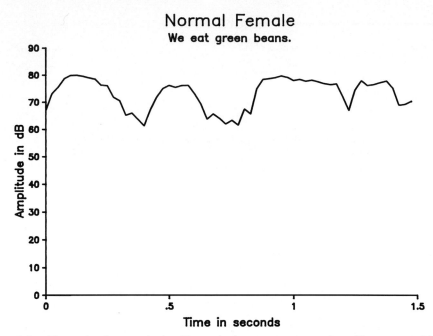

Figure 2.3. Example of an analysis of intensity in a sentence produced by a normal female speaker. In general, the humps in the figure correspond to the production of the words in the sentence. The valleys correspond to the gaps between words or very slight pauses.

in muscle function, and variations in the motor control of the muscles controlling the vibration. Thus, perturbation may not be useful for differentiating among etiologies but may reflect the extent of a pathology (Colton, Reed, Sagerman, and Chung, 1982).

Amplitude

There are several acoustic variables that reflect the amplitude or strength of the tone produced by the vocal folds. Many are expressed in decibels. Overall sound pressure level (SPL) refers to the average level of an utterance (sustained vowel, spontaneous sentence, or paragraph). Amplitude standard deviation is simply a measure of amplitude variability, whereas dynamic range reflects the range of vocal amplitudes an individual can produce. Finally, amplitude perturbation reflects the short-term variation of amplitude from one glottal period to the next.

Overall SPL.   The average or overall sound pressure level in decibels provides an indication of the strength of the vocal fold vibration. If a person speaks softly, the overall SPL will be low. Conversely, if a person speaks loudly, the overall SPL will be high. Everyday conversational speech may exhibit sound pressure levels between 75 and 80 dB (Baken, 1987). Sound pressure levels as a function of time for a normal speaker's production of a simple sentence are shown in Figure 2.3. The mean SPL was 69.01 dB.

Amplitude Variability.   During speech or a reading passage, the amplitude of speaking will vary depending on the sounds spoken and the message. Variability of amplitude during speech would be expressed as a standard deviation. The standard deviation of SPL for the normal speaker in Figure 2.3 was 5.4 dB.

Dynamic Range.   This is the range of vocal intensities that a person can produce. Normal persons should be able to produce minimum intensities of around 50 dB and maximum intensities of around 115 dB; intensities for males are slightly higher than for females (Coleman, Mabis, and Hinson, 1977). Figure 2.4 presents the mean dynamic ranges as a

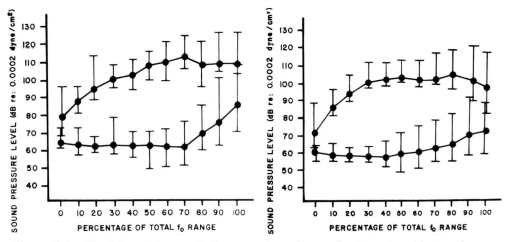

Figure 2.4. The left panel presents the average and range for 10 male subjects, whereas the right panel presents the average and range for 12 female subjects. Each subject produced a sustained vowel at 10% increments of their fundamental frequency ranges and at minimum and maximum SPL. (From Coleman, Mabis, and Hinson, 1977.)

function of fundamental frequency for the normal subjects in the Coleman, Mabis, and Hinson study. Note how the sound pressure levels at the extremes of the fundamental frequency range are much smaller than the dynamic ranges at the mid frequencies.

Perturbation. As was the case for fundamental frequency, it is possible that the amplitude of the vocal fold tone will vary from one cycle to the next. This characteristic is called amplitude perturbation or shimmer. Growths on the vocal folds or poor neural control of the vocal folds would be expected to affect the stability of the vocal folds. Therefore, shimmer should reflect the kind and degree of pathology that a speaker might exhibit. Chapter 13 summarizes some of the available data on shimmer for normal speakers.

Spectral Noise

Noise is random, aperiodic energy in the voice. It may occur throughout the entire frequency range of the voice, or it may be located in certain frequency bands. Normal voices have low levels of noise, whereas abnormal voices show greater noise levels (Yanagihara, 1967; Emanuel and Sansone, 1969; Wolfe and Steinfatt, 1987). Two general approaches have been developed for the analysis of noise components in voice.

The first, reported by Yanagihara (1967), uses spectrograms to classify voices, using the level of noise near the second formants of several vowels. As such, the system is qualitative although based on objective data. It cannot provide data that might differentiate subtle differences among patients, differences that might assist in diagnosis.

The second approach analyzes the level of noise directly. An example of this approach is the harmonics-to-noise ratio (Yumoto, Gould, and Baer, 1982; Yumoto, Sasaki, and Okamura, 1984). Harmonics-to-noise ratios greater than 1 mean that the harmonic energy was greater than the noise energy. Normal speakers are expected to have harmonics-to-noise ratios greater than 1.

Noise may be generated in two ways. First, there may be a noise source at or near the vocal folds (e.g., air rushing against the open vocal fold). Second, greater aperiodicity of vibration may show up as greater noise in the spectrum (Klingholz and Martin, 1985). Most procedures for the measurement of noise would not be able to distinguish between these two sources. Nevertheless, increased noise levels would be associated with problems that affect the vibrating frequency of the vocal folds or create additional, unwanted sources of sound at the level of the vocal folds.

Vocal Rise or Fall Time

The ability of the vocal folds to start tone production quickly or to stop phonation quickly may be impaired by pathology. The time it takes to produce a tone of full amplitude is referred to as rise time. The time it takes for the vocal folds to stop producing a tone is called fall time. Rise time is also associated with vocal attack. It has been shown that some pathologies will affect the time it takes the vocal folds to attain their amplitude (Koike, 1967b).

Pathologies affecting the neural control of laryngeal muscles would theoretically be expected to have a pronounced effect on the rise or fall time of glottal amplitude, although little work has been reported on these relationships.

Voice Tremor

Tremor refers to a regular variation in the fundamental frequency or amplitude of the voice (Aronson, Brown, Litin, and Pearson, 1968a; Hatcinski, Thomsen, and Buch, 1975; Izdebski and Dedo, 1979; Ludlow, Bassich, Connor, and Coulter, 1986). As a patient attempts to sustain a tone at a constant frequency, there is a slow variation of frequency around the desired constant frequency. Usually, this variation is between 3 and 5 Hz, about the mean, although it could be higher or lower than these limits. Tremor may also be exhibited by slow variation in the amplitude of the voice signal. Tremor is usually associated with variations in muscle activity levels or the control of the muscles used in phonation. As such it is usually associated with central nervous system dysfunction and not impaired peripheral motor control or vocal fold pathology.

Figure 2.5 presents an example of tremor on a sustained vowel. Note the slow oscillations of SPL during the production. Measuring the distance between the peaks of the SPL oscillations would yield the tremor rate, which in this example was about 5 Hz.

Phonation Time

Maximum phonation time refers to the maximum time a subject can sustain a tone on one breath. As a rule of thumb, one would expect normal adult male subjects to produce a vowel for about 20 seconds, adult female subjects about 15 seconds, and children about 10 seconds (Kent, Kent, and Rosenbek, 1987). However, these values may vary considerably between people and among age groups. Phonation time may vary as a function of trials. With proper instruction and practice, as few as three trials may be sufficient (Sawashima, 1966; Bless and Hirano, 1982). Short maximum phonation times reflect inefficiency of the phonatory or respiratory system.

Another measure of phonation time is what is referred to as the s/z ratio (Eckel and Boone, 1981; Boone, 1983), or the maximum sustained phonation time of /s/ divided by the maximum sustained phonation time of /z/. A normal speaker would be expected to sustain both the voiceless /s/ and the voiced /z/ for approximately equal durations, resulting in a ratio of 1. However, in the presence of a disturbance of vocal fold vibratory behavior and/or ability to close the glottis, the duration of sustained voicing for /z/ would be expected to suffer. The resulting s/z ratio becomes increasingly larger as the discrepancy between sustained productions of these sounds (z shorter than s) becomes greater. For a group of normal subjects, Eckel and Boone (1981) reported average s/z ratios between 0.4 and 2. Based on the results of their statistical tests between normal and pathological speakers, they suggest that any s/z ratio greater than 1.3 may indicate a vocal pathology.

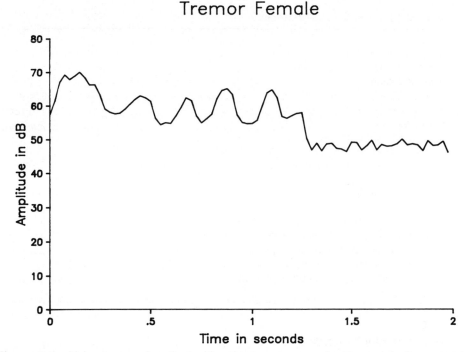

Figure 2.5. Voice tremor. A patient with voice tremor was asked to sustain the vowel /ee/. The variation of SPL accompanying the tremor during the vowel production is evident in this figure. Toward the end of phonation, the patient produced a low-level, harsh phonation.

S/z ratios for children were similar (Tait, Michel, and Carpenter, 1980; Shearer, 1983; Fendler and Shearer, 1988).

Voice Stoppages

Normal speech consists of phonation, noises, and silences. The latter are usually brief. When silences become longer than normally expected or appear unexpectedly during phonation, they call attention to themselves, disrupt intelligibility, and are considered abnormal. In some disorders, the voice may suddenly stop for a brief period of time and then revert to its previous level. These interruptions would be observable in the spectrum of the sound.

Frequency Breaks

Frequency breaks refer to sudden shifts of fundamental frequency either upward or downward. One would expect that these would be related to the perceptual pitch breaks often reported in the literature in the speech of patients with certain vocal pathologies.

Normal Acoustics

Finally, it is possible that a patient with a phonatory problem will exhibit acoustic features typical of a normal voice. In other cases, the differences between a normal and abnormal voice may be so subtle that they are not manifested in these acoustic signs.

Table 2.4.
Physiological Signs of Voice Problems

Aerodynamics
   increased or reduced airflow
   increased or reduced air pressure
   variability of airflow
     periodic
     aperiodic
Vibratory behavior
   aberrant glottal pulse shape
   slowed opening and closing phases of vocal folds
   inadequate or excessive closed times
   irregularity or asymmetry of vocal fold motion
   mucosal wave changes
Muscle activity
   absent,reduced, or excessive levels
   involuntary rhythmic variations of level
   sudden, unexpected bursts of activity
   slow rise or fall in signal amplitude
   diminution of level with sustained phonation
   imbalance of paired muscle activity

Physiological Signs

The physiological signs that may be affected by pathology include aerodyamic features (airflow and pressure), vibratory behavior (contact area, waveform shape), and muscle activity (as recorded by electromyography). These are summarized in Table 2.4.

Aerodynamics

Airflow.   During normal speech, airflow may range between 50 and 200 ml/sec, with males producing higher flows than females (Hirano, 1981a). Usually, the measurement of airflow represents the average flow over several glottal cycles. It is possible to measure the peak flow that occurs during a vibratory cycle. If possible, one should differentiate the peak flow measures from the steady airflow rates that occur during speech. The steady airflow rates for speakers with various vocal fold pathologies are greater than those for normal speakers. Normal speakers exhibit a small amount of airflow when the vocal folds adduct, whereas speakers with vocal pathology may produce large airflows during the closed phase of the vocal folds. If closure of the vocal folds is compromised by a lesion or poor muscular or neural control, airflow rates will be greater than normal.

Air Pressure.   The magnitude of air pressure beneath the vocal folds is important in producing vibration and determining the intensity of the sound. Typical pressures beneath the vocal folds (subglottal air pressure, lung pressure or alveolar pressure) range from about 2 to 20 cm H_2O, depending on the loudness of the sound. Pressures between 3 and 7 cm H_2O would be expected for conversational speech levels (Shipp and McGlone, 1971; Brodie, Colton, and Swisher, 1988). Higher than normal levels may indicate either excessive lung pressures or inefficient valving of the vocal folds.

Variability of airflow or pressure may be important to measure in persons with vocal pathology. Excessive variation could be associated with poor motor control of the vocal folds or of the respiratory system.

Vibratory Behavior

Vibratory characteristics of the vocal folds are important in determining the final acoustic output of the vocal folds. Many of these characteristics have been studied using high speed films. Information about some of the vibratory characteristics can be obtained from stroboscopic examinations or by using indirect techniques for assessing laryngeal function. Some of the more popular systems include (*a*) electroglottography (EGG), (*b*) inverse filtering of the oral airflow waveform, and (*c*) photoglottography.

During normal voice function, the shape of the airflow pulse or the shape of the area pulse is different depending on the mode of vibration (Timcke, von Leden, and Moore, 1958; Colton and Estill, 1981). Similarly, the shape of the airflow pulse through the glottis is different (Rothenberg, 1981). In pathology, the pattern of glottal opening becomes irregular and distorted (von Leden, Moore, and Timcke, 1960), as does the airflow pulse (Colton and Brewer, 1985; Colton, Brewer, and Rothenberg, 1985). Thus, analysis of glottal area from high speed films or airflow waveform shape can help to describe the vibratory characteristics of voice-disordered patients.

Muscle Activity

Pathology may affect the muscles that control vocal function directly by affecting peripheral function or indirectly by affecting the central nervous system. Clinically, muscle function could be assessed by observing the movements of the structures themselves (i.e., vibration of the vocal folds) or by recording the electrical activity of the muscles (electromyography, or EMG). Faaborg-Andersen (1957) was among the first to use EMG in the analysis of muscle function in the larynx. Many studies since that initial work have been concerned with various muscles of the larynx in healthy subjects as well as subjects with voice disorders. EMG is an invasive technique and should be performed only by those skilled in its application. EMG cannot and should not be performed on every patient (Basmajian, 1979). But for a few patients, EMG can be a valuable technique to assess laryngeal function.

When a muscle is activated for a task, an EMG recording will show a fairly rapid rise in the amplitude of the signal, followed by a consistent level of activity. When muscle activity ceases, the recording will show a fairly rapid fall in amplitude to a low level of baseline activity adequate to maintain the tonus of the muscle (Kotby and Haugen, 1970; Basmajian, 1979). Pathology may severely reduce or increase the background levels as well as the muscle levels during contraction (Sawashima, Sato, Funasaka, and Totsuk, 1958; Kotby and Haugen, 1970b). Muscles may be slow to become activated and slow to turn off, or a sudden unexpected burst of muscle activity may be superimposed on steady activity during muscle contraction, or muscles may show normal levels of activity when first contracted but with continued contraction, diminishing levels. There may also be differences of level between pairs of muscles controlling the vocal folds, suggesting a difference of activity between the two muscles (Hiroto, Hirano, and Tomita, 1968). Normal EMG levels, onsets, and offsets will be found in those patients whose laryngeal pathology does not affect muscles or their neural control.

Stroboscopic Signs

The stroboscope has found increased usage in the diagnosis and treatment of voice problems. Recent models are relatively easy to use and provide sharp imaging (Hirano, 1981a; Hirano, Feder, and Bless, 1983; Kitzing, 1985).

The stroboscope flashes a light at a rate equal to or approximating the vibrating rate of the vocal folds (Alberti, 1978). If the flash rate is equal to the vibrating rate of the vocal

Table 2.5.
Stroboscopic Signs of Voice Problems

Degree of glottal closure
Phase closure
Vertical level of vocal folds
Amplitude of vibration
Mucosal wave
Vibratory behavior of vocal folds
Phase symmetry
Periodicity

folds, they appear to stand still since they are illuminated at the same phase of their vibratory cycle. If the rate is slightly different from the vibration rate of the vocal folds, they are illuminated at different phases of their vibratory cycle. The effect is a slowing of the vibratory motion of the vocal folds, permitting observation of vibratory details.

The strobe must measure the fundamental frequency of the vocal folds in order to function. This measure is available to determine the regularity of vocal fold vibration.

The stroboscopic signs of laryngeal pathology are obtained from the recordings of the strobe images (Kallen, 1932; Fex, 1970). They, like many of the signs previously discussed, depend on the knowledge and skill of the examiner. The signs listed in Table 2.5 are based on those presented by Bless (unpublished technical manual, B&K Stroboscope Course) and Hirano (1981a).

Glottal Closure

The degree of glottal closure can be determined from strobe images. Glottal closure may range along a continuum from complete to incomplete. Moreover, patterns of closure may differ.

Phase Closure of the Vocal Folds

Do the vocal folds have a predominately open phase during vibration, as in a whisper, or do they have a predominately closed phase, as evident in a hypertense voice?

Vertical Level of the Vocal Folds

Are both vocal folds equal vertically? Or does one consistently appear lower than the other?

Amplitude of Vocal Fold Movement

The horizontal extent of vocal fold movement can be determined from stroboscopic recordings and may be altered by the loudness of phonation.

Mucosal Wave

A wave-like motion of the vocal folds is seen on the superior surface in normal speakers. This wave-like motion reflects their complex structure and movement. Any change in the normal movement patterns will be reflected in the appearance of the mucosal wave.

Vibratory Behavior

In the context of these signs, vibratory behavior refers to its presence or absence, or the extent of its presence or absence. Vibration may be observable throughout the entire length of the vocal folds, or there may be segments that are adynamic.

Table 2.6.
Laryngoscopic Signs of Voice Problems

Variations of vocal fold approximation
Vocal fold movement
Tissue change of vocal folds
Lack of change in appearance of pyriform sinuses
Anteroposterior laryngeal dimensions
Ventricular fold activity
Anatomical malformations
Vocal fold lengthening
Vertical laryngeal position
Involuntary laryngeal activity
Phonatory apraxia

Phase Symmetry of the Vocal Folds

This sign refers to differences in appearance between the moving vocal folds. For example, do the folds appear similar to each other in configuration?

Periodicity of the Vocal Folds

Periodicity is determined by comparing the image of the vocal folds when the strobe flash is controlled by the fundamental frequency of the vocal folds to the image when it is not. The vocal folds will appear static in the image when vibration is periodic and will appear to move under the stroboscopic light flashes when aperiodic.

Laryngoscopic Signs

In this section, we will describe those signs that can be visualized through a variety of techniques, including indirect mirror examination, flexible fiberoscopy, and examination with a rigid endoscope. Other means of laryngeal visualization include direct laryngoscopy under anesthesia and ultra-high speed photography. The following listing (see Table 2.6) and explanation reviews the observations that can help to establish a diagnosis. The ability to make these observations may vary with the visualization technique used.

Vocal Fold Approximation

Variations of vocal fold approximation may include (*a*) incomplete closure along the length of the one or both vocal folds; (*b*) bowing of the vocal folds, seen as a central gap; and (*c*) lack of approximation of the vocal processes, resulting in a posterior chink.

Vocal Fold Movement

Movement of one or both vocal folds may be reduced or absent due to a variety of conditions. The vocal folds may (*a*) not adduct (move to the midline), (*b*) not abduct (move away from the midline), or (*c*) adduct excessively or abduct involuntarily and at inappropriate times during phonation.

Tissue Changes

There are a host of changes that can affect the vocal fold mucosa. These include edema, inflammation, and benign, malignant, or premalignant lesions. Each has a characteristic appearance and/or site of occurrence (see Chapter 3).

Pyriform Changes

The opening of the pyriform sinuses usually increases with adductory movement of the vocal folds. Lack of aperture variation of the pyriform sinus cavity is usually a sign of laryngeal paralysis and is a significant sign to note when attempting to differentiate between paralysis and arytenoid ankylosis or dislocation (Brewer and Gould, 1974).

Anteroposterior Laryngeal Dimensions

During phonation, the distance between the epiglottis and arytenoids (anteroposterior dimension) is sufficient to allow visualization of most of the length of the vocal folds in most normal speakers. The extent of the visualization will depend on the phonatory conditions produced by the patient (i.e., pitch, loudness, and vowel). However, in some persons, the epiglottis and arytenoids can be seen to approach each other during phonation, thereby shortening this anteroposterior dimension and obscuring visualization of the vocal folds.

Ventricular Folds

The ventricular folds are usually seen superior and lateral to the true vocal folds, and there is variation in the degree of their movement. During phonation they are usually seen to maintain their position relative to the edge of the true vocal folds. However, sometimes they appear to move toward the midline, obscuring all or part of the true vocal folds (Freud, 1962). They may even approximate each other during phonation. Furthermore, their movements may not always be symmetrical.

Anatomical Malformations and Congenital Anomalies

Structures may be malformed as the result of a congenital anatomic deformity or the result of abnormal growth and development. Laryngomalacia, a softness or abnormal flaccidity of the laryngeal cartilages, is the most common congenital laryngeal anomaly and may resolve by 1 to 2 years of age (Hollinger and Brown, 1967; Cotton and Richardson, 1981). In this condition, there is a characteristic movement pattern of the larynx involving a downward and anterior displacement and a bowing of the aryepiglottic folds during inspiration. Other congenital problems include (a) subglottal stenosis, a thickening of subglottal tissues that may be sufficient to obstruct the airway; (b) vocal fold paralysis, often a temporary condition lasting about 4 weeks (Cotton and Richardson, 1981), and (c) laryngeal web, a band of tissue (which may vary in extent) joining the two vocal folds at the anterior commissure.

Vocal Fold Lengthening

Vocal fold lengthening is usually observed as vocal pitch is raised. This is seen fiberoptically as a lengthening of the distance between the arytenoid cartilages and the epiglottis as the vocal folds elongate. In some persons, the elevation of pitch does not produce this effect.

Vertical Laryngeal Position

The larynx is able to move in the vertical dimension. This can be visualized in laryngoscopic examination as a rising of the larynx as pitch is raised and a descent below resting level as pitch is lowered. Degree of movement varies among individuals and between trained and untrained singers (Shipp, 1975; Shipp and Izdebski, 1975). For a further discussion on vertical laryngeal position, please see Chapter 4, "High Laryngeal Position."

Involuntary Laryngeal Activity

Rhythmic involuntary movement of laryngeal structures in the resting state, in the absence of phonation, is often seen accompanying neurologically based disorders (Parnes, Lavarato, and Myers, 1978). Another common observation is the movement of the arytenoids toward the midline. In voluntary effort closure, a medial squeezing and "closing down" of the entire larynx ocurs. On occasion, such a movement occurs involuntarily and is described as hyperadduction. The normal larynx, when viewed at rest, maintains a relatively static posture with a fully open glottis. In some individuals, random, arrhythmic movement of various structures may be observed.

Phonatory Apraxia

Phonatory apraxia is an inability to produce phonation volitionally. Although seemingly normal movement of the vocal folds and other laryngeal structures may be observed during swallow and reflexive activities, it is absent when the person is asked to phonate voluntarily (Aronson, 1985).

Normal-Appearing Larynx

Despite the perception of a vocal abnormality, the larynx may appear to be normal in structure and function.

Interrelationships of Physiological, Acoustic, and Perceptual Signs

The signs of voice problems are not independent of one another. That is, there are interrelationships among the physiological, acoustic, and perceptual signs. Simply stated, movements of the vocal folds (physiology) create pressure disturbances in the air (acoustics) that are received by the ear and processed (perception).

A change in the structure of the vocal folds (e.g., a lesion, a tissue change) or a change in their manner of use (e.g., excess tension, inadequate energy) will affect the acoustic signal produced, which in turn will alter the perception of the voice. For example, a mass on the vocal folds may interfere with their closure. Consequently, air will continue to flow during that part of the vibratory cycle in which the vocal folds should be completely closed. This disturbed physiology will create a weak acoustic disturbance. Furthermore, due to the constant flow of air through a small glottal opening, there may be an increase of noise level. The weaker acoustic signal in combination with noise from the air striking the vocal folds will create the perception of breathiness.

As another example, the fundamental vibrating rate of the vocal folds is determined by their mass, length, and tension. If there is a mass on the vocal folds (e.g., a polyp or nodule), the basic vibrating rate will be altered. Vocal folds with a large mass would vibrate at a lower rate, producing a lower fundamental frequency and the perception of a lower pitch (Isshiki, Tanabe, Ishizaka, and Board, 1977). Masses on both vocal folds that are asymmetrical in size will each vibrate at a different rate, producing greater aperiodicity of vibration and increased frequency and amplitude perturbation. Greater perturbation usually is associated with the perception of greater roughness or hoarseness in the voice.

Signs cannot be viewed in a vacuum. Signs interrelate within a domain (physiology, acoustics, or perception) and across these domains. Some are redundant and assist in the confirmation of other signs. Patterns of signs accompany different voice problems and when considered in combination with laboratory tests, physical examination, and the patient's history assist in the accurate diagnosis of the voice disorder.

Differential Diagnosis of Voice Problems Demonstrated in Eight Case Studies

In the previous sections we have defined the terminology used to describe the symptoms and signs of voice disorders. In the following sections, each of the eight symptoms will be explored in further detail in the manner of the differential diagnosis process, using case studies. The first case will be presented and followed by a discussion of the process of differential diagnosis as it applies to that case. For each of the other cases, we will present only the case study, with questions designed to guide the reader's thinking. Tables providing those signs that are consistent with each major symptom are also provided throughout the text. Please keep in mind that an individual patient would not necessarily present all of the signs listed in the tables.

Hoarseness

J. H., a 37-year-old woman, was referred for voice therapy by an otolaryngologist who had made a diagnosis of vocal nodules. The history she presented included the following: (*a*) She teaches seven to nine elementary school classes of physical education per day; (*b*) She owns and teaches in a gymnastics school for 3 to 4 hours per day after the school day and often on weekends; (*c*) this business requires that she spend much time on the phone; (*d*) she is married and has two teenage sons at home; (*e*) she neither smokes nor drinks; and (*f*) she describes herself as a very active and vocal person. J. H. reports that she has noticed increased hoarseness for a number of years but that during the past year this hoarseness has worsened in degree and in constancy. She is aware that the hoarseness increases following extended voice use and that she also experiences periods of vocal fatigue, occasional soreness in the throat, and the need to strain to produce voice loud enough to be heard. She sought medical attention at the point when her voice was severely hoarse all the time, her students were unable to hear her, and the fatigue she felt at the end of the day became intolerable.

In the differential diagnosis processes, the clinician should now be asking, is this history consistent with a diagnosis of vocal nodules? In view of the gradual onset, increased worsening, and excessive voice usage, a probable cause of her vocal difficulties could be expected to be vocal nodules. However, prior to laryngoscopic examination, the possible diagnoses that would be entertained, based on the history, include polyps, cancer, keratosis, chronic laryngitis, edema, and intracordal cyst.

At this point, the clinician should be concerned about the compatibility of the perceptual signs and symptoms noted above with the stated history and presenting diagnosis.

Perceptual signs noted at the initial evaluation included hoarse/rough quality, increased breathiness, episodic aphonia, and excessive throat clearing. Increased tension was observed as J. H. worked at producing voice. Acoustic signs included a fundamental frequency of 195 Hz, a phonation range of less than one octave, an s/z ratio of 1.9, and a maximum phonation time of 6 seconds. Her airflow data showed good closure of the vocal folds but with high peak flows. Vocal fold contact area measurements (EGG) showed a brief closure period but normal opening and closing characteristics.

No additional examinations were recommended at that time, and J. H. began a course of voice therapy. Although it was difficult for her, she began to make significant changes in her voice use habits. A plan was devised whereby she could continue to work but would cease abusing her vocal folds. Throat clearing was eliminated quickly, as were all attempts at loud voice use. J. H. became more dependent on the use of her whistle in place of her voice. She began to demonstrate for her students rather than explain verbally. And her voice improved. Almost immediately she reported that the symptoms of soreness and fatigue abated.

A school vacation allowed J. H. to really "rest her voice" for a week. She talked minimally, without strain and with reduced intensity. At the end of that week, further improvement was noted in her voice. Phonational range was significantly increased, aphonic episodes were no longer present, voicing occurred with minimal effort, and hoarseness was reduced. J. H. returned to her teaching but was extremely careful about voice use. Nevertheless, her voice showed marked deterioration within a week. This rapid vocal worsening raised questions in the clinician's mind.

This rapid vocal worsening was unexpected because J. H. had made significant progress and had engaged in no activities that would be expected to adversely affect the condition of the vocal folds. When such an unexpected change occurs in a patient's condition, the clinician should review the diagnosis and the ensuing therapy. This may lead to the recognition of the need for further examination. In this case, J. H. was scheduled for fiberoptic and stroboscopic examination.

Visualization of the vocal folds utilizing fiberoptic and stroboscopic techniques revealed the presence of a vocal fold cyst. No nodules were apparent. J. H. was scheduled for laryngeal surgery with a recommendation for a course of voice therapy postoperatively.

This case study is an example of the process of differential diagnosis. The questions raised at critical points in the history suggest the thinking process that is essential to the understanding of voice problems and their management. The nature of this particular case also makes it quite clear that the process of differential diagnosis is ongoing throughout the treatment program. A patient's response to treatment (or lack of response) is meaningful information that must become a part of the understanding of the problem. It may, as it did in this case, point to the need for further testing and perhaps a changed diagnosis.

The patient in this case was referred to the speech pathologist with a stated diagnosis, vocal nodules, made by an otolaryngologist. The primary symptom expressed by the patient, hoarseness, was consistent with that diagnosis. An examination of Table 2.7 reveals the perceptual signs that may accompany the symptom of hoarseness. A number of these signs were noted in this case during the initial voice evaluation, for example, hoarse voice quality, increased breathiness, episodic aphonia, excessive throat clearing, and increased tension.

Table 2.7 lists those acoustic signs that would be consistent with the symptom and the perceptual signs. In other words, our ears hear certain vocal characteristics, some of which are accessible to measurement, thereby providing an independent corroboration of our perception. We would therefore expect to find a certain degree of match between the perceptual and the acoustic signs. In this case, we find reduced phonation range, a significant s/z ratio, and reduced phonation time.

Let us examine these factors a little more closely. Remember that hoarseness was given as a perceptual sign. A lesion, such as a nodule, on the vibratory edge of the vocal fold mucosa will disrupt vibratory behavior by adding mass at a specific location on the vocal fold. Addition of the same amount of mass distributed along the entire length of the vocal fold would most likely reduce fundamental frequency. In the case of a nodule, the extra mass loads down the vocal fold and affects its periodicity. Stiffness of the vocal folds is also increased due to the biomechanical characteristics of the nodule. This disruption results in a disturbance of the periodicity of the signal, creating a noisier signal that results in a perception of hoarseness. The increased mass and stiffness of the folds will also interfere with their ability to stretch and vibrate at a more rapid rate, which normally results in pitch elevation. Thus, the phonational range would be decreased.

The s/z ratio is based on the theory that vocal fold vibration sufficient to produce phonation (z) can be maintained for a time period equal to the time that airflow can be maintained without vocal fold activity. When a lesion is present on the vocal folds, there is incomplete glottal closure, resulting in a loss of air and a reduction in the ability to sustain

Table 2.7.
Signs that may be associated with symptom of Hoarse voice

Typical complaint: "My voice is hoarse or froggy. People think I have laryngitis."

Perceptual signs
  hoarseness/roughness
  breathiness
  laryngeal tension
  inappropriate pitch
  excessive throat clearing
  episodic aphonia
  pitch breaks
Acoustic signs
  restricted phonational range
  restricted dynamic range
  excessive spectral noise
  greater perturbation
  greater shimmer
  reduced maximum phonation time and high s/z ratios
  reduced fundamental frequency variability
Laryngoscopic signs
  anteroposterior shortening
    functional
  increased ventricular fold activity
    functional
    compensatory
      paralysis
      fixed cord
      inadequate closure
  tissue change
    nodules
    polyps
    carcinoma
    papilloma
    leukoplakia
    edema
    cyst
  color change
    burns
      heat
      chemical
    other vocal fold lesions
  variations of vocal fold approximation
    posterior chink
      functional
    bowing
      reduced muscle tonus
      keyhole
      aged voice
    incomplete anteroposterior approximation
      paralysis
      functional
      ankylosis
      dislocation
  anatomical malformation
    congenital

Table 2.7.—continued

     malacia
     stenosis
     web
    trauma
     blunt
     pentrating
     surgery
  normal larynx
    functional
     psychogenic
     misuse
    neurological
    minor or hidden tissue change

Physiological signs
  aerodynamics
    increased flow
    increased air pressure
  vibratory
    aberrant glottal pulse shape
    irregularity or asymmetry of vocal fold motion
    muscosal wave changes
  muscle activity
    higher than normal levels
    imbalance of paired muscle activity
    normal activity

phonation. The resulting s/z ratio becomes significantly greater than 1 to 1.4, which is reported to be the normal range (Eckel & Boone, 1971). Similarly, the maximum time that phonation can be sustained is reduced. When air leakage during phonation is of a sufficient degree, there will be a perception of breathiness.

Excessive throat clearing is a common observation in patients who have vocal nodules or other lesions. These patients report the sensation that something is in the way of their being able to talk and that they must first attempt to dislodge it by clearing the throat, often quite strenuously. Unfortunately, this leads in a cyclical fashion to increased vocal abuse, which results in an exacerbation of the symptoms, which leads to an increased feeling of the need to clear the throat, and so on.

When a vocal fold lesion is present and maximum phonation time is reduced, it is not unexpected to find momentary episodes of absence of voicing. This occurs because the patient is unaccustomed to the reduction in the ability to sustain phonation or because there was insufficient effort, air pressure, or vocal fold approximation to compensate for the extra demands placed on the system by the presence of the lesion.

We would expect that breathiness would be reflected in greater than expected airflow during phonation. Indeed, when this patient was seen for further examination, one of the physiological aerodynamic signs (see Table 2.7) was increased flow. The glottal pulse shape was aberrant, revealing the poor glottal closure. It should be noted, however, that at the time of the reexamination, the amount of breathiness perceived in the voice was considerably reduced from that present at the initial evaluation. This could be due to reduction of general irritation and edema of the vocal folds in response to a marked reduction in abusive and excessive voice use.

Stroboscopic examination, which was helpful in making the diagnosis of a vocal fold cyst, revealed reduced mucosal wave in the area of the cyst (see Table 2.5). The laryngoscopic signs noted on fiberoptic examination revealed some tissue change, which appeared as a lesion on the superior surface of the vocal fold mucosa at a midway point along its length (see Table 2.6).

During the differential diagnosis process, the pieces must fit together. The process can work from a starting point of the patient's complaint, or it can work backward, as it were, from a previously arrived at diagnosis. It is typical for speech pathologists to be in the position of having patients referred with a stated diagnosis. In certain cases, however, the observations and perceptions of the speech pathologist and information about the acoustic and physiological signs do not seem to be consistent with the diagnosis. Further examination is often warranted in such cases. On other occasions, as typified by the case of J. H., the symptoms and signs may be consistent with the diagnosis, yet the patient's treatment course suggests the need for reexploration of the case. It is especially important to recognize that in the case of J. H., all the perceptual, acoustic, and physiologic signs could have been consistent with the original diagnosis. The stroboscopic and laryngoscopic signs were the determining factors in making the diagnosis, and the suspicion of the speech pathologist, based on sudden and unexpected worsening of a condition, was the catalyst for reexamination of the original diagnosis.

Although some case history material was provided in the description of J. H., that part of the diagnostic process has been only briefly considered in this chapter. We do not mean to suggest that it is not an essential part of the process. Indeed, a thorough case history is essential and will be fully covered in Chapter 6.

We will explore the other primary symptoms of voice problems and the differential diagnosis process in the remainder of this chapter. Each will begin with a case study. However, we will not explain each one in the same amount of detail provided for J. H. Consult the tables for listings of all the various signs that we believe to be consistent with the symptom. Following the process should lead the reader to an understanding of the interrelatedness of the various factors, that is, perception, acoustics, and physiology, and the need for complete evaluation. In turn, this understanding should help to eliminate the cookbook approach to voice problems and replace it with the ability to follow the process of differential diagnosis thoughtfully.

Vocal Fatigue

S. D., a 45-year-old first grade teacher and mother of nine children, complained of feeling vocally tired at the end of each day. She could not identify any recent changes at home, at work, or in her personal health status that might account for the vocal fatigue she was experiencing. However, further discussion revealed that the aide in her classroom had become sick in November and had not been able to return to work. The symptoms had begun in early December, and at the time we saw her, they had persisted for 3 months. When questioned about the specific symptoms of this vocal fatigue, she described a tired feeling in the throat; a feeling of not wanting to talk and, if required to talk, a feeling of having to work to do so; sometimes a feeling of tightness in the throat and chest; and a rough-sounding voice quality that seemed to get worse as the day progressed. She also complained that it was difficult for her to produce a loud voice.

Q. What are the possible diagnoses that you might begin to consider on the basis of this limited information?

Although S. D. must use her voice extensively both at work and at home, she reports that she rarely shouts. She does not sing, smoke, or drink. She does not talk on the telephone except when necessary.

Table 2.8.
Signs That May Be Associated with the Symptom of Vocal Fatigue

Typical complaint: "My voice gives out at the end of the day."

Perceptual signs
  monopitch
  tension
  breathiness
  hoarseness
Acoustic signs
  restricted phonational range
  reduced variability of fundamental frequency
  normal acoustics
Laryngoscopic signs
  variations of vocal fold approximation
    functional
  tissue change
    color
    nodule
  change of laryngeal position
    muscle tension
  normal appearing larynx
    neurological
    myasthenia gravis
Physiological signs
  aerodynamic
    increased airflow
  vibratory
    inadequate closed time
  muscle activity
    muscle imbalance
    excessive levels
    variation of level

Perceptually, we noted a tendency toward a monopitch voice, with little pitch variability during general conversation (see Table 2.8). Voice quality was judged to be only mildly to moderately rough, with an apparent increase in the degree of roughness occurring at the end of sentences or breath groups. Voice production seemed unchanged perceptually when S. D. was asked to talk to us as she might to her class or to her children. We also observed what might best be described as a low energy level, as if all systems were working at 50% power.

S. D.'s measured speaking fundamental frequency was found to be 205 Hz, but the variability of fundamental frequency around this mean was limited to three to four semitones. Phonational range was found to be within normal limits when measured, but it was necessary to work with S. D. first on a pitch-matching task in order to begin to get some variability in frequency.

Fiberoptic laryngeal examination revealed a structurally normal larynx. Visualization of the vocal folds during speech was often obscured, however, due to approximation of the arytenoid cartilages and the epiglottis. This anteroposterior "squeezing" was marked throughout speaking tasks. When this squeezing is present in a patient, it is not possible to view the vocal folds with a rigid endoscope. With the flexible fiberscope in place, we engaged S. D. in a short period of "diagnostic therapy" in which we asked her to engage in a variety of vocal maneuvers. We began by having S. D. match a very high-pitched vocalization on the vowel /ee/. As we watched her do this, we noted that the vocal folds appeared to lengthen and their full length became visible. The anteroposterior "squeezing" was not visible. We were then able to help S. D. bring the vocal pitch down gradually while maintaining this "open" laryngeal posture. As she approached speaking fundamental frequency, we became aware of a perceptual difference in vocal quality from what had been heard initially.

The videotaped fiberoptic examination of this patient was used in a study of changes in laryngeal physiology resulting from voice therapy techniques (Casper, Brewer, and Conture, 1981). The visible vocal fold length was measured in the production of a word in the patient's typical phonatory behavior and again when the identical word was produced following the period of diagnostic therapy when perceptually the voice quality was judged to be improved.

Based on the findings of the extended evaluation, a diagnosis of "hyperfunctional voice use" without any laryngeal tissue changes was made, and a period of voice therapy was recommended.

Breathiness

Thirteen-year-old K. B. was referred for voice therapy with the description of a hoarse voice. No diagnosis per se was provided by the referring otolaryngologist. K. B. had been taken to this physician by her mother because of an earache. During the examination the physician had noted the aberrant voice quality and had made the referral for voice therapy. Mrs. B., the mother, reported that she had never been particularly aware of K.'s voice because K. had always sounded this way. Furthermore, none of K.'s doctors, teachers, or other school personnel had ever raised any concern about it.

Despite the mother's lack of awareness of a problem, K. B. was very much aware of her voice being "different." She reported being called derogatory names by other children and being made fun of by them because of the sound of her voice. In addition, she had difficulty in making herself heard in the classroom and was often told to "speak up" by her teachers. Indeed, this had become so distressing to her that she rarely volunteered to speak in class and worried about when she might have to do so.

The rest of the history was essentially negative. K. B. had experienced no serious illnesses, nor had she had any surgery. She had never been involved in an accident, and she had normal hearing and normal intelligence.

Q. What possible diagnoses begin to be suggested?

Perceptual signs included marked breathiness, reduced loudness, and hoarseness and were consistent with the acoustic findings of reduced dynamic range, restricted phonational range, and reduced maximum sustained phonation time (see Table 2.9).

Q. How do these findings affect the diagnoses you entertained above?

Attempts to alter voice quality through a variety of vocal maneuvers were unsuccessful. At no time during the voice evaluation was there any significant change in K. B.'s voice quality. K. B. was then scheduled to be seen in the voice laboratory for physiological and fiberoptic evaluation. Physiologic signs included a large amount of airflow leakage and low peak flows. Her electroglottogram showed irregular pulses, suggesting random variations in opening and closing of the vocal folds.

Q. Does this added information narrow your diagnostic choices?

Most revealing, and corroborative of the findings reported thus far, were the stroboscopic and laryngoscopic signs (Table 2.9). K. B.'s larynx was difficult to visualize due to an omega-shaped epiglottis that was oriented in such a way as to frequently obscure the larynx. The larynx was noted to be asymmetric, with the left side appearing to be smaller

Table 2.9.
Signs That May Be Associated with the Symptom of Breathy Voice

Typical complaint: "My voice is weak, I run out of air. People can't hear me."

Perceptual signs
  breathiness
  too soft loudness variation
  hoarseness/roughness
  episodic aphonia
Acoustic signs
  restricted phonational range
  restricted dynamic range
  reduced sustained phonation time
  increased s/z ratio
  excessive spectral noise
  increased perturbation
  increased shimmer
Laryngoscopic signs
  variation of vocal fold approximation
    incomplete a-p approximation (most prevalent)
      paralysis (adductor)
      functional
      ankylosis
      dislocation
      neurological
        ALS
        Parkinson's
        myasthenia gravis
    posterior chink
      functional
    bowing
      aging
      reduced muscle tonus
  lack of movement of one or both vocal folds
    paralysis
    ankylosis
    dislocation
    carcinoma
  lack of change in appearance of pyriform sinuses
    paralysis
  anatomic malformation
    congenital
      laryngomalacia
    trauma
      blunt
      penetrating
      surgery
    tissue change
      burns
        heat
        chemical
Physiological signs
  aerodynamic
    increased airflow
    increased air pressure
  vibratory

Table 2.9.—*continued*

aberrant glottal pulse shape
inadequate closed time
irregularity and asymmetry of vocal fold motion
mucosal wave changes
muscle activity
absent or reduced levels
imbalance of paired muscle activity

and less well developed than the right. Left unilateral vocal fold paralysis was observed and glottal closure was never obtained. The stroboscopic examination revealed reduced muscosal wave on the left fold. The diagnosis of congenital vocal fold paralysis was made.

Q. Can you explain how all the symptoms and signs reported in this case are consistent with this diagnosis?

Reduced Phonational Range

M. L. is a 39-year-old woman referred to the voice lab by her choir director for an inability to produce her upper vocal range with clarity. Four months previously she had had an upper respiratory infection (URI) during the course of which she had coughed a great deal. She also experienced what she described as acute laryngitis. The symptoms of the URI resolved, including the acute laryngitis, but the coughing persisted for about 2 months. She has continued to note mild hoarseness. Her main concern, however, is that she appears to be unable to produce the top of her range with clarity. Indeed, there have been times when she has been unable to produce the highest notes at all.

Q. What conditions accompanying an upper respiratory infection or presenting as its sequelae would be important to consider?

M. L. has been singing in a choir for many years and has also performed both as a soloist and with another singer for local events such as weddings, funerals, and other social gatherings. She had minimal vocal training, many years ago. She neither smokes nor drinks, nor does she perform in loud or smoke-filled settings. She is married and has several grown children. She does not describe herself as either a loud or a constant talker. She is employed at a job that does not require much talking, and all of it is done in a relatively quiet environment. She denies any allergies, takes no medicines, and has no known medical problems.

Perceptually M. L. presented with an essentially normal-sounding speaking voice (see Table 2.10). Although she complained of a mild hoarseness, we found this to be extremely mild and inconsistently present. M. L.'s singing voice was marked by occasional pitch breaks within the upper third of her range. We observed a "reaching" for the high notes with upward and forward tilting of the chin, wrinkling of the forehead, and a generalized body tension, especially the upper body.

Q. What do these observations suggest to you?

M. L.'s phonational range was found to be 2.5 octaves at best, which she claims is reduced by at least half an octave from her optimal vocal production. In addition, the highest notes were not produced with what she described as her usual clarity of tone. Her speaking fundamental frequency was 205 Hz. Airflow data revealed elevated peak flows and a small leakage but was otherwise normal. Her electroglottogram showed very brief closed times with an unusual break in the closing phase of the signal, suggesting irregular closing patterns.

Fiberoptic examination revealed an essentially normal-appearing larynx. There was the suggestion of some roughness along the edge of the right vocal fold, and a mucus

Table 2.10.
Signs That May Be Associated with the Symptom of Reduced Phonational Range

Typical complaint: "I am not able to produce the high notes of my range during singing."

Perceptual signs
  tension
  pitch breaks
  normal-sounding voice
Acoustic signs
  restricted phonational range
  restricted dynamic range
Laryngoscopic signs
  tissue change of vocal folds
    nodule
    color
  normal appearing larynx
    functional
      misuse
      improper vocal technique
    minor or hidden tissue change
Physiological
  muscle
    excessive levels
    normal physiology

strand formed and broke at about the junction of the anterior one-third and posterior two-thirds of the vocal folds. Her stroboscopic examination was normal.

Q. What do the laryngoscopic signs suggest?

A period of diagnostic therapy was provided during which M. L. was instructed to consciously use good breath support, to allow sound to be produced easily without the "reaching" tensions, and to use the type of imagery she recalled from her vocal training in producing the high pitches. The ease of sound production was emphasized, rather than the beauty of the sound. It was gratifying to observe the change in phonatory behavior and to hear the difference in the resulting sound.

The diagnosis in this case seemed to involve a combination of factors. Because some of the precipitating conditions were no longer present, judgments had to be made based on history and current findings. The history of excessive coughing combined with acute laryngitis suggests that the mucosa was sufficiently irritated to begin to show some changes. The slight suggestion of roughness along the vocal fold edge and the presence of the strand of mucus forming and reforming may be evidence of a resolving problem or of an ongoing problem. Although M. L. does not seem to be abusing her voice significantly in speaking, her singing technique is very poor, and there is obvious strain and tension in attempts to produce the upper frequency range. In view of her positive response to diagnostic therapy, at least some of the difficulty she is encountering may be the result of the psychological fear that she has built up concerning her inability to produce those notes. We recommended a resumption of vocal training with periodic monitoring of the condition of the vocal folds.

Aphonia

P. M., a 32-year-old woman, was referred for voice therapy with a very involved history. She presented for the voice evaluation seated in a wheelchair and with no voice.

Indeed, she was so aphonic that she was not even producing a whisper, nor were the voiceless consonants audible.

Q. Can you explain how a person could be so aphonic?

Her history was exceedingly lengthy, often vague, and difficult to follow. Key points seemed to be that she was quite sick for a period of time as a small child and was not expected to survive; she has had frequent upper respiratory problems since then; she had a father who had had tuberculosis; and she claimed to have severe asthma attacks and breathing problems (which had never been observed by anyone else despite numerous hospitalizations). She had been married for a period of time, but the marriage was terminated after she was involved in an automobile accident that left her confined to a wheelchair. This accident resulted in cervical spine nerve root avulsions, but the main reason for use of the wheelchair was her reported "dizziness" and subsequent fear of falling. P. M. lived alone in a trailer. She reported an episode in which a young man broke into her trailer and attempted to strangle her. She denied being raped but stated that he knocked her down and twisted her neck. She began to have some difficulty with her voice following that, but this became worse after she was involved in another automobile accident 3 years later. She did not suffer any injuries in this accident. P. M. wore a hearing aid with a moderate degree of gain for several years. However, a subsequent audiological examination revealed essentially normal hearing sensitivity and showed that she did as well without amplification as she did with it.

P. M. had consulted and been treated by numerous specialists for a variety of problems. She claimed that she was told that her phrenic nerve was damaged and that this was the reason she was unable to speak.

Q. What does the phrenic nerve innervate, and what effect would damage to this nerve have on voice production?

During the history taking, P. M. continued to be totally aphonic. Her affect was very pleasant and strangely cheerful given her condition. Some voicing was noted in the voluntary production of a coughing sound, although much support and encouragement were necessary in order to elicit a "fake" cough.

Q. What diagnoses would you consider at this point?

Observation of P. M.'s breathing at rest showed normal abdominal and chest movements. During her attempts at speech, we observed adequate inhalatory behavior, but P. M. seemed to hold her breath while her mouth was moving and expel it at the end of a soundless utterance.

Q. Are these observations consistent with phrenic nerve damage?

Because there was no voice production, no acoustic measures could be made (see Table 2.11). The airflow trace showed large amounts of airflow unmodulated by the vocal folds. Laryngoscopic examination using the fiberscope revealed a normal-appearing larynx. Vocal fold movement was observed during reflexive behaviors and also during nonphonatory whistling. The movement was noted to be symmetric and quite normal. Since there was no phonation, stroboscopy was not indicated.

A diagnosis of a psychogenic voice disorder was made. P. M. was seen for two sessions of trial voice therapy. During each of these sessions we were able to elicit entirely normal voice quality. Despite the normal sound of the voice and her ability to produce complete sentences naturally and without effort, P. M. was unable to accept return of voicing. She did not acknowledge the presence of voice when she first produced it, and when it was noted by the examiner, she continued to ignore it. P. M. was referred for psychiatric consultation and treatment. She followed up on the consultation but refused

Table 2.11.
Signs That May Be Associated with the Symptom of Aphonia

Typical complaint. "I lost my voice" or "My voice is gone."

Perceptual signs
  breathiness
  consistent aphonia
Acoustic signs
  excessive spectral noise
Laryngoscopic signs
  variations in vocal fold approximation
  incomplete vocal fold approximation
  bilateral adductor paralysis
  lack of movement of vocal folds
  phonatory apraxia
  CNS lesion
Physiological
  aerodynamics
    increased airflow
    increased air pressure
  vibratory
    not applicable
  muscle activity
    unknown

treatment. Although she has experienced full return of voice, she continues to have many other problems, both physical and psychosocial.

Pitch Breaks or Falsetto

When S. P., a 20-year-old man, was referred for voice therapy, the referring otolaryngologist reported that examination had revealed a normal larynx but the voice was hoarse. S. P., however, complained that his voice often sounded "squeaky" and that he was aware that his voice was different from that of his friends. He also complained of difficulty in making himself heard at work, where there was often much loud noise.

S. P. was employed as a garage mechanic, had completed high school, shared an apartment with a friend, had never smoked, drank no more than two to three beers a week, and had a steady girlfriend. He had never sustained an injury to his neck, did not believe he had been exposed to any noxious fumes, had experienced no serious illnesses, denied allergies, and was in general quite happy with his life.

Concerning his voice, S. P. reported that he had no memory of ever sounding different. He denied any recent change in his voice and reported that his friends never commented on how he sounded. He believed that they were all simply used to hearing his voice.

Q. What would be your next question?

Our next question was to wonder about the motivation for this consultation, given a situation that seems to have been status quo for a long time and has not had any significantly negative effect on his life. In response, S. P. stated that he just knew that something was wrong and that he had indeed been worried about this for a number of years but did not know what to do about it. The opportunity to do something came about when he sought medical attention for an earache.

Q. Are any possible diagnoses coming to mind?

Table 2.12.
Signs That May Be Associated with the Symptoms of Pitch Breaks or Inappropriately High Pitch

Typical complaint: "My voice sounds squeaky."

Perceptual signs
  inappropriate pitch level
  pitch breaks
Acoustic signs
  higher than expected speaking fundamental frequency
  rapid shifts of fundamental frequency
  restricted phonational range
  restricted dynamic range
  reduced maximum phonation time
Laryngoscopic signs
  normal-appearing larynx
    functional
  anatomical malformations
    hormone imbalance
    web
Physiological signs
  aerodynamics
    decreased airflow
  vibratory
    inadequate closed times
    mucosal wave changes
  muscle activity
    excessive levels

S. P. presented as a handsome, strong, and muscular young man. Perceptually, however, he had a nonresonant, thin, rather high pitched voice that sounded somehow out of control (see Table 2.12). There were frequent pitch breaks. These were documented acoustically, with rapid shifts of frequency, averaging an octave. Average speaking fundamental frequency was measured at 175 Hz.

Q. With this additional information, what would your differential list consist of?

Additional acoustic signs included a very restricted total phonational range as well as restricted dynamic range (Table 2.12). The referral source had indicated a normal laryngeal examination, and no further laryngeal examination was done. The stroboscopic examination revealed small lateral excursions of the vocal folds, and the mucosal wave was suggestive of stiff vocal folds. Such a finding would be expected in falsetto voice phonation due to the high laryngeal tensions and small mass of the vocal folds. Physiologic signs included decreased airflow and an inadequate closed phase was seen on the electroglottographic waveform.

The working diagnosis that seemed to be consistent with all of the signs and symptoms was that of puberphonia. With that as a base, it was hypothesized that S. P. should be capable of producing a modal voice of a more appropriate pitch. S. P. was asked whether he had ever produced a different voice even momentarily, and he responded affirmatively. It was found that he could produce a relatively low pitched (125 Hz) and very resonant voice at will and with ease. Although he had been aware of his ability to do this, he was concerned that this "other voice" sounded very strange and would subject him to ridicule. A short period of using the voice in the clinic setting with reassurance, support, and encouragement was all that was necessary to help S. P. cross that barrier.

Strain/Struggle

R. O., a 45-year-old man who was in a management position with a small industrial firm, was referred for otolaryngological examination by his family physician after a 4-year period of voice difficulty. He had already been seen by several physicians and had also been through a course of voice therapy with no relief of his symptoms. Indeed, he felt that his voice was becoming worse.

R. O. recalls that his initial voice difficulty seemed to be "laryngitis," following which he began to notice "voice breaks." As his symptoms worsened, he found that he began to experience a tightness in his throat as he was speaking, and this did not seem to be related to the length of the utterance. He also reports that he has been unable to detect any pattern related to the severity of his symptoms. Although he thinks that the voice is worse when he is tired or under stress, he can't decide whether the symptoms are actually worse or whether he just becomes more aware of them.

A variety of diagnoses and recommendations for treatment had been made up to this time. These included a bowed vocal fold, requiring teflon injection; overuse of the voice, requiring an extended period of vocal rest; an unexplained problem but one that should be helped by speech therapy; and a psychiatric problem. Voice therapy, as noted, had been tried for a period of 3 months. By his report, the therapy included a variety of relaxation exercises and breathing exercises. R. O. reports that during therapy and during practice, he was occasionally able to produce a very short sentence without difficulty but that otherwise there was no change in his voice.

Q. What possible diagnoses might be entertained at this point as part of the differential?

We found R. O.'s speech difficult to understand (see Table 2.13). There was the perception of much vocal tension; sudden interruption of voicing occurred within words, with aphonia extending over a syllable or over several words; initiation of sentences was sometimes louder than the rest of the utterance and seemed somewhat explosive, as if much effort had been required to produce voicing; and there were periods of increasing tightness in the voice as a sentence progressed. Slight tremor was heard only on vowel prolongation.

Acoustic analysis gave evidence of voice stoppages, and maximum sustained phonation time was 8 seconds, a value well below the norm for an adult man. The electroglottographic trace was aberrant, revealing excessively long closed times during the vibratory cycle. Airflow was decreased while air pressures were increased.

Q. Does this additional information shorten the differential diagnosis list, and if so, how and why?

This patient was not subjected to electromyography. However, based on the findings from others with similar symptoms and based on other physiological signs, we would expect to find sudden, unexpected bursts of muscle potentials, slow rise or fall of signal amplitude, and excessive levels of muscle activity.

Fiberoptic laryngoscopic examination revealed rhythmic, involuntary laryngeal movement (particularly of the arytenoid cartilages) at rest, effort closure of the larynx at unexpected and unpredictable moments during speech, and occasional apparent anteroposterior shortening of the vocal folds as the epiglottis and arytenoids moved toward each other (Table 2.13). It was not possible to obtain good stroboscopic pictures due to the aperiodicity of phonation.

The working diagnosis made in this case was spasmodic dysphonia. In order to more fully examine this diagnosis, the right recurrent laryngeal nerve was anesthetized by injection of lidocaine. This procedure was carried out in the voice laboratory with the fiberoptic

Table 2.13.
Signs That May Be Associated with the Symptom of Strain/Struggle

Typical complaint: "My voice just stops. I can't get anything out."

Perceptual signs
  strain/struggle voice
  tension
  sudden interruption of voicing
  loudness variation—uncontrolled
  tremor
Acoustic signs
  unexpected voice stoppages
  spectral interruptions
  reduced sustained phonation time
Laryngoscopic signs
  effort closure of the larynx
    spasmodic dysphonia
    myoclonus
    hyperkinetic dysarthria
    mixed dysarthria (ALS)
    functional
  anteroposterior shortening of the vocal folds
    spasmodic dysphonia
    functional
  rhythmic movement of laryngeal structures
    spasmodic dysphonia
    ALS
    essential tremor
    myoclonus
  arhythmic movements of laryngeal structures
    spasmodic dysphonia
Physiological signs
  aerodynamic
    decreased airflow
    increased air pressure
  vibratory
    excessive closed times
    aberrant glottal pulse shape
  muscle activity
    excessive levels
    sudden, unexpected bursts of activity
    involuntary rhythmic variations of level
    slow rise or fall of signal amplitude

laryngoscope in place. This permitted visualization of the activity of the vocal folds and verified the temporary paralysis of the right vocal fold induced by the injection. The patient was able to speak during this procedure, and it was noted that in the paralyzed condition his voice was produced without strain or sudden voice interruptions but with a breathy quality. R. O. and those present during this procedure found this voice to be a significant improvement.

Q. What is the purpose in anesthetizing the recurrent laryngeal nerve? Why should paralysis of one cord have had this effect on R. O.'s voice?

    The results of this procedure were felt to be consistent with the diagnosis of spasmodic dysphonia.

Tremor

We met C. W. in a very interesting way. Her niece had sought assistance for her voice problem and was referred to the voice lab. During the course of the diagnostic process it was learned that there seemed to be a family history of voice difficulties. C. W. was the one surviving family member known to have this problem who lived in the area. She was most interested in coming to the voice lab for examination.

C. W., 78 years old and in generally good health, states that her voice began to get shaky and wobbly when she was in her early 60s. Although the symptoms were mild at the outset, she reports that they have become gradually worse over the past 18 years. For the past 2 to 3 years she has found that people often have difficulty understanding her. Her voice has never been free of the wobbliness since it first began, and she reports that stress makes the wobbliness much more pronounced. C. W. recalls that her mother, who lived to be 90, began having a similar problem with her voice when in her 70s. The severity of the problem increased over the span of those years.

Until 2 years ago, C. W. was never aware of shakiness of any other part of her body. She states that her mother never showed the symptom anywhere but in the voice. However, C. W. now notices that both of her hands become shaky as she engages in an activity, such as bringing food to her mouth. She has no difficulty with activities such as driving her car. Most recently, she has become aware of some slight shakiness in her jaw.

The most prominent perceptual impression is that of vocal tremor (see Table 2.14). Beyond that, there is little if any change in pitch to mark for stress or meaning. The vocal tremor is noted in regular and predictable changes in the acoustic signal and occurs about five times per second. Phonational range is restricted to less than one octave. Variations in airflow are found that coincide with the tremor rate, and the glottal pulse shape is aberrant.

The fiberoptic bundle was passed through the nose and was held above the soft palate. Constant rhythmic movement of the palate was observed even though C. W. was not phonating. The fiberscope was advanced, and observation of epiglottis and laryngeal structures revealed similar involuntary movements. While at rest, the arytenoids were observed to rhythmically adduct. During phonation we observed tremor of the larynx. The stroboscope was of limited value with this patient because of the tremor in her voice and the inability of the strobe to lock on to the acoustic signal.

Q. What do you think is the nature of this problem, and how do the signs and symptoms fit with your understanding?

The diagnosis in this case was familial essential tremor. Attempts with experimental therapy were completely unsuccessful in changing any of the characteristics of this speech pattern. C. W. is unable to exert voluntary control over this disorder.

Summary

In this chapter, a basic approach to the diagnosis of voice problems is presented. The approach, based on the medical model of differential diagnosis, carefully considers the patient's symptoms (complaints) and relates them to the signs of the patient's voice problem. There are five categories of signs: perceptual, acoustic, physiological, stroboscopic, and larynoscopic.

Table 2.14.
Signs That May Be Associated with the Symptom of Tremor

Typical complaint: "My voice wobbles. My voice is unsteady."

Perceptual signs
  tremor
  monopitch
  monoloudness
  loudness variations—uncontrolled
Acoustic signs
  voice tremor
  restricted phonational range
  restricted dynamic range
  less variability of
    fundamental frequency
    intensity
  slow rise or fall in signal amplitude
Laryngoscopic signs
  rhythmic movements of laryngeal structures
    essential voice tremor
Physiological signs
  aerodynamics
    periodic variations of airflow
  vibratory
    aberrant glottal pulse shape
  muscle activity
    involuntary rhythmic variations of level

Eight primary symptoms are presented: hoarseness, vocal fatigue, breathiness, loss of range, aphonia, pitch breaks, strain/struggle, and tremor. These are defined and discussed within the context of case studies of individual patients.

Signs can be observed and tested independently of the patient's report. The major perceptual signs associated with voice problems include those related to pitch, loudness, and quality, as well as aphonia and nonphonatory signs. Acoustic signs include reduced phonation and dynamic range, higher or lower fundamental frequency, perturbation, low or high sound pressure level, and spectral noise. Physiological signs include reduced or excessive airflow and pressure, aberrant airflow or electroglottographic waveform, reduced or excessive muscle activity, and unusual muscle activity. Stroboscopic signs include mucosal wave, level of folds, symmetry of vocal folds, and amplitude of vocal fold motion. Laryngoscopic signs include tissue change, vocal fold approximation, anteroposterior approximation, movement of the vocal folds, and anatomic malformations. Table 2.15 presents a summary of the relationships between symptoms and signs discussed in this chapter.

Case studies have been presented to illustrate the symptoms of a voice problem and the signs associated with each symptom. The process by which the symptoms and signs are considered in the making of the diagnosis of a voice problem is emphasized in this chapter.

The diagnosis of a voice problem is an ongoing, dynamic process. It is incumbent on those who work with patients with voice disorders to continue to ask questions about the nature of the problem and the treatment approach.

Table 2.15.
Summary of Perceptual, Acoustic, and Physiological Signs That May Accompany the Eight Major Voice Symptoms

Symptom[a]								Perceptual Signs
1	2	3	4	5	6	7	8	
	X[b]							Monopitch
							X	Monoloudness
X	X	X						Hoarseness
X	X	X						Breathiness
X	X		X			X	X	Tension
						X	X	Tremor
						X	X	Strain/struggle
X			X					Inappropriate pitch
		X				X	X	Loudness variation
								Stridor
X	X							Throat clearing
X		X	X					Aphonia—consistent
X		X			X	X		Aphonia—episodic
X			X		X			Pitch breaks
							X	Sudden interruptions
			X					Normal

1	2	3	4	5	6	7	8	Acoustic Signs
X				X				Mean frequency
X	X						X	variability
X	X							perturbation
				X				shifts
X	X	X	X		X		X	Phonational range
X	X	X						Mean intensity
X	X						X	variability
X	X	X						perturbation
X	X	X	X		X		X	dynamic range
								Spectrum
X		X		X				noise
	X							harmonic energy
					X			interruptions
								Phonation time
X	X	X			X	X		maximum
X		X						s/z ratio
					X			Unexpected pauses
							X	Tremor
	X							Normal

1	2	3	4	5	6	7	8	Physiological Signs
X	X	X		X	X	X	X	Airflow
X		X		X		X		Air pressure
X		X				X	X	Glottal pulse shape
	X	X				X		Open/closed phases
X		X						Vibratory behavior
								Muscle
X	X	X	X		X	X		levels
	X				X	X		rate changes
					X			bursts
								onset/offset
					X			level decay

Table 2.15.—*continued*

1	2	3	4	5	6	7	8	Physiological Signs
X	X	X						paired muscle activity
X			X					Normal

1	2	3	4	5	6	7	8	Laryngoscopic Signs
X	X	X		X				Variation of VF approx.
		X		X		X		Vocal fold movement
X	X	X	X					Tissue changes
		X						Pyriform sinuses
X						X		AP laryngeal dimension
								Ventricular fold act.
X		X			X			Anatomical malformation
								Vocal fold length
X	X							Vertical laryngeal pos.
						X	X	Rhythmic movements
						X		Effort closure
						X		Arrhythmic movements
				X				Phonatory apraxia
X	X		X		X			Normal

1	2	3	4	5	6	7	8	Stroboscopic Signs
+[b]	−	−	+	*	+	+	**	Glottal closure
+	?	−	+	*	+	+	**	Phase closure
+	+	+	+	*	+	+	**	Vertical level
−	+	+	+	*	−	−	**	Amplitude
−	+	−	+	*	−	−	**	Mucosal wave
−	+	−	+	*	−	?	**	Vibratory behavior
−	+	+	+	*	+	?	**	Phase symmetry
−	+	−	+	*	+	−	**	Periodicity

[a]Symptom key
  1 = Hoarseness
  2 = Vocal fatigue
  3 = Breathy voice
  4 = Reduced phonational range
  5 = Aphonia
  6 = Pitch breaks, inappropriately high pitch
  7 = Strain/struggle voice
  8 = Tremor

[b]Table entry key
  X = Presence of sign
  + = Greater than normal activity
  − = Less than normal activity
  *   = Difficult to strobe because of the lack of vibration of the vocal folds
  ** = Difficult to strobe because of the tremor
  ? = Unknown

3

Laryngeal Histopathology

Histology of the Normal Human Larynx: Overview

Histologically, the larynx consists of cartilages, muscles, and mucous membrane or mucosa.

Cartilage

There are four major cartilages and two adjunct cartilages. The former are the cricoid, thyroid, arytenoid, and epiglottic cartilages, while the latter are the corniculate and cuneiform cartilages. The arytenoid, corniculate, and cuneiform cartilages are paired, whereas the other three are single structures.

The thyroid and cricoid cartilages are composed of hyaline cartilage; the epiglottic, corniculate, and cuneiform cartilages are made of elastic cartilage. The arytenoid cartilage is composed of both hyaline and elastic cartilaginous material. The main portion of the arytenoid cartilage is composed of hyaline cartilage, while the portion that meets its contralateral counterpart, including the vocal process, is made of elastic cartilage.

Cartilage is made of cells called chondrocytes and an intercellular substance containing mucopolysaccharide sulfate and fibers. Hyaline and elastic cartilage are most markedly differentiated by the type of fibers of which they are made. Hyaline cartilage has very thin, dense collagenous fibers, while elastic cartilage contains dense elastic fibers.

Muscle

There are five major muscles in the larynx: the cricothyroid, the thyroarytenoid, the lateral cricoarytenoid, the interarytenoid, and the posterior cricoarytenoid. The interarytenoid muscle is a single muscle; the other four are paired. In addition, there are two thin,

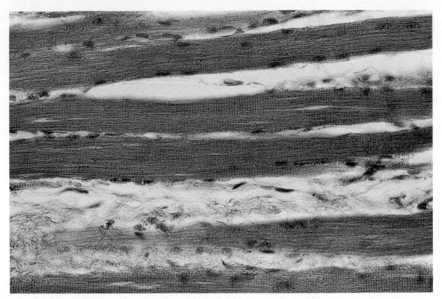

Figure 3.1. Histological picture of the mucosa of striated muscle (a part of the vocalis muscle). Note the existence of fine striations.

paired muscles: the thyroepiglottic and aryepiglottic muscles. Part of the thyroarytenoid muscle is located in the vocal fold and is called the vocalis muscle. All these muscles are striated (Fig. 3.1).

Mucosa

The mucosa of the alimentary canal typically consists of four layers: the epithelium, the lamina propria, the lamina muscularis mucosa and the tela submucosa. In contrast, the laryngeal mucosa lacks the lamina muscularis mucosa. As a result, the lamina propria and the tela submucosa cannot be differentiated, and the entire mucosa beneath the epithelium is called the lamina propria.

The epithelium in the larynx is basically pseudostratified ciliated epithelium. The exceptions to this include the membranous vocal fold and the inner aspect of the arytenoid cartilage, where stratified squamous epithelium covers the structures. Metaplasia of pseudostratified ciliated epithelium into stratified squamous epithelium occasionally takes place throughout the larynx.

Histological structure of the mucosa, especially that of the lamina propria, varies among the various structures of the larynx. In the following paragraphs, the structure of the mucosa at different areas of the larynx will be described.

Epiglottis

Figure 3.2 shows a histological photograph of the laryngeal aspect of the epiglottis. The epithelium is basically pseudostratified ciliated epithelium. The lamina propria is loose and thin. Underneath the mucosa lies the epiglottic cartilage, which consists of elastic cartilage.

Ventricular Fold (False Vocal Fold)

Figure 3.3 depicts a histological picture of the ventricular fold. The ventricular fold is covered with pseudostratified ciliated epithelium. The lamina propria has many glands and is very thick.

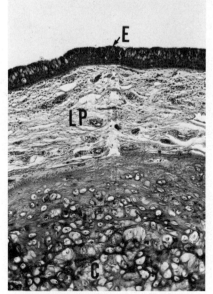

Figure 3.2. Histological picture of the mucosa of the laryngeal surface of the epiglottis. *E*, epithelium; *LP*, lamina propria; *C*, cartilage.

Posterior Wall of the Glottis

Figure 3.4 shows a histological picture of the mucosa of the posterior wall of the glottis. The mucosa has pseudostratified squamous epithelium. The tissue of the lamina propria is loose at the thin superficial layer but dense with elastic and collagenous fibers and glands in the thick deep layer. Underneath the mucosa lies the cricoid cartilage.

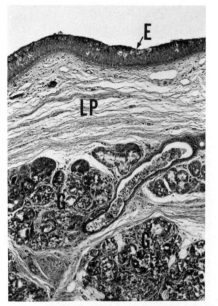

Figure 3.3. Histological picture of the mucosa of the ventricular fold. *E*, epithelium; *LP*, lamina propria; *G*, gland.

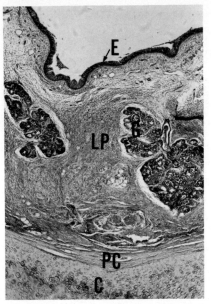

Figure 3.4. Histological picture of the mucosa of the posterior wall of the glottis. *E*, epithelium; *LP*, lamina propria; *G*, gland; *PC*, perichondrium; *C*, cartilage.

Subglottic Region

A histological photograph of the mucosa of the subglottic region is shown in Figure 3.5. The epithelium consists of pseudostratified squamous epithelium. The lamina propria is loose and contains some glands. The cricoid cartilage underlies the mucosa.

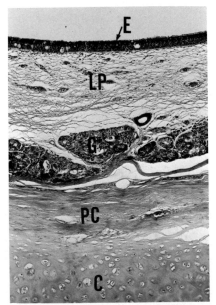

Figure 3.5. Histological picture of the mucosa of the subglottic region. *E*, epithelium; *LP*, lamina propria; *G*, gland; *PC*, perichondrium; *C*, cartilage.

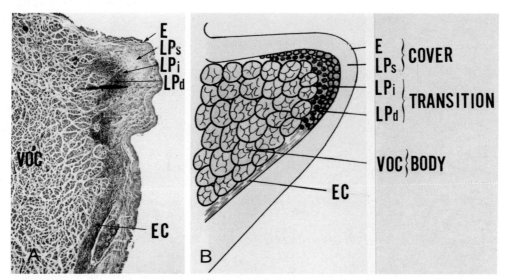

Figure 3.6.   A, Histological picture of a frontal section of an adult human vocal fold (from Hirano, 1981b). **B**, Schematic presentation of the layer structure. *E*, epithelium; *LP*, Lamina propria; *LPs*, superficial layer of the lamina propria; *LPd*, deep layer of the lamina propria; *VOC*, vocalis muscle; *EC*, elastic conus.

The mucosa of the vocal fold, the sound generator, will be described in detail in the following sections.

Vocal Fold in Adults

Basic Structure at the Vocal Fold Edge

From the viewpoint of vocal function, the most important concept about vocal fold structure is that the vocal fold is a multilayered vibrator. Figure 3.6 consists of a histological picture of a frontal section of an adult human vocal fold (A) and a schematic presentation of the layered structure (B).

The vocal fold is composed of mucosa and muscle. The mucosa in turn consists of the epithelium and the lamina propria. The epithelium is stratified squamous cell epithelium around the vocal fold edge, as described earlier, and from a mechanical point of view, it can be regarded as a thin capsule of the vibrator. At the vocal fold edge, the lamina propria displays a unique structure. It can be divided into three layers: superficial, intermediate, and deep.

The superficial layer, often referred to as Reinke's space, is loose and pliable and can be likened to a mass of soft gelatin. It is this layer that vibrates most markedly during phonation. If it becomes stiffened by pathologies, including inflammation, tumors, or scar tissue, its vibratory movements are disturbed, resulting in dysphonia. The intermediate layer consists primarily of elastic fibers that are something like soft rubber bands, whereas the deep layer consists chiefly of collagenous fibers that can be likened to cotton thread. The vocal ligament is the name given to the structure that comprises the intermediate and deep layers of the lamina propria. Thus, the tissue in the lamina propria becomes stiffer as the muscle is approached.

The vocalis muscle forms the main body of the vocal fold and from a mechanical point of view, when contracted it is like a bundle of stiff rubber bands.

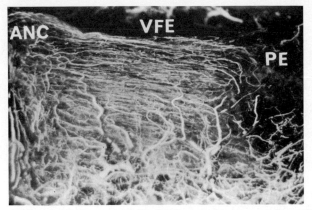

Figure 3.7. Blood vessels of the vocal fold. *ANC*, anterior commissure; *PE*, posterior end of membranous vocal fold; *VFE*, vocal fold edge. (From Kurita, 1980.)

The superficial layer of the lamina propria is clearly delineated from the intermediate layer. The border between the intermediate and deep layers, however, is not very clear. In the vocal ligament, elastic fibers decrease while collagenous fibers increase as the muscle is approached. The border between the lamina propria and the muscle is not clearly delineated at the vocal fold edge. Some fibers of the deep layer of the lamina propria insert into the muscle layer.

From a mechanical point of view, the five layers described above can be reclassified into three sections: the *cover*, consisting of the epithelium and the superficial layers of the lamina propria; the *transition*, composed of the intermediate and deep layers of the lamina propria, or the vocal ligament; and the *body*, composed of the vocalis muscle (Fig. 3.6B).

Around the vocal fold edge, the elastic and collagenous fibers in the lamina propria as well as the muscle fibers of the vocalis muscle run roughly parallel to the edge. This arrangement of fibers facilitates vibratory movements.

Blood vessels in the mucosa of the vocal fold edge come from both the anterior and posterior ends of the membranous vocal fold and run roughly parallel to its edge (Fig. 3.7). All of the blood vessels are very small, and few vessels enter the mucosa directly from the underlying muscle. This blood vessel arrangement is also advantageous to the maintenance of vibration.

No glands that give marked resistance to vibratory movement are found in the mucosa around the vocal fold edge.

Variation of the Structure along the Length of the Vocal Fold

The layered structure around the vocal fold edge varies along the length of the vocal fold. Figure 3.8A is a schematic drawing of a horizontal section of an adult human vocal fold and Figure 3.8B is a histological section of a vocal fold.

At the anterior end of the vocal fold, the intermediate layer of the lamina propria becomes thick, forming an oval mass called the anterior macula flava, which is composed of a fine mesh of elastic fibers, fibroblasts, and stroma. Anterior to the anterior macula flava lies another mass consisting primarily of collagenous fibers, called the anterior commissure tendon. This tendon is connected to the deep layer of the lamina propria lateroposteriorly, to the anterior macula flava posteriorly, and to the thyroid cartilage anteriorly. Thus, the stiffness of the tissue changes gradually from the pliable membranous vocal fold to the stiff thyroid cartilage.

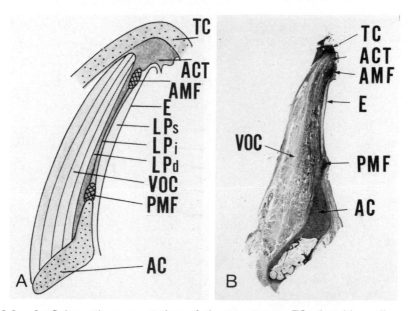

Figure 3.8. **A**, Schematic presentation of the structures. *TC*, thyroid cartilage; *ACT*, anterior commissure tendon; *AMF*, anterior macula flava; *PMF*, posterior macula flava; *AC*, arytenoid cartilage; *E*, epithelium; *LPs*, superficial layer of lamina propria; *LPi*, intermediate layer of lamina propria; *LPd*, deep layer of lamina propria; *VOC*, vocalis muscle. **B**, Histological picture of a horizontal section of an adult human vocal fold. (from Hirano, 1981b).

At the posterior end of the membranous vocal fold, the intermediate layer of the lamina propria forms another oval mass, which is referred to as the posterior macula flava. Its structure is similar to that of the anterior macula flava. It is connected to the vocal process of the arytenoid cartilage with a small intervening transitional area. The transitional area is stiffer than the macula flava but less stiff than the cartilage. The tip of the vocal process is composed of elastic cartilage, which is less stiff than the hyaline cartilage that constitutes the main portion of the arytenoid cartilage. Thus, again, the stiffness of tissue changes gradually from the pliable membranous vocal fold to the stiff arytenoid cartilage.

The structures at both ends of the membranous vocal fold appear to have a roll of tissue designed possibly to protect the ends from mechanical injury caused by the vibration of the folds during phonation.

Vocal Fold Structure in Newborns

The structure of the vocal fold edge in newborns differs greatly from that in adults, with the most marked differences occurring in the lamina propria of the mucosa. Figures 3.9A and C are histological pictures of the vocal fold of a newborn; Figures 3.9B and D are schematic presentations of the structures.

The epithelium at the vocal fold edge is squamous cell epithelium that does not significantly differ from that in adults. The lamina propria is very thick relative to vocal fold length, and it is rather uniform in structure. There is no ligamentous structure. Almost the entire lamina propria is rather loose and pliable. However, some fibrous tissue, which appears to be the immature maculae flava, is aggregated at the anterior and posterior ends of the membranous vocal fold.

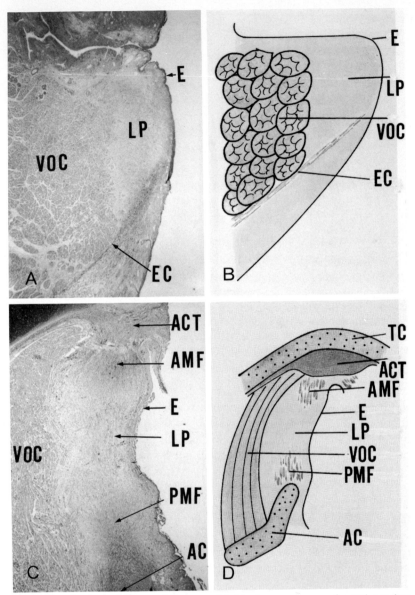

Figure 3.9.   Histological pictures of the vocal fold of a newborn , frontal section (**A**) and horizontal section (**C**), schematic presentations of these structures, frontal section (**B**) and horizontal section (**D**). *E*, epithelium; *LP*, lamina propria; *VOC*, vocalis muscle; *EC*, elastic conus; *TC*, thyroid cartilage; *ACT*, anterior commissure tendon; *AMF*, anterior macula flava; *PMF*, posterior macula flava; *AC*, arytenoid cartilage. (From Hirano, Kurita, and Nakashima, 1983.)

Development of Vocal Fold Structure

An immature vocal ligament appears between the age of 1 and 4 years. In this stage, however, the ligament is very thin and does not touch the vocalis muscle. There is no differentiation between the layer of elastic fibers and the layer of collagenous fibers. In other words, during this developmental stage the lamina propria does not yet have the three-layer structure. Differentiation of the two layers in the vocal ligament begins sometime between 6 to 12 years of age, and the ligament becomes thicker. After the age of 15 years, a clear three-layer structure of the lamina propria is consistently observed. Maturation of this layered structure of the vocal fold seems to be completed around the end of adolescence.

Vocal Fold Structure in the Geriatric Population

There are great individual differences in changes in vocal fold structure as a function of aging. Certain tendencies have been observed, though. The epithelium does not show any consistent and significant changes with aging. The superficial layer of the lamina propria tends to become edematous and thicker with age (Fig. 3.10A). The density of fibroblasts, collagenous fibers, and elastic fibers in this layer tends to decrease. These changes are more marked in men than in women.

Age-related changes in the intermediate layer of the lamina propria are noted in men, but seldom occur in women. These changes include a loosening and atrophy of elastic fibers in the intermediate layer (Fig. 3.10B). As a result, this layer tends to become thinner. Occasionally, deterioration of the contour of this layer occurs, caused chiefly by a fibrotic change in the deep layer of the lamina propria.

Changes in the deep layer of the lamina propria also take place more markedly in aged men than in aged women. Collagenous fibers tend to become thicker and denser with aging, which results in the deep layer becoming thicker. Occasionally, collagenous fibers increase locally and run in various directions, displaying a condition referred to as fibrosis (Fig. 3.10C). The muscle tends to become atrophied with age.

Histopathology of Non-Neoplastic Diseases of the Mucosa

Epithelial Hyperplasia and Dysplasia

The term ''epithelial hyperplasia'' implies any kind of pathology in which hyperplastic thickening of the epithelium is the primary lesion (Fig. 3.11A). When the lesion is associated with atypia of cells, it is called epithelial dysplasia (Fig. 3.11B). Lesions such as leukoplakia, hyperkeratosis, pachydermia, and acanthosis fall into this category.

Lesions of the hyperplastic and dysplastic type are regarded as precancerous conditions. As a matter of fact, carcinoma occasionally develops from hyperplastic or dysplastic epithelium. Clinically, it is often difficult to differentiate carcinoma in situ or very early invasive carcinomas from epithelial hyperplasia or dysplasia.

The lesions in this category originate from the epithelium and may enter the superficial layer of the lamina propria (Fig. 3.12). The lesion never invades the vocal ligament unless it becomes malignant. It may be unilateral or bilateral. It is usually asymmetrical and is not uniform within the affected vocal fold. Glottic closure is occasionally disturbed. From a mechanical point of view, the mass and stiffness of the cover increase, whereas the mechanical properties of the transition and the body are not affected. The lesion occasionally interferes with the vibratory movements of the contralateral vocal fold.

Vocal Fold Nodules

Vocal fold nodules develop around the vocal fold edge at the middle of the membranous vocal fold. They are whitish, tiny sessile bumps and are usually bilateral. The lesion is located in the superficial layer of the lamina propria and consists primarily of edematous tissue and/or collagenous fibers (Fig. 3.13). The lesion is usually symmetrical and may prevent the glottis

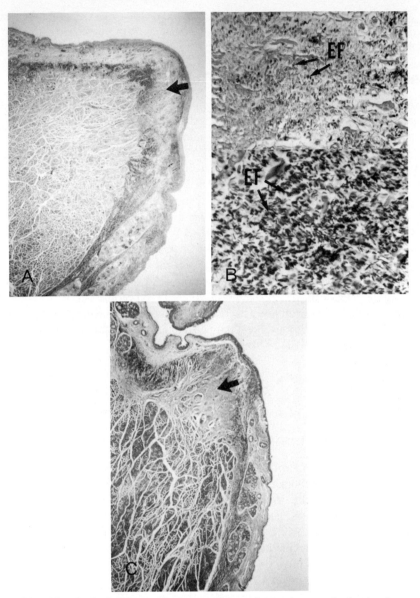

Figure 3.10.   Histological pictures demonstrating geriatric changes in the lamina propria of the mucosa of the vocal folds. **A**, Edema (*arrow*) in the superficial layer (a 61-year-old man). **B**, Atrophy of elastic fibers (*EF*) in the intermediate layer (a 47-year-old man, upper figure; the lower figure is a control, a 27-year-old man). **C**, Fibrotic changes (*arrow*) in the deep layer (a 53-year-old man). (From Hirano, Kurita, and Nakashima, 1983.)

from closing completely during phonation. The mass and stiffness of the cover are slightly increased, whereas the mechanical properties of the transition and body are not affected. The lesion may slightly interfere with vibratory movements of the contralateral vocal fold.

Vocal Fold Polyp

Vocal fold polyps usually develop around the vocal fold edge at the middle of the membranous vocal fold. They may be reddish or whitish, small or large, sessile or pedun-

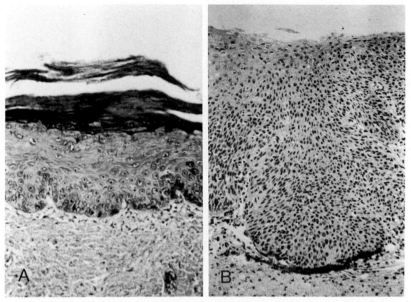

Figure 3.11.   Epithelial hyperplasia (**A**) and dysplasia (**B**). (From Hirano, 1983.)

culated, unilateral or bilateral; usually they are asymmetrical. The lesion is located in the superficial layer of the lamina propria. The histological features of the lesion are edema (Fig. 3.14A), intratissue bleeding, hyaline degeneration, thrombosis (Fig. 3.14B), proliferation of collagenous fibers, and/or cell infiltration. Glottic closure is impeded. The mass of the cover is increased, but the stiffness of the cover varies depending on the pathology. It is increased when bleeding, hyaline degeneration, thrombosis, proliferation of collagenous fibers, and/or cell infiltration is the main pathology. When edema is the primary pathology, the stiffness of the cover decreases. The mechanical properties of the

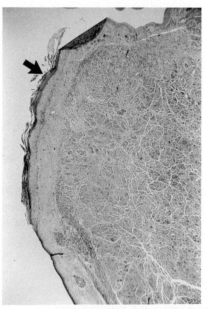

Figure 3.12.   Histological picture of a vocal fold with epithelial hyperplasia (*arrow*). (From Hirano, 1981b.)

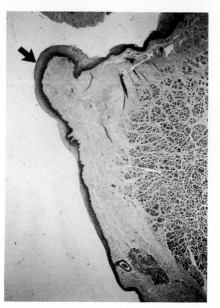

Figure 3.13. Histological picture of a vocal fold with nodule (*arrow*).

transition and the body are not affected. Polyps interfere with vibratory movements of the contralateral vocal fold.

Reinke's Edema

There are several different terms for Reinke's edema: polypoid degeneration, chronic polypoid corditis, chronic edematous hypertrophy, and polypoid vocal fold. Histologically, one finds primarily edema in the superficial layer of the lamina propria (Fig. 3.15). It is neither degeneration, inflammation (–itis), nor hypertrophy. The membranous vocal fold is edematous and swollen along its entire length. The lesion is usually bilateral and is asymmetrical in most cases. The glottis usually closes completely during phonation. The mass of the cover is increased while the stiffness of the cover is usually decreased. The mechanical properties of the transition and body are not affected. The edematous lesion interferes with vibration of the contralateral counterpart.

Epidermoid Cyst

Epidermoid cysts are basically located in the superficial layer of the lamina propria (Fig. 3.16). Occasionally they have a tiny opening to the laryngeal lumen and/or they insert partly into the vocal ligament (Fig. 3.17). The cystic wall is lined with thin squamous cell epithelium. Cysts contain caseous material and may be compared to a balloon full of fluid. The lesion may be unilateral or bilateral and small or large. The vibrating structures are usually asymmetrical. Glottic closure is often impeded. The mass and stiffness of the cover are increased. The mechanical properties of the transition and the body are usually not affected. The cyst often interferes with vibratory movements of the contralateral vocal fold.

Nonspecific Granuloma

There are three types of nonspecific granulomas that develop within the glottic region: intubation granulomas, contact granulomas and granulomas caused by gas-

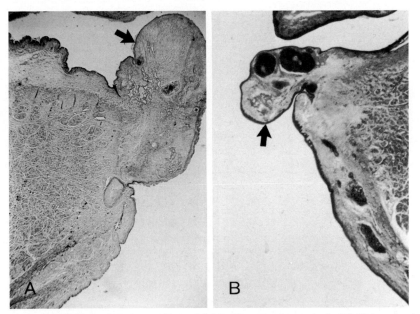

Figure 3.14. Histological pictures of vocal fold with polyp (*arrow*). **A**, Whitish polyp in which edema is the dominant pathology (from Hirano, 1981). **B**, Reddish polyp in which intratissue bleeding, hyaline degeneration, and thrombosis are the dominant pathologies (from Hirano, 1975).

troesophageal reflux. Granulomas are located at the vocal process of the arytenoid cartilage or on the lateral wall of the posterior glottis (Fig. 3.18). The membranous vocal fold is not affected. Histologically, granulomas consist chiefly of proliferated capillaries, fibroblasts, collagenous fibers, and leukocytes (Fig. 3.19). They may or may not be cov-

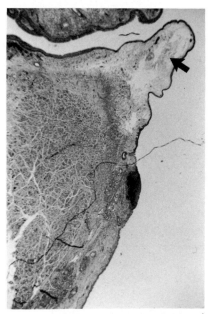

Figure 3.15. Histological picture of a vocal fold with Reinke's edema (*arrow*). (From Hirano, 1981b.)

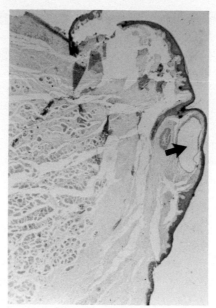

Figure 3.16.   Histological picture of a vocal fold with epidermoid cyst (*arrow*). (From Hirano, 1981b.)

ered with epithelium. The lesion may be unilateral or bilateral. Granulomas impede glottic closure only when they are very large. There is no effect on the mechanical properties of any layer of the membranous vocal fold.

Sulcus Vocalis

The term ''sulcus vocalis'' refers to a furrow along the entire length of the edge of the membranous vocal fold. The vocal fold edge is bowed to a greater or lesser extent. Al-

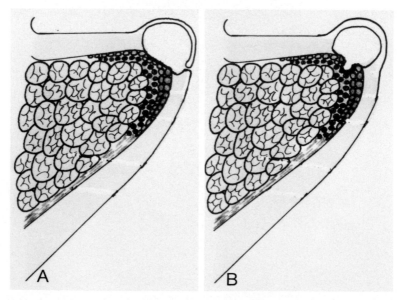

Figure 3.17.   Variations of epidermoid cyst of the vocal fold. **A,** A tiny opening to the laryngeal lumen. **B,** Partial insertion into the vocal ligament.

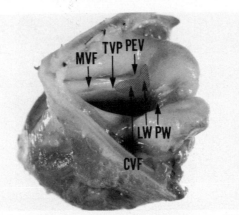

Figure 3.18. Location of nonspecific granuloma (*dotted area*). *PW*, posterior wall of the glottis; *LW*, lateral wall of the posterior glottis; *PEV*, posterior end of the ventricle; *CVF*, cartilaginous portion of the vocal fold; *TVP*, tip of the vocal process; *MVF*, membranous portion of the vocal fold. (From Hirano, Kurita, Kyokawa, and Sato, 1986.)

though the lesion may occasionally be unilateral, in most cases it is bilateral and roughly symmetrical. The glottis does not close completely during phonation. Histologically, the sulcus is located in the superficial layer of the lamina propria (Fig. 3.20). The epithelium in the sulcus is occasionally thickened. Collagenous fibers are frequently increased, and capillaries are poor around the sulcus. From a mechanical point of view, the mass of the cover is reduced whereas the stiffness of the cover is increased. The mechanical properties of the transition and the body are not affected.

Vocal Fold Scar

Scarring can occur any place on the vocal fold as a result of trauma, surgery, burn, or inflammation. Scar tissue consists of dense collagenous fibers and is much stiffer than the normal tissue of the vocal fold mucosa and the muscle. The glottis often does not close completely during phonation. The mass of each layer varies, depending upon the amount of scarring, whereas the stiffness of the layer(s) involved is increased.

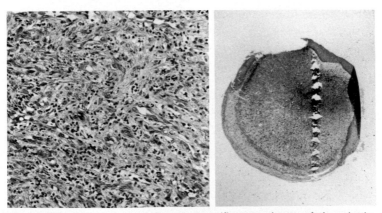

Figure 3.19. Histological pictures of a nonspecific granuloma of the glottic area. **Left,** Entire view. **Right,** Greater magnification.

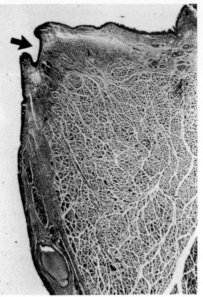

Figure 3.20. Histological picture of a vocal fold with sulcus vocalis (*arrow*). (From Hirano, 1975.)

Histopathology of Neoplastic Diseases

Carcinomas

Most carcinomas of the vocal fold are squamous cell carcinoma. They originate from the epithelium and invade the deeper structures, including the lamina propria and the muscle (Fig. 3.21). The lesion is originally unilateral, but it can extend to the contralateral side. The vocal fold tissue is asymmetrical and glottic closure is usually disturbed. Both the mass and the stiffness of the cover are increased. The mass and stiffness of the transition and the body are increased when these structures are involved. The carcinomatous mass interferes with vibration of the contralateral vocal fold.

Papilloma

Papillomas originate from the epithelium and may invade the lamina propria and the muscle. The lesion may be unilateral or bilateral, and it is usually asymmetrical. Histologically, papillomas consist of proliferated neoplastic epithelial cells growing in a papillary shape (Fig. 3.22). The lesion impedes complete glottic closure during phonation. The mass and stiffness of the cover are increased. The mass and stiffness of the transition and the body are increased when these structures are affected. The papilloma mass interferes with vibratory movements of the contralateral vocal fold.

Histopathology of Neuromuscular Diseases

The most frequent neuromuscular disease of the vocal fold is paralysis caused by recurrent laryngeal nerve (RLN) lesions.

From a neuropathological point of view, there are three types of paralysis: neuroapraxia, axonotmesis, and neurotmesis (Fig. 3.23). In neuropraxia, conduction of

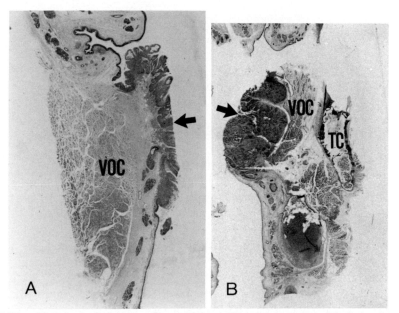

Figure 3.21.   Histological pictures of vocal folds with carcinoma (*arrow*). **A**, Lesion confined to the mucosa (from Hirano, 1981b). **B**, Lesion involving the muscle. *VOC*, vocalis muscle; *TC*, thyroid cartilage.

nerve impulses is temporarily blocked. It is caused, for example, by injection of local anesthetics. It does not cause muscle atrophy, and the neuromuscular system recovers to its normal state. Axonotmesis is a condition in which the axons of the nerve are sectioned, and neurotmesis refers to a condition in which the nerve fibers are entirely cut. In both conditions, the portion of the nerve peripheral to the site of lesion degenerates, and the muscle becomes denervated. The nerve may or may not regenerate, and the muscle may or

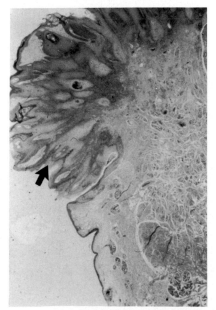

Figure 3.22.   Histological picture of vocal fold with papilloma (*arrow*). (From Hirano, 1975.)

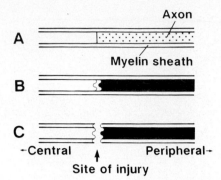

Figure 3.23.   Three types of paralysis. **A**, Neuropraxia. **B**, Axonotmesis. **C**, Neurotmesis. *Dotted area*: Conduction of neural impulses is temporarily blocked. *Solid area*: Axon is degenerated.

may not be reinnervated accordingly. When the muscle is not reinnervated, it becomes atrophied. In many clinical cases, the RLN is only partly affected, meaning that some motor units are affected while others are not.

Vocal fold paralysis is unilateral in most cases. Glottic closure is usually disturbed because of lack of adduction of the affected vocal fold. Figure 3.24 shows a histological picture of a vocal fold in which marked atrophy of the vocalis muscle has resulted. In cases of vocal fold paralysis associated with muscle atrophy, the mass and stiffness of the body are decreased. Paralysis without muscle atrophy results in a decrease in the stiffness of the body, and the mass of the body may be slightly decreased. In any case, the mechanical properties of the cover and the transition are basically not affected.

Summary of Implications for Vocal Physiology

In understanding the effect of various pathologic conditions on the sound generation properties, the vibratory behavior of the vocal folds, it is important to consider the following parameters:

1. Localization of the pathology
2. Symmetry of both vocal folds

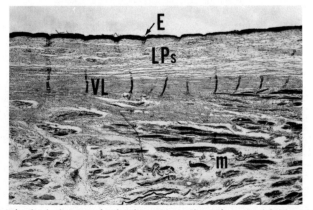

Figure 3.24.   Histological picture of a horizontal section of a vocal fold with RLN paralysis, demonstrating muscular atrophy. *E*, epithelium; *LPs*, superficial layer of lamina propria; *VL*, vocal ligament; *M*, atrophic muscle.

3. Uniformity within each vocal fold
4. Glottic closure
5. Layered structure
6. Mass and stiffness of each layer
7. Interference with vibratory movements of the contralateral vocal fold

Table 3.1 summarizes these aspects for varying pathological conditions. Each parameter can vary from case to case for a given pathology. In Table 3.1, the most typical states are described for each pathology.

Table 3.1.
Summary of Various Pathological Conditions[a]

Pathology	Location of pathology	Symmetry	Uniformity	Glottic incompetence	Layer structure	Cover		Transition		Body		Interference
						Mass	Stiffness	Mass	Stiffness	Mass	Stiffness	
Epithelial hyperplasia and dysplasia	Epithelium → Superf. layer of lamina propria (Cover)	Deteriorated	Deteriorated	Occasionally	Frequently deteriorated	Increased	Increased	Normal	Normal	Normal	Normal	Varying
Nodule	Superf. layer of lamina propria (Cover)	Maintained	Deteriorated	Partly	Maintained	Increased (slightly)	Increased (slightly)	Normal	Normal	Normal	Normal	Slight
Polyp	Superf. layer of lamina propria (Cover)	Deteriorated	Deteriorated	Partly	Maintained	Increased	Varying	Normal	Normal	Normal	Normal	Marked
Reinke's edema	Superf. layer of lamina propria (Cover)	Deteriorated	Usually maintained	None	Maintained	Increased	Decreased	Normal	Normal	Normal	Normal	Marked

Disease	Location											
Epidermoid cyst	Superf. layer of lamina propria (Cover)	Deteriorated	Deteriorated	Partly	Partly deteriorated	Increased	Increased	Normal	Normal	Normal	Normal	Marked
Granuloma	Posterior glottis	Maintained	Maintained	None	Maintained	Normal	Normal	Normal	Normal	Normal	Normal	None
Sulcus vocalis	Superf. layer of lamina propria (Cover)	Maintained	Maintained	Entire length (slight)	Partly deteriorated	Decreased	Increased	Normal	Normal	Normal	Normal	None
Scar	Varying	Deteriorated	Deteriorated or maintained	In varying degree	Deteriorated	Varying	Increased	Varying	Normal or increased	Varying	Normal or increased	None
Carcinoma	Epithelium → Superf. layer of lamina propria → Vocal ligament → Muscle (Cover → Body)	Deteriorated	Deteriorated	Partly	Deteriorated	Increased	Increased	Increased	Increased	Increased	Increased	Marked

Table 3.1.—continued

Pathology	Location of pathology	Symmetry	Uniformity	Glottic incompetence	Layer structure	Cover		Transition		Body		Interference
						Mass	Stiffness	Mass	Stiffness	Mass	Stiffness	
Papilloma	Epithelium → Superf. layer of lamina propria → Vocal ligament → Muscle (Cover → Body)	Deteriorated	Deteriorated	Partly	Frequently deteriorated	Increased	Increased	Occasionally increased	Occasionally increased	Occasionally increased	Occasionally increased	Marked
Vocal fold paralysis	Muscle	Deteriorated	Maintained	Entire length (marked)	Deteriorated	Normal	Normal	Normal	Normal	Decreased	Decreased	None

[a]Adapted from Hirano, 1981.

4

Voice Misuse and Abuse: Effects on Laryngeal Physiology

Vocal misuse and abuse are frequently claimed to be the causes of voice problems. Furthermore, they are thought to contribute to the laryngeal tissue changes that result in the formation of such lesions as nodules, polyps, contact ulcers, and others. What do these terms mean? What kinds of vocal activities can be properly deemed to be abusive or somehow improper or unhealthy? When does misuse become abuse? How much abuse or misuse can laryngeal tissues tolerate? How do patterns of misuse evolve, and what maintains them? How do misuse and abuse create voice problems? These questions must be asked, and answers must be sought. In this chapter we will discuss our current state of knowledge about vocal misuse and abuse.

Misuse

Misuse suggests voice production behaviors that distort the normal propensity of the phonatory mechanism to work effectively and efficiently. An efficient system produces its best results with a minimum of effort. A car engine whose various components are in top working condition so that its operation is smooth and uses the least energy is said to be operating efficiently. Similarly, with the voice, a phonatory system whose individual components are healthy and whose coordination and interaction with all of its supporting parts and systems is in tune produces voice in an efficient manner.

There are a number of ways in which that smooth operation of the voice may be altered. Each of us can voluntarily produce voice in a variety of different ways, some of them efficient, some inefficient. Those who work with disordered voices should be able to produce inefficient as well as efficient voice in order to get a better understanding of and feel for how various changes in voice production can be made. For example, take a breath,

Table 4.1.
Characteristics of Vocal Behaviors Categorized as Misuse

A. Increased tension/strain
   1. Hard glottal attack
   2. High laryngeal position
   3. Anteroposterior laryngeal squeezing

B. Inappropriate pitch level
   1. Puberphonia
   2. Persistent glottal fry
   3. Lack of pitch variability

C. Excessive talking

D. Ventricular phonation

E. Aphonia, dysphonia of psychological origin

and as you begin to speak tighten your chest to the point of almost holding your breath. How does it feel to talk like that? Where do you feel the tensions? What changes did it make in how your voice sounds? As another example, try to squeeze your larynx tightly and speak in a hoarse voice. Think about how that feels and what you have done to change the sound of your voice. As a final experiment, pick a pitch about two tones above your present pitch level and try to converse, and then do this at a pitch about two tones lower than your comfort level. Has your larynx height changed? What does it feel like to try to do this? What does it do to your breathing, your degree of tension, your inflection patterns?

All of the activities you have engaged in could be categorized as examples of vocal misuse, yet all are within the ability of each of us to produce. In Table 4.1 we have identified some of the behaviors that when used habitually constitute misuse. Each of these will be discussed in the following sections.

Increased Tension/Strain

Descriptions of what is meant by increased vocal tension abound but frequently lack specificity. The judgement of vocal tension is most frequently made on a subjective basis. The subjectivity may be the reporting by the patient of the sensation of tension, or sometimes even pain, accompanying speaking, or it may be the judgement of the voice clinician based on auditory and visual observations. There are few objective methods of documenting tension, and there are none that can be put to routine clinical use to provide measurement of specific muscle tensions. Biofeedback using externally placed electrodes has been attempted, but it is not at all clear what specific muscles are being tapped, nor is there sufficient information available to identify which muscles are the most significant in assessment of vocal tension.

In cases of vocal misuse, the laryngologic examination is usually reported to be negative, with perhaps a suggestion of increased redness or slight swelling of the vocal folds. In some cases it is noted that a strand of mucus forms and reforms between the vocal folds at the nodal point, a sign thought by some to be an early indication of nodule formation. We have found fiberoptic examinations to be of significant help in identifying patterns of excessive laryngeal tension in some patients. The specific observable signs of that tension will be discussed under their appropriate categories.

Hard Glottal Attack/Glottal Coup

The hard glottal attack describes a manner of initiating vowels, usually characterized by rapid and complete adduction of the vocal folds prior to the initiation of phonation. This adducted state, which may be accompanied by considerable muscle tension, requires that subglottal pressure be increased in order to overcome vocal fold resistance and initiate phonation. The audible characteristic of an abrupt, explosive, and hard-edged onset of phonation results. This form of voice initiation is often visible fiberoptically, especially when subjects are asked to produce isolated vowel sounds (Casper, Colton, Brewer, and Woo, 1989), and appears to be produced in at least two ways. In one method, medial compression of the vocal folds is observed almost simultaneously with the onset of phonation. The second variation is characterized by prephonatory laryngeal constriction in which the ventricular folds approach each other, as do the arytenoids and the epiglottis, obscuring visualization of the true vocal folds. As phonation is initiated, there is a reduction in the forced adduction and a sudden springing open of the larynx as the true vocal folds become visible. It is important to add a note of caution. We have observed occasional fiberoptic evidence of this hard glottal attack in speakers who were judged to have normal voices and who were experiencing no voice problems. It is a behavior that may occur on occasion in most speakers. Whether or not this particular behavior is identified as evidence of misuse must depend in part on the degree of its presence. In general, when the hard glottal attack is present to a significant degree, it is but one of several behaviors that give evidence of increased tension and strain.

High Laryngeal Position

Vertical laryngeal height has been the subject of study and of some controversy. It has been reported that untrained singers show greater laryngeal elevation with increased pitch level than do trained singers (Shipp and Izdebski, 1975; Shipp, 1987). There are different schools of thought among singers, singing coaches, and voice scientists relative to the benefits of maintaining a low laryngeal position. Many believe that raising laryngeal height with elevation of pitch is improper singing technique and detrimental to the voice (Sundberg and Askenfelt, 1983). However, more recently Sundberg reported that an x-ray study of two well-trained female singers revealed an increase in vertical laryngeal height with an increase in pitch, in what he described as a "very elegant" and "well-trained" behavior (Shipp, Guinn, Sundberg, and Titze, 1987). It was suggested that varying laryngeal position may be useful and that raising the larynx during singing may not be abusive.

There are many differences between singing and speaking that make it difficult to suggest that a particular behavior in one activity is the same or has the same effect in the other activity. Raising the larynx results in (a) a shortening of the vocal tract, with a subsequent raising of all formant frequencies; (b) a stiffening of vocal fold tissues that alters the vibratory pattern and increases fundamental frequency; and (c) an increased tendency for tight vocal fold closure. This tight adduction is a desirable and essential part of the swallowing process wherein the larynx elevates and a tight valving maneuver ensues, thereby protecting the lower airway. In speaking, it is not variability of laryngeal height that is suggestive of excessive tension but rather a speaker's tendency to consistently speak with the larynx in an elevated position. Titze states (Shipp et al., 1987) that the human body seems naturally to do that which is easiest to do, and it seems to optimize itself for a given task. Further, he suggests that the speaker who constantly maintains a low laryngeal posture may be using more energy in doing so than the speaker who allows the mechanism the freedom to do what it wants to.

Vocal tension is characterized by increased tension in both the intrinsic and extrinsic laryngeal muscles. However, we are not yet able to isolate the contributions of each muscle group to a voice problem. Indeed, the system as a whole is so interactive that when excessive tensions exist in one muscle, they will probably occur also in some other muscles. Thus, although laryngeal height is affected by the extrinsic laryngeal muscle activity, we cannot attribute a voice disorder to that condition alone and must recognize the total physiological disturbance. A high laryngeal position may be related to excessive tension in both extrinsic and intrinsic muscle groups, or it may be related to a disturbance in the functioning of the intrinsic muscles. Sundberg and Askenfelt (1983) stated that "the muscles used for raising the larynx also may affect the way in which the vocal folds vibrate" (p. 307), which underscores the relationship between larynx height and the voice source. Shipp (1987) also addresses this relationship and reports that increased stiffening of the vocal fold margin results from the upward stretch of tissues created by laryngeal height elevation.

It is not unusual for patients with this particular pattern of hyperfunction to report sensations of pain or soreness in the neck lateral to the larynx, sometimes radiating upward or downward. These patients also report that their voices tend to become worse with increased use and that by the end of the workday they feel it takes too much effort to bother to talk.

Anteroposterior Laryngeal Squeezing

In the fiberoptic examination of voice-disordered patients, we have often observed (usually in the absence of observable pathology) a "squeezing" of the larynx in which the epiglottis and the arytenoids approach each other during phonation. A similar but not identical movement is typical in the production of the low back vowels (e.g., /ah/), when the tongue position dictates a posterior movement of the epiglottis. That movement is a natural one in which none of the "squeezing" elements are present. During production of the vowels /ee/ and /oo/, the epiglottis is normally expected to be pulled somewhat anteriorly and superiorly, making the vocal folds fully visible. This does not occur in patients with a "squeezed" larynx. These patients, even in the production of the /ee/ and /oo/ vowels, as well as other stimulus materials heavily loaded with these vowels, demonstrate anteroposterior "squeezing" behavior to the extent that visualization of the true vocal folds along their full length is often obscured.

Another vocal maneuver that is normally expected to "open" the larynx when it is being viewed fiberoptically is pitch elevation. Patients who tend to habitually use very tight laryngeal posture with anteroposterior shortening do so even as they raise pitch. In fact, they often encounter difficulty in raising pitch and may exhibit a reduced phonational range. We believe that this vocal behavior is an indication of disturbed phonatory physiology, probably due to excess strain and tension.

Inappropriate Pitch Level

A common concept in the voice literature is that of optimum pitch. Clinicians are instructed that the use of a too high or a too low habitual pitch level is a frequent cause of voice disorders. Much therapy time is spent in identifying what is purported to be an individual's optimum pitch, and therapy is then directed toward teaching the patient to use that pitch. We have difficulty with this approach for a number of reasons (see Chapter 9).

The physiological approach to voice disorders, based on an understanding of vocal fold physiology and acoustics, suggests that a disturbance of physiology due to mass lesions, manner of use, or abnormal motor control will result in acoustic changes. Thus, an inappropriate pitch level, if indeed it is present, may well be a sign of a problem rather than the cause of the problem. Attention needs to be paid to the underlying cause of the problem, and when the physiology is normalized or improved, then the pitch level of the voice will also improve or normalize. Indeed, it is quite possible for a person to speak at a totally appropriate pitch level and yet do so in an abusive way.

Judgments of the pitch of a voice should not be made subjectively. Perception of pitch levels can be quite erroneous, especially in the presence of hoarseness or excess noise energy in the voice. Objective measurement of fundamental frequency rather than casual judgments of pitch may be easily made using methods described in Chapter 7 and should always be done before any judgments about the acceptability of this parameter are considered.

If the fundamental frequency of a person's voice is altered by pathology, for example, it seems to us that attempts to "measure" an optimum pitch are immediately flawed. The most common methodology espoused for obtaining the so-called optimum pitch is described by Fairbanks (1960) and involves obtaining a measure of phonational range. Recall, however, that phonational range is often reduced in the presence of certain laryngeal pathologies and voice disorders. It is important to recognize that despite the apparently widespread use of the concept of optimum pitch, there are no data to demonstrate or document its validity nor its therapeutic efficacy.

Inappropriate pitch is typically the hallmark of the voice problems discussed in the following sections. It is necessary to recognize, however, that inappropriate pitch may be only one sign of an underlying problem.

Puberphonia

This category is referred to in the literature by a number of names: adolescent falsetto, pubescent falsetto, incomplete mutation, and mutational falsetto. Although we have difficulty with all of these terms, the one we have chosen to use, puberphonia, is the least objectionable. The term "falsetto" in these cases is rarely correct. Furthermore, falsetto is a normal although atypical mode of phonation in normal voices. The word "mutation," which means "changed," does not tell us anything about what has or has not changed, as in incomplete mutation, or it suggests that falsetto is characteristic of the state of change, as in mutational falsetto. The term "puberphonia" suggests the developmental stage at which this problem is encountered and tells us that this has to do with voice (phone). Rather than add yet another term, we prefer to describe the nature of the problem.

Puberphonia most simply refers to the persistence of a high pitched voice beyond the age at which the male voice change is expected to have occurred. This is a problem very specific to men. Although some women continue to have very high pitched and childlike voices into their adult years, there is little stigma attached because the lowering of the fundamental frequency in women as a result of laryngeal growth (3 to 4 semitones) is not as marked as for men (one octave) and because women are expected to have higher pitched voices. Thus, the presence of a high pitched voice in a woman does not carry the social stigma or appear as inappropriate or unusual as in a man.

In cases of puberphonia it is important that, first, a determination be made as to whether an organic abnormality is present. The adequacy of laryngeal growth must be assessed, and endocrinological problems must be ruled out. The laryngeal examination and the history may provide sufficient information regarding these concerns. The vocal symptoms include not only the high pitched voice but also often hoarseness and some degree of breathiness. The voice tends to sound unstable and uncertain, and the patient's reporting often confirms that perception in comments such as "It sounds funny, and I never know what it is going to sound like.'' Pitch breaks may also be heard. Although the onset of the problem is, by definition, during the adolescent growth spurt and the emergence of secondary sex characteristics, it may persist for a considerable length of time before any treatment is sought.

Psychosocial factors, such as difficulty with male identification or with the acceptance of emerging adulthood, are most often cited as the primary etiological factors. Our experience, however, suggests that if present, these factors are not overwhelming in their expression. It seems quite logical to us that a certain percentage of young boys may have fairly traumatic voice change experiences not only in the psychological sense but also in the physical sense. Pitch breaks may be frequent and extreme, and the lack of control over the voice may be pronounced. Feelings of embarrassment would result and be aggravated by a lack of understanding of what is happening. An understandable reaction to such feelings might be an attempt to hold on to the voice that is known (the child voice) and to attain control of what otherwise seems to be an uncontrollable behavior. In many cases, when asked if they have another voice, young men with this problem will answer in the affirmative. In some patients, we have observed a profound sense of relief when this admission has been made and reassurance has been provided about the normalcy of the ''hidden'' voice. Indeed, for many, little additional treatment has been necessary beyond providing a period of practice in using the new voice, coupled with encouragement and guidance. In others, the process of ''releasing'' the adult voice (see Chapter 9) is usually very effective in producing a more typical adult voice within a short time period. We are not aware, either through personal experience or perusal of the literature, of posttherapy failures wherein there is a regression to the high pitched voice. We also have not been impressed that the young men who have presented with this problem in our clinic have had difficulty with male identification. Indeed, we would not describe the sound of their voices as ever having been effeminate. The characteristics of an effeminate voice are comprised of speech mannerisms and suprasegmental differences that go well beyond just the presence of a higher than expected pitch level. We believe that the theory of the domineering mother figure with, of course, a weak father figure as the primary underlying cause for the maintenance of the inappropriately high pitch level should either be supported by appropriate data or laid to rest.

Persistent Glottal Fry

Glottal fry, or pulse register, is described as one of the three normal voice registers, the other two being loft (falsetto) and modal. These registers are characterized by a change in the mechanical mode of vibration (Hollien, 1974), and there is usually a little overlap in the frequency of phonation between adjacent registers. Daniloff, Shuckers, and Feth (1980) state that the physiologically complex larynx ''can vibrate in three (or more) relatively different ways, giving rise to airflow modulation that yields acoustically and perceptually distinct vocal quality'' (p. 209). Glottal fry is the register lowest in fundamental frequency and the least flexible. The vocal folds are noted to close quickly, and the closed phase of the vibratory cycle is very long relative to the length of the entire period. Moore and von Leden (1958) described the occasional occurrence of two open phases during one vibratory cycle. Zemlin (1968) reported that the closed phase occupies about 90% of the cycle. In describing the characteristics of glottal fry as seen in high speed motion pictures, he observed tightly approximated vocal folds whose free edges, however, appeared flaccid. Zemlin further noted that air seemed to ''bubble up'' between the folds near the junction of the anterior two-thirds of the glottis. Glottal fry is produced with greater glottal impedance than the other registers, and air is released in irregularly timed bursts. Pulsated voice, according to Perkins (1983), allows the production of only very low fundamental frequencies, with a decay of energy in every glottal cycle.

Glottal fry has a very characteristic sound, which has been described variously as similar to the popping of corn, the sound of an imitation of a motor boat engine, or a creaky voice. The vibratory pattern is so slow that individual vibrations of the vocal folds are heard. The amplitude of vocal fry sound is very low.

Although glottal fry is a normal mode of vibration, its consistent and habitual use is atypical and may be considered misuse of the voice. It is difficult to produce glottal fry with adequate volume for many speaking situations. A person using this mode of phonation will show increased tension when attempting to increase vocal loudness. The lack of flexibility of pulse register makes it difficult to achieve variation of fundamental frequency and results in monotonic voice. Complaint of a sense of vocal fatigue and a constant awareness of vibration even below the larynx are typically heard from speakers who habitually use glottal fry.

Lack of Pitch Variability

There are some individuals who speak in a monotone with barely perceptible variations in fundamental frequency, as corroborated by acoustic analysis. A monotonic voice may be a sign of neurological dysfunction affecting the ability to control pitch, or it may be a sign of misuse. We have been impressed with the presence of this problem in untrained speakers who lecture or frequently address large groups. They do not know how to modulate their pitch level for maximum communication effectiveness. In this type of pattern, the phonatory mechanism establishes a "set" that rarely varies. This set includes a certain configuration of the vocal folds, with the adductory and contact forces occurring with the same strength and in the same area over and over again. This behavior fails to take advantage of the flexibility of the phonatory mechanism and tends to become fatiguing. It is not unusual to find that persons with this pattern allow their voices to drift into vocal fry at the end of utterances. The delivery usually is perceived as lacking in energy, vitality, and interest.

Excessive Talking

Each individual larynx has a physiological limit that varies not only from person to person but also intraindividually as influenced by numerous factors. A healthy, well-rested, well-nourished, emotionally stable individual may encounter no vocal difficulties despite heavy voice use demands. However, should that same person be physically exhausted, eating poorly, and perhaps taking some medication, the same amount of demand on the larynx, or even less, may result in phonatory problems. Factors of individual selectivity are involved in determining the physical tolerance limits of body structures and systems. Therefore, it is not possible to predict whether excessive talking per se will result in a problem or, if a problem does result, how severe the impairment will be.

Excessive talking may result in vocal fatigue. The voice quality may be reported to become slightly rough or hoarse, the voice may sound weak, and the person may report that talking requires effort. Frequently, those who have such complaints in the presence of a chronic pattern of excessive voice use report that a night's rest or a weekend with fewer vocal demands may temporarily restore the voice to normal but that the symptoms recur with the next period of excessive voice use. It is also important not to lose sight of the fact that patterns of misuse do not always occur as single, isolated behaviors. It is, of course, quite possible that the excessive talker is also engaging in other patterns of vocal misuse or abuse.

Ventricular Phonation

The diagnosis of ventricular phonation is usually made when laryngologic examination reveals greater than expected movement of the ventricular folds toward the midline. Visualization of the true vocal folds is often largely obscured by the compression of the ventricular folds, particularly in indirect mirror examination. Fiberoptic studies often permit visualization of some part of the true vocal folds or of their adductory and abductory movements. Stroboscopic examination can document whether or not there is actual ventricular fold vibration present. Videofluoroscopic examination, particularly in the anteroposterior orientation, can also be helpful in observing the presence or absence of true vocal fold adduction and abduction, as well as ventricular fold movements.

Ventricular fold phonation has been described as being low in pitch, very hoarse in quality, rattling, rumbling, cracking, reduced in intensity, diplophonic (Case, 1984; Aronson, 1985). However, acoustic data to support these perceptual descriptors are not available. The pathophysiology of ventricular phonation is not well understood (see Chapter 9 for further discussion). We have observed it as a manifestation of a psychogenic dysphonia (Brewer and McCall, 1974), as a compensatory behavior in the absence of adequate vocal fold movement, as one component in a pattern of hyperfunction, and as an unexplained phenomenon. Furthermore, in a study of normal nonsymptomatic speakers, Casper, Brewer, and Colton (1987) observed much variability in the degree of medial movement of the ventricular folds accompanying adduction of the true vocal folds.

Therapeutically we have found ventricular phonation to be reversible when its etiology is psychological or when it is a manifestation of hyperfunction. Its use as compensatory behavior may well be very functional and therefore an appropriate behavior requiring neither change nor elimination. However, in instances when the etiology is unclear, we have found this increased ventricular fold activity to be very resistant to change through behavioral therapy.

In instances when excess medial compression of the ventricular folds is present in the absence of laryngeal pathology, and when a voice problem seemingly related to this ventricular fold activity is present, ventricular phonation may be considered vocal misuse.

Aphonia and Dysphonia of Psychological Origin

There is no single way to characterize the patterns of misuse of the phonatory mechanism exhibited by persons whose voice problems are psychogenic. In our experience, we have encountered a wide diversity of patterns, including (a) total aphonia in which even the voiceless consonants were inaudible and the vocal folds were maintained in an abducted posture; (b) dysphonia in which the laryngeal mechanism was held in a tension equal to that of very forceful effort closure, with episodic bursts of explosive vocalization alternating with extreme hoarseness; (c) dysphonia in which the ventricular folds appeared to adduct; (d) dysphonia so variable that it encompassed normal voicing, aphonia, hoarseness, and very strained phonation, all within two or three sentences; and many other patterns. In all of these instances, when the physiology was normalized, so too was the voice. Therapeutic approaches to achieve normalization are discussed in Chapter 9.

Prior to discussing vocal abuse, it is appropriate to return to some of the questions posed in the first paragraph of this chapter. We have thus far discussed the vocal behaviors that we believe constitute misuse. However, the line between misuse and abuse is a very thin one, and perhaps rather than there being a division between the two, the behaviors might be thought of as existing along a continuum. Bear in mind, however, that a continuum is only a scale. It is usually thought to represent lesser or greater degrees of a behavior (in this case), but it does not necessarily imply progression of a behavior or disorder along the continuum. Thus, a pattern of misuse such as puberphonia can remain misuse and will not necessarily develop into a problem of greater severity. We are unable to predict if or when misuse may become abuse and lead to tissue change. It is logical to assume that excessive talking, for example, might at some point result in actual tissue changes. Indeed, many patients with lesions such as nodules or polyps admit to being incessant talkers. A distinction should be made between amount of talking and manner of talking (i.e., is it at a very high pitch, loud, tense?).

How patterns of misuse evolve is often difficult to determine or track down. One of the most frequently asked questions we have encountered clinically, and often a difficult one to answer, is the patient's incredulous wonderment about how it is possible, after several decades of presumably talking correctly, to no longer be doing so. We have no prospective information about this and can therefore only theorize retrospectively, using the information provided by patient recall. There are inherent dangers in doing this because most people are usually unaware of their speaking patterns until they encounter difficulty. To speak, to produce voice, is so innately human that very little conscious effort or thought is involved. Furthermore, memory is often flawed. The tendency to date the onset of a problem to a coincident event or one closely related in time is sometimes very useful, but it may also be totally misleading.

The most common antecedents to vocal misuse that seem to have validity include periods of increased personal tension or of greater than usual demands on the voice. Patients frequently report an episode of what they describe as laryngitis as the precipitating event. This laryngitis is reported to have been but one symptom of a more extensive upper respiratory infection, or it may have been an isolated symptom. Some patients recall periods of voice difficulty in the past that they ascribed to laryngitis and that had always resolved spontaneously within a short period of time. On occasion they may report that these episodes had become increasingly frequent and that each one had taken longer to resolve. Because producing voice is such a "natural" phenomenon, and because sensory feedback from the larynx is so limited, it is possible to change phonatory behavior with little awareness of having done so. In the presence of laryngitis, whether due to infection or to vocal fold edema resulting from misuse, adjustments in phonatory behavior need to be made in order to produce any voice. It is conceivable that these changes may go unrecognized and persist after the precipitating condition has resolved, or may contribute to maintaining the condition. One other factor that is often neglected must be considered. That is, we are not the same person from moment to moment or day to day. Our bodies are constantly changing and reacting to nutritional status, to drug intake, to environmental factors, to emotional state. A behavior that may have been present for many years and tolerated by the body may, due to some of the above factors, become intolerable and create what appears to be a sudden change in body function. It is also possible that the body reaches a threshold of tolerance for a certain behavior, the effects of which may have been minimal but cumulative. The changes may have been so gradual as to have gone unnoticed until the cumulative effect reached threshold level.

Abuse

Recognizing the fine distinction between misuse and abuse and the possibility of misuse becoming abuse, behaviors that we categorize as abuse tend to be harsher than those described above, with a greater likelihood of causing trauma to the laryngeal mucosa. Table 4.2 presents vocal behaviors that we categorize as outright abuse of the mechanism. Each will be discussed in the following sections.

Table 4.2.
Abusive Behaviors

A. Excessive, prolonged loudness

B. Strained and excessive use during period of swelling, inflammation, or other tissue change

C. Excessive coughing, throat clearing

D. The screamer and noise maker

E. The sports and exercise enthusiast
   1. Observer
   2. Participant

Excessive, Prolonged Loudness

In this category we would include persons who have habituated patterns of excessively loud voice use, those who spend much time talking above high environmental noise levels, teachers who have come to depend on loudness as a means of capturing and maintaining attention and discipline, cheerleaders, some ministers, sports coaches, and untrained or poorly trained singers, speakers, or actors whose activity requires loud voice usage, often in environments not conducive to good voice production.

The mechanism for loudness requires the creation of increased resistance of the laryngeal valve until an appropriate level of air pressure is produced and released. The vocal folds must be adducted strongly to create the increased medial compression required for this valving capability. Awareness of this mechanism results in an understanding of the abusive nature of excessive or prolonged loudness. The laryngeal mucosa, especially along the glottal edge, may become irritated, inflamed, and swollen. This may result in altered mass and affect the stiffness of the cover of the vocal folds. Vibratory behavior is changed and reflected in the sound of the voice. Continued use of the voice in this abusive manner may lead to further tissue changes, resulting in organized local lesions at the point of the greatest force of contact of the vocal folds, that is, the midpoint of the vibratory portion of the vocal folds (or in more generalized pathology, a greater extent of the vocal folds may be affected). The ability to fully adduct the vocal folds may be altered by mass lesions, and this will change the sound of the voice. Leakage of air through an incompletely closed glottis is heard as noise and adds a breathy component to the voice. As changes in phonatory function occur, there is a natural tendency on the part of the speaker to make compensatory adjustments. However, these attempts often constitute further abuse and result in greater tissue damage.

Daniloff et al. (1980) have pointed out that untrained speakers and singers have difficulty changing vocal parameters (e.g., pitch, loudness) independently of one another. Thus, as loudness is increased, the increased air pressure produces faster vocal fold vibration, resulting in an elevation of pitch. This may put additional strain on the mechanism.

Strained and Excessive Use during Periods of Swelling, Inflammation, or Other Tissue Changes

In the previous section we mentioned the negative effect of continued use of excess and prolonged loudness after such behavior had already resulted in irritation of the vocal fold mucosa. There are other times when similar caveats must be recognized. Edema of the vocal folds may result from infection, allergic reaction, or noxious environmental agents. Other conditions, such as chronic sinusitis with purulent drainage and gastroesophageal reflux, may serve to irritate and inflame the mucosa. Excessive drying of the tissues, resulting from certain drugs (see "Drugs and the Voice," below), extreme dryness of heated buildings (especially due to the use of woodburning stoves for heating), excessive use of alcohol, or reduced function of mucus glands can also increase the vulnerability of the mucosa. The chances of creating further damage to the vocal folds are increased if abusive vocal behaviors occur in the presence of any of these conditions. Tissues that are not in their healthiest and strongest condition are unable to withstand added stress.

It is not at all unusual for a patient to report that a voice problem seemed to begin with an episode of laryngitis of the bacterial type, but that normal voice did not return after the infection had cleared. Persons who rely heavily on voice use are often the most likely to engage in abusive behavior by continuing to use their voices during periods of laryngeal irritation. They tend to strain and exert greater effort in order to produce as much voice as possible, and in so doing increase the abuse.

Excessive Coughing and Throat Clearing

It is a normal occurrence for all of us to cough and clear our throats. Coughing may be in response to a local irritation or to infection and serves a life-sustaining purpose in guarding the airway against the entry of foreign objects. The cough reflex evokes a blast of air at high pressure as a mechanism for expelling anything that has attempted to pass through the larynx. The sensation of needing to clear the throat may result from momentary collection of mucus on the vocal folds that interferes with phonation. For some people, certain foods may create a reaction of increased mucus secretions (dairy foods seem to be the most common culprits) and an increased need to clear the throat. During upper respiratory infections or other illnesses, or as a reaction to drugs or treatment such as radiation therapy, the mucus tends to thicken and become tenacious. The sensation this arouses is again such that clearing the throat seems necessary. Inadequate laryngeal lubrication may result from drug effects, from emotional reactions such as stage fright, from excessive smoking or drinking, or from poorly functioning mucus glands.

Occasional coughing and throat clearing are not of concern. It is when these behaviors become excessive or habitual that they can be abusive. The entire larynx and supraglottal structures are involved in a cough. High speed films of coughing behavior reveal wide glottal opening first, followed by firm and protracted glottal closure during which large lung pressures build up, and ending in a complex expulsive phase (von Leden and Isshiki, 1965). The vocal folds and supraglottal structures, including the posterior pharyngeal wall, are all involved in that final vibratory phase and show periodic undulations of a violent nature. Very vigorous laryngeal activity has also been described during throat clearing (Timcke, von Leden, and Moore, 1959). An understanding of the "violent" nature of these behaviors makes it clear that both excessive coughing and habitual throat clearing can be damaging to the sensitive laryngeal mucosa.

An inventory of abusive behaviors frequently reveals habitual throat clearing as one such behavior. It is not uncommon to find the pattern so habituated that it is almost at an involuntary level and the patient's general level of awareness of it is limited. Most patients who exhibit this behavior report sensations of something in the throat that they feel they must dislodge in order to begin to speak. A habitual, hacking cough and frequent throat clearing are recognized hallmarks of the cigarette smoker and occur in response to the mucosal irritation caused by the noxious agents and the heat of the inhaled substances. They may also be symptomatic of an allergic reaction or other laryngeal irritation.

The Screamer and Noise Maker

Some young children are the prime exhibitors of these behaviors. They tend to be aggressive youngsters who talk a lot, habitually using loud voice in most situations and engaging in much yelling and screaming in interactions with family and friends, be it in anger or in play (Barker and Wilson, 1967; Wilson and Lamb, 1973; Toohill, 1975). Parents frequently report that a child has been a "screamer" since infancy, being perhaps the only one in the family to be so categorized. On other occasions the report implicates other family members who also tend to be "loud" in their vocal behavior. Because of factors of individual selectivity coupled with amount and degree of excessive screaming, a child may begin to exhibit a voice problem. Vocal nodules are often referred to as "screamer's nodes" due to their frequent occurrence in association with excessive screaming and yelling behavior.

Another manifestation of abuse of the voice most frequently noted in young children is that of using the voice to make a variety of sound effects. Not all such behavior need be abusive; however, many of the sounds typically produced by these children tend to involve strained vocalizations. Some children take special delight in producing the most unusual sounds they can devise. Others tend to supply all of the sound effects during play, not only for themselves but also for their friends.

There are many more boys implicated in screaming and noise making than girls. The incidence of vocal nodules is similarly greater for boys than girls (Senturia and Wilson,1968; Moore, 1986). Aronson (1985) assigns the "abnormal speaking behavior" of these youngsters to personality or emotional factors. Barker and Wilson (1967) studied the amount and type of voice use in the classroom of children with hoarse voices and compared them to a group of children with normal voices. They noted that those with hoarseness produced almost three times as many vocalizations within a 2-hour period than did those with normal voices. These dysphonic children were also observed to be more behaviorally active during unstructured classroom time than the control group of children. A further finding of interest was that 65% of the hoarse children came from families in which there was much intrafamily conflict, while only 35% of the nondysphonic children had such a family background.

Chronic Laryngitis

Chronic laryngitis is a condition in which the vocal fold mucosa is persistently inflamed and thickened. It is not to be confused with acute laryngitis that is the direct result of infection, or with an acute episode of "functional" laryngitis following a single episode of excessive voice use. Chronic laryngitis is thought to be related to cigarette smoking, environmental pollutants, alcohol, and vocal abuse. An acute episode may become chronic if abuse is added to other contributory factors. For further discussion of chronic laryngitis, see "Vocal Pathologies Secondary to Vocal Abuse/Misuse," below.

The Sports and Exercise Enthusiast

The Observer

Prime demonstrations of vocal abuse may be seen at many sporting or political events. The roar of the crowd is made up of many individual roars. In concert with the crowd noise, it becomes difficult to monitor the loudness of an individual voice. In the heat of the moment, and in keeping with socially accepted behavior, the louder the scream or yell, the better. These loud yells are usually produced with great tension and with elevated pitch, which adds to the degree of tension under which the laryngeal mechanism is held. This behavior and its results are so commonly known that lay people talk about screaming till the voice is gone. Indeed, even Shakespeare commented on this phenomenon in *Henry IV* with the exclamation, "For my voice, I have lost it with halloing and singing of anthems."

The delicate vocal fold mucosa becomes edematous and irritated in response to this abuse, thereby increasing the mass of the folds. The severity of the vocal symptoms will be related to the extent of this irritation and the tissue reaction to it. However, return to normal or slightly reduced vocal use plus a good night's rest will usually suffice to restore the vocal folds to their normal condition. But should the person continue to use the voice abusively, or place greater demands on it than the weakened mucosa can withstand, further deterioration of both the condition of the mucosa and the dysphonia may occur.

The Participant

A number of sports or fitness exercises by their very nature may set the stage for vocal abuse. Whenever it becomes necessary to build intrathoracic pressure, the laryngeal valve is involved, and effort closure of the glottis often results. Producing voice under this condition is very stressful. When lifting weights, for example, it is necessary for the person to build and maintain lung pressure as a ballast against which the weight may be lifted. This is a reflexive behavior when attempting to lift any heavy weight. Weightlifters often produce grunting sounds during the actual lift. With the larynx and vocal folds in tight adduction and great subglottal pressure present, it is not difficult to recognize the abusive nature of phonation in that mode. Similar effort closure of the glottis occurs accompanying a tennis serve or a golf drive.

In other types of sports, it is often necessary for team members to yell to one another above the noise of the spectators. Aerobics instructors who not only participate in the routine but also verbally cue the class above the sound level of the music are a new group of voice abusers to encounter voice problems. Persons who use motorized sports equipment such as snowmobiles and talk above the noise of the engines may also find themselves having repeated episodes of dysphonia.

When dealing with vocal misuse or vocal abuse, it is essential to pursue an exhaustive history of voice use. Patients do not readily identify behaviors other than the obvious ones, such as screaming, excessive talking, and loud singing. It is necessary for the clinician to explore the full range of potentially abusive vocal behaviors. Although we have attempted to highlight many such behaviors, our listing is probably not all inclusive. Each voice clinician will be able to add to it from personal experience.

Drugs and the Voice

This section of the chapter will deal with the known and potential effects of drugs on the voice. Although the taking of drugs does not come under the category of a vocal behavior, the effects of drugs are potentially damaging to the mucosa and disruptive to phonation. For these reasons, we have chosen to place this material in this chapter.

Research on the effects of various drugs on the laryngeal mucosa and laryngeal physiology is almost nonexistent. Therefore, in discussing the effects of drugs on voice, we are talking about expected effects based on an understanding of drug action and laryngeal anatomy and physiology. The following summary is based on the work of pharmacologist

F. Gene Martin (1983, 1984, 1988), who presents five basic pharmacological principles to keep in mind when discussing the general effects of drugs:

1. There is wide biological variability in individual response to drugs, based on a large variety of factors including age, body composition, kidney function, genetic inheritance, biochemistry, stress level, disease, drug/drug interaction, and nutritional status. Responses may differ both quantitatively and qualitatively.

2. The placebo effect, (the expectation of an effect) may influence the type and degree of effect obtained. This is a poorly understood but generally accepted phenomenon.

3. The intensity of the effect of a drug is usually expected to be proportional to the dose administered or taken; that is, the larger the dose, the greater the effect, proportionally. However, the dose-response relationships of most drugs form sigmoid-shaped curves rather than straight lines, when their effects are plotted against dosage. Such curves indicate that the intensity of a drug increases gradually at first, then rapidly, and then gradually again, eventually reaching a ceiling or plateau level as the dose is increased incrementally (step-wise). Increasing the dose after the ceiling effect has been obtained produces no further enhancement of effect and may only produce undesirable toxic side effects. Allergic reactions to drugs may appear with any dose, no matter how small, and the intensity of such allergic effects is not related to the magnitude of the dose.

4. Drugs may have a multiplicity of effects. Those that are not the specifically intended effect are usually referred to as side effects. These are the effects that most frequently have ramifications for voice production.

5. The efficacy of a drug is of more concern than its potency. Thus, if drug A produces a desired level of response at a lower dose than drug B does, it does not necessarily mean that drug A is better than B. Drug A may, in fact, be worse, if even at its lower dose it produces more undesirable side effects than drug B does. It matters little to the patient whether the pill swallowed contains 5 mg or 200 mg of a drug. What matters is the production of an adequate therapeutic effect and the absence of unacceptable side effects with a given reasonable dose.

To those basic principles an additional caution should be included concerning the geriatric population. Elderly people may respond differently, quantitatively or qualitatively, than younger persons do to the same dose of the same drug. This difference in response is due to the loss, reduction, or alteration of certain body structures and functions with aging, as for example a reduced ability to metabolize or absorb certain drugs.

The voice-related effects of drugs may be classified in the following seven categories: (a) coordination and proprioception, (b) airflow, (c) fluid balance, (d) secretions of the upper respiratory tract, (e) structure of the vocal folds, (f) hearing, and (g) miscellaneous. Each of these areas will be discussed.

Coordination and Proprioception

Any agent that is stimulating or depressing to the central nervous system has the potential to affect coordination, including the fine motor control of phonatory behavior. Central nervous system stimulants include amphetamines, dextroamphetamine sulfate (Dexedrine), cocaine, caffeine, and phenylpropanolamine (PPA), the active agent in over-the-counter diet aids. Stimulants are used primarily as recreational drugs and appetite depressants. Their adverse effects may include nervousness and tremor. Central nervous system depressants include alcohol, barbiturates, tranquilizers such as diazepam (Valium) and chlordiazepoxide hydrochloride (Librium), and chloral hydrate. They are used primarily as antianxiety agents and produce a sedating effect that in high enough doses may have a negative influence on muscle coordination. For example, slurred and slowed speech are well-recognized hallmarks of the person who has had too much to drink.

Diazepam (Valium) is often prescribed for patients with a variety of voice disorders. However, administration of diazepam is usually unproductive of any beneficial change in voice production or in the alleviation of voice symptoms. In a study of the effect of diazepam on respiratory and laryngeal muscle activitation, Ludlow, Schulz, and Naunton, (1988) report strong interindividual respiratory and phonatory effects, which may be age related. Laryngeal activation decreased in their older subjects, while it increased in their younger subjects. The authors caution that use of diazepam as a treatment for spastic dysphonia or other movement disorders affecting the voice may, in some individuals, result in a worsening of symptoms. Furthermore, they call attention to the not uncommon administration of diazepam or other such medications to subjects in studies of laryngeal muscle activity during speech, suggesting that this practice may significantly alter the results of such studies.

Another group of drugs that affect the central nervous system are those that produce an anesthetic effect. Local anesthetics such as benzocaine (Americaine), lidocaine (Xylocaine), procaine hydrochloride (Novocain), or phenol may be the primary ingredients in over-the-counter lozenges and sprays used to treat a sore throat. These agents are capable of blocking nerve impulse conduction and reducing pain sensation. Pain serves as an alarm system, indicating the presence of a problem somewhere in the body. The usual response to throat or laryngeal pain is to reduce voice usage. Reduction of pain by the use of these analgesic agents masks the presence of the problem, and the individual may then be prone to overstressing voice use. Leonard and Ringel (1979) reported some changes in laryngeal behavior following the dripping of a local anesthetic onto the vocal folds.

Airflow

Drugs that either dilate or constrict the bronchioles will affect the movement of pulmonary air through the larynx. Bronchodilators, such as albuterol (Proventil, Ventolin), metaproterenol sulfate (Alupent), and others are used primarily as antiasthma agents. Negative side effects may be nervousness and tremor. Bronchoconstrictors potentially have a more adverse effect on voice production. Drugs cause bronchoconstriction most often as an allergic reaction. The effects may vary from very mild discomfort and wheezing to a significant, even life-threatening effect on respiratory function. Many environmental irritants, such as dust, pollen, and molds, produce similar effects.

Fluid Balance

Fluid balance in the mucosa of the vocal folds may have a very significant and direct effect on voice production. There are many drugs that, either as a consequence of their primary intended effect or as their side effect, work in such a way as to reduce edema. Diuretics, which reduce the formation of edema, are commonly used in the treatment of high blood pressure and heart or kidney failure. Perhaps the most widely used group of agents with the effect of reducing edema are the decongestants, many of which are sold as over-the-counter preparations in tablet, capsule, or liquid form or as topical sprays (e.g., oxymetazoline hydrochloride (Afrin), pseudoephedrine hydrochloride (Sudafed, etc.). These are used in the treatment of the symptoms of cold, cough, allergy, or sinus problems.

Vocal fold edema, under most circumstances, is the result of protein-bound water (Lawrence, 1987; Sataloff, 1987a) and will not be responsive to diuretic agents. Corticosteroids, often used as drying agents in the treatment of vocal fold edema in performers following vocally abusive episodes, affect protein-bound water directly. Although they are often effective, they offer only a palliative, not a curative, effect. A patient may be using a diuretic agent for a number of reasons not directly related to vocal fold edema. In such instances, the danger of reducing the normally desirable fluid level in the laryngeal mucosa must be kept in mind. Long-term use of decongestants may cause a rebound effect wherein, as the vasoconstrictive effects of the drug wear off, there is a return of the edema and congestion to a greater degree than was previously present. As a result, a vicious cycle may be established in which the patient must continue to take the decongestant in an attempt to counteract the side effect that is being caused by the drug itself. The long-term effects of vasoconstriction and the adverse effects from the loss of adequate fluid balance include a reduction in blood flow to the mucosa; loss of electrolytes with concomitant decrease of potassium level, leading to a decrease in energy and a sedating effect; increased nervousness and tremor; and potential damage to the mucous membranes. Edema formation in reaction to drugs occurs primarily in the form of an allergic response. Agents that cause an allergic reaction in a patient may have more than a single effect. While bronchoconstriction may be one effect, edema of the mucosa may occur simultaneously. Edema of the laryngeal mucosa may also occur in response to vocal abuse, trauma, infection, and environmental allergens.

Steroid inhalants are used in the treatment of asthma. Their effect on voice is not entirely clear. Williams, Baghat, DeStableforth, Shenoi, and Skinner (1983) reported dysphonia and bilateral vocal fold bowing in patients using an inhaled corticosteroid. The vocal fold bowing appeared to be related to the dose and potency of the drug used and was believed to represent a local steroid myopathy. The bowing and concomittant dysphonia were reversed in all patients after cessation of use of the steroid inhalant. Watkin and Ewanowski (1979) reported that prolonged administration of aerosol-delivered triamcinolone acetonide (Kenalog), a drug used by chronic asthmatics, results in significantly altered vocal tract functioning and an elevation of fundamental frequency of approximately 20 Hz. They reported that changes were evident after 1 year of use, with a cumulative effect described after 2 years.

Secretions of the Upper Respiratory Tract

According to Martin (1983,1984,1988), exposure to agents that affect upper respiratory tract secretions occurs with great frequency. Many drugs act as drying agents by causing a reduction in secretions of the salivary and mucus glands. Furthermore, Martin states, a major portion of our lives "is spent in buildings with very low humidity, and we are continuously breathing air with moisture levels similar to that of the Sahara" (Martin, 1983, p. 127–128). A vicious cycle ensues in which breathing dry air results in dryness and irritation of the mucosa, which leads to coughing, which serves to further irritate and dry the mucosa.

Among the drugs creating a drying effect, the most common are the antihistamines used in the treatment of allergy, cold, cough, sinus, motion sickness, and insomnia. Drugs functioning as antispasmodic agents (e.g., atropine, scopolamine, diphenoxylate hydrochloride [Lomotil], etc.) used in the treatment of diarrhea also create a reduction in glandular secretions. The action of antitussive drugs such as codeine and dextromethorphan hydrobromide (Benylin DM), used in cough remedies, is drying, and a side effect is sedation. Antipsychotic agents such as chlorpromazine hydrochloride (Thorazine) and haloperidol (Haldol) and antidepressant agents such as amitriptylene (Elavil) and lithium carbonate (Lithane, Lithobid) cause drying and sedation. The last group of drying agents is the antihypertensive drugs used in the treatment of high blood pressure, such as methyldopa (Aldomet), reserpine (Sandril, Serpasil), and captopril (Capoten).

The most effective wetting agent is water, abundantly available and easily consumed. Ambient humidity may be voluntarily controlled, as may the amount of water consumed. Expectorants, used in the treatment of cough, are agents that increase secretions. However, many of these products contain other drugs that have the opposite effect. Guaifenesin (Robitussin, Glycotuss) is the most commonly used expectorant drug and can be obtained as the only drug in a product. Saliva substitutes (e.g., dibasic sodium phosphate [Moi-stir], sodium carboxymethlcellulose [Salvart], etc.) have recently become available and appear to be very helpful as wetting agents. They are used primarily by persons who have salivary gland pathology but can be effectively used to combat the dry mouth caused by the use of drying agents and also by preperformance anxiety.

Changes in Structure of the Vocal Folds

Agents that create change in the actual structure of the vocal folds are the androgens, which are structurally related to the male hormone testosterone. They are used in the treatment of hormonal imbalance (frequently in postmenopausal women) and by body builders seeking to increase muscle mass. Androgens cause an increase in the mass of the vocal folds, which, of course, results in a change in the voice, referred to as the virilization of the voice. Once this change has occurred, it is irreversible (Damste, 1967). A synthetic androgen, danazol androgen (Danocrine), is commonly used in the treatment of benign fibrocystic breast disease, although a side effect of voice change occurs in about 10% of the patients treated. It is not yet clear whether these voice changes are reversible (Martin, 1988).

Hearing

A number of drug groups are known to be potentially ototoxic. Some of these are aminoglycoside antibiotics, such as amikacin sulfate (Amikin) and tobramycin sulfate (Nebcin), which are used intravenously in life-threatening disease states. Certain diuretics, referred to as "loop" or "high ceiling" diuretics, such as furosemide (Lasix) or bumetanide (Bumex), used in the treatment of heart failure and high blood pressure, also have the potential to create hearing loss. Some drugs used in chemotherapy for cancer are also suspected to have ototoxic side effects, and their use should be monitored closely. Obviously the loss of hearing will not have a direct effect on laryngeal anatomy, and perhaps not an immediate effect on laryngeal physiology. Indirectly, however, loss of hearing may affect vocal production, and it is likely that vocal physiology may be altered over time.

Miscellaneous Agents

Martin notes additional agents that are thought by some to have an effect on voice production and on performance, although they do not specifically fit any of the previous categories. These include herbal teas, aspirin, beta blockers, and tobacco and other smoked or inhaled drugs.

Herbal Teas

Certain varieties of these herbal mixtures are reported to have a soothing effect on the respiratory tract mucosa. They have not been shown to have any medicinal value. In general, it is well to exercise care in the use of any herbal mixtures and to know exactly what they contain.

Aspirin

Aspirin has anticoagulant properties that are not usually of consequence to the average voice user unless that individual has a bleeding disorder or is taking other anticoagulant medication. Because the professional voice user is called upon to use the voice strenuously, the risk of vocal fold hemorrhage may be somewhat increased, and particularly so if that person is taking aspirin or any preparations containing acetylsalicylic acid.

Beta Blockers

During times of stress and fear, the adrenal glands release the chemicals epinephrine and norepinephrine. It is the increased level of these chemicals that results in rapid heart beat, tremor, elevated blood pressure, sweaty palms, dry mouth, respiratory tension, nausea, and an urge to urinate. These are also the well-known symptoms of the phenomenon known as stage fright. Beta blockers, of which propranolol (Inderal) is the most common, act to block the effect of epinephrine on glands, smooth muscles, and the heart, thereby reducing the symptoms described above. Whether or not the reduction of symptoms produces enhanced performance has not been determined. Instrument musicians have been reported to demonstrate improved performance and a lessening of subjective stage fright symptoms with the use of beta blockers (Liden and Gottfries, 1974; James, Pearson, Griffith, and Newburg, 1977; Brantigan, Brantigan, and Joseph, 1982). Evidence of their effectiveness in singers is less conclusive. Gates and Montalbo (1987) suggest that low-dose (20 mg) beta blockade had no significant effect on singers' performance. In an earlier study, Gates, Saegert, Wilson, Johnson, Sheppard, and Hearne (1985) reported a deleterious effect on singing quality with the administration of beta blocker in high doses (40 to 80 mg). There does not appear to be strong evidence that beta blockers significantly enhance performance. Indeed, it has been suggested by some that heightened preperformance anxiety serves a useful purpose in that it lends a degree of intensity and excitement to the performance that might be lost if beta blockers were used. Data to support this contention or its corollary are not yet available.

Tobacco and Other Smoked or Inhaled Drugs

We should not leave this section on the effect of drugs on the voice without some direct mention of tobacco, marijuana, and other drugs that are smoked or inhaled. There is very convincing evidence (Hammond, 1966; Kahn, 1966; Wynder, Covey, Mabuchi, and Mushinski, 1976; Wynder and Stellman, 1977; Burch, 1981) that smoking cigarettes is closely related to laryngeal cancer. The vast majority of individuals who present with laryngeal carcinoma have a history of heavy smoking. Precancerous conditions such as leukoplakia and hyperkeratosis are also closely linked to smoking. Some smokers present with very boggy, polypoid vocal folds, a condition that is benign but usually results in significant dysphonia and can be extensive enough to compromise the airway. Redness and generalized irritation of the mucosa of the upper respiratory tract and the larynx are often present in persons who use tobacco, marijuana, and other inhaled substances. A recent study reports on the harmful effects of inhaling environmental smoke (U.S. Department of Health and Human Services, 1986). Lung cancer and emphysema are also known to be directly related to smoking. When the respiratory system is compromised, there is a direct effect on voice production. Thus, even in the absence of actual laryngeal pathology, the effects of smoking on lung function are sufficient to produce a broad effect on phonation.

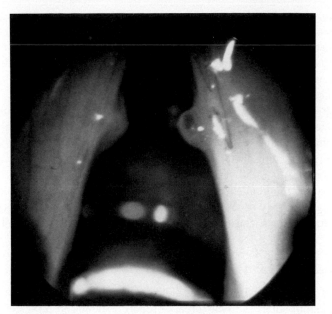

Figure 4.1.   Vocal fold nodules. (Color photograph on page xiii by Eiji Yanagisawa, M.D.)

Vocal Pathologies Secondary to Vocal Abuse/Misuse

Nodules

Primary Voice Symptom

The primary voice symptom is hoarseness.

Description and Etiology

Nodules are localized benign growths on the vocal folds that are usually thought to be the result of vocal abuse. They are a reaction of the tissue to the constant stress induced by frequent, hard oppositional movement of the vocal folds. In the initial stages of the formation of a nodule, the trauma causes localized edema on the vocal fold edge. Early or acute nodules are fairly soft and pliable; they may be reddish in appearance and are mostly vascular and edematous. The remainder of the vocal fold may also be edematous, and the entire larynx may be slightly inflamed. In this early stage, the nodule may be evident only on one side and may easily be mistaken for a polyp. With continued trauma, the tissue undergoes hyalinization and fibrosis and becomes firm. Chronic nodules are usually hard, white, thick, and fibrosed. Arnold (1962, 1980) reported that at this chronic stage of nodule development, the epithelium may show hypertrophy, horny or very rough surfaces, and a change in the type of cells present. Chronic nodules are usually bilateral and not always symmetrical in size. Figure 4.1 is an illustration of a pair of vocal nodules. (Also note the small hematoma on the right fold.)

There is some controversy about the distinction between nodules and polyps. A polyp is a projecting mass with a central core of fibrous tissue of greater density than the lamina propria and covered by a normal or slightly hyperplastic epithelium. Clinically, there are times when the distinction is very clear and other times when the difference is minimal. Histologically, the situation is not much clearer. Fitz-Hugh, Smith, and Chiong (1958) reviewed the histological findings of 300 consecutive cases of benign tumors of the vocal folds. They commented on the difficulty of distinguishing among nodules, polyps, and polypoid degeneration. Many nodules were classified as polyps and vice versa, on review. They eventually concluded that a nodule was a trauma-related lesion consisting of a local nodular or polypoid degeneration of the lamina propria. They state that a polyp has its origin in the subepithelial (or Reinke's) space.

Luchsinger and Arnold (1965) consider general physical constitution, personality, and local laryngeal signs to be important predisposing conditions for nodules (or polyps). Allergies or thyroid imbalances may contribute to precipitating factors; tobacco and alcohol use may be aggravating factors. In adults, nodules occur most frequently in women between the ages of 20 and 50 years.

Nodules may be found in children who are prone to excessive loud talking or screaming. In this age group, they occur most frequently in boys. They usually occur in children who have a history of loud, constant voice usage in conversation, in school, at home, and at play.

Perceptual Signs and Symptoms

Hoarseness and breathiness are the major perceptual signs of a nodule. An individual may also complain of soreness in the throat or report difficulty in producing pitches in the upper third of their range. This is especially true for singers. The degree of hoarseness or breathiness present is usually dependent on the size of the nodule and may vary from slight to moderately severe.

Acoustic Signs

Acoustically, a patient with a nodule will exhibit increased frequency and amplitude perturbation (jitter and shimmer) with a normal fundamental frequency. Davis (1981) reported pitch perturbation quotient (PPQ) values of 2.61% and 1.87% for two patients with nodules, compared to a PPQ of 0.42% for normal speakers. Others have reported similar greater than normal frequency perturbation measurements in the presence of nodules. Takahashi and Koike (1975) reported a mean relative average perturbation (RAP, see Chapter 2) of 0.0084, whereas Ludlow, Coulter, and Gentges (1983) reported a mean jitter of 9.26 microseconds, compared to a normal value of 5 microseconds. Davis also reported an amplitude perturbation quotient (APQ) of 9.07% and 15.33% for the nodule cases, compared to a normal APQ of 6.14%.

Phonational range may be markedly reduced, especially at the upper end. The patient may also show reduced dynamic range, with an inability to produce high sound pressure levels. Eckel and Boone (1981) reported an average s/z ratio of 1.65 for their group of 28 patients with nodules and polyps. Normal subjects produced an s/z ratio of 0.99.

Spectrum analysis of a patient's phonation will show evidence of noise in the spectrum (Yanagihara, 1967; Arnold and Emanuel, 1979), the degree of which depends on the severity of hoarseness and lesion size. Interestingly, nodules seem to produce little effect on fundamental frequency of phonation (Murry, 1978).

Physiological Signs

Airflows in a patient with a nodule may be equal to or slightly higher than normal (Iwata, von Leden, and Williams, 1972; Iwata, Esaki, Iwami, and Takasu, 1976). Tanaka and Gould (1985) reported a mean value of 275 ml/sec for their two patients with nodules. Normal male subjects produce flows of about 125 ml/sec. Woo, Colton, and Shangold (1987) reported a mean flow rate of 265 ml/sec for their combined polyp and nodule group, collapsed across 14 male and 18 female subjects. In their study, normal speakers produced a mean flow rate of 144 ml/sec. The magnitude of the increase of airflow rates appears to depend on the severity of the lesion (Shigemori, 1977). Lung pressures may also be high because of the tendency for an individual to increase the driving force to overcome incomplete glottal closure (Tanaka and Gould, 1985). Unfortunately, there are few data reported in the literature to support this conclusion. In our experience, vibratory flows may show marked offset flow, with normal and slightly increased peak flow measures. Electroglottograms will show decreased closing times of the vocal folds and an irregular pattern. Normal electromyogram levels would be expected, although it is possible for these to be elevated if the patient shows excessive laryngeal tension.

Laryngoscopic Signs

Nodules usually occur at the midpoint of the vibrating vocal folds because it is there that the forces encountered during vibration are the largest (Luchsinger and Arnold, 1965). It is not uncommon, however, for nodules to be reported at the junction of the anterior one-third and posterior two-thirds of the vocal folds. It must be remembered that the posterior one-third of the vocal fold is composed of stiff cartilage that does not vibrate. The remaining two-thirds of the vocal folds vibrate, and it is at the midpoint of this vibrating portion that the contact forces will be the greatest. Laryngoscopically, there may be evidence of incomplete closure of the vocal folds, especially in the area surrounding the nodule.

Vocal fold vibratory patterns of patients with nodules also vary. Moore, Cannon, and Wilson (1979) studied five female patients with nodules and reported that the size of the nodule varied among the subjects, as did the size of the nodule on one fold versus the other. More important, they found seven closure patterns of the vocal folds, each somewhat dependent on the size and precise location of the lesion on the vocal fold. Some patients were able to achieve complete closure (pattern I), whereas others showed a small posterior opening (pattern II). Others showed a greater amount of posterior opening of the vocal folds (patterns III and IV), and in the three remaining patterns (V, VI, VII) a small amount of opening was apparent anteriorly in addition to varied amounts of opening posteriorly (similar to patterns II, III, and IV).

Stroboscopic Signs

According to Kitzing (1985), the vocal folds will show normal symmetry and periodicity but reduced amplitudes and mucosal waves at the nodule site and reduced glottal closure. In view of the greater frequency perturbation found in patients with vocal nodules (as reported in "Acoustic Signs," above), the stroboscopic finding of normal periodicity is questionable. It is possible that a small nodule may have a minimal effect on the vibratory frequency of the vocal folds.

Pathophysiology

A nodule will increase the mass of the cover of the vocal fold. The stiffness of the cover will be increased by a hard and firm nodule and decreased by a soft and pliable one (Hirano, 1981b). The mechanical properties of the transition layers and the muscle will not be affected by the nodule. Because the mechanical properties of the cover are very important in determining the vibratory characteristics of the vocal folds, a nodule may have a pronounced effect on the mechanics of vibration. The extra mass at the midpoint of the vibrating vocal folds results in increased aperiodicity of vibration, greater frequency perturbation, and greater hoarseness. Depending on the size of the nodule, glottal closure will

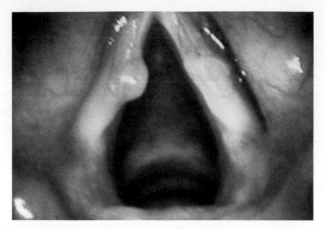

Figure 4.2. A single vocal fold polyp. (Color photograph on page xiii by Eiji Yanagisawa, M.D.)

also be affected. Incomplete closure will permit increased air escape, resulting in the perception of breathiness.

Polyps

Primary Voice Symptom

The primary voice symptom is hoarseness.

Description and Etiology

Polyps, like nodules, are caused by excessive voice use and abuse. Luchsinger and Arnold (1965) consider that polyps and nodules have the same etiology and differ only in degree. According to Jackson (1941), a polyp is larger and more vascular, edematous, and inflammatory than a nodule, which is described as a more organized mass of tissue (Fig. 4.2). It is easy to see how an acute nodule can be mistaken for a polyp. Polyps usually occur in Reinke's space (the superficial layer of the lamina propria) and may consist of dilated blood vessels, fibrotic tissue, and small hemorrhages.

The distinction between polyp and polypoid degeneration is sometimes confusing. According to Lowenthal (1958), they are very similar in that they are a localized or diffuse inflammatory tumor involving the space of Reinke. If the tumor is localized, it may show up as pedunculated (on a stalk) or sessile (closely adhering to mucosa). If the lesion is diffuse, it may cover one-half to two-thirds of the entire length of the vocal fold. Histologically, however, both types are very similar.

Polyps usually result from a period of vocal abuse, although they can occur as the result of a single traumatic incident, as, for example, yelling at a basketball game. Polyps are usually unilateral, although sometimes a small polyp can be found on the contralateral side. Although polyps usually occur on the free margin of the vocal folds,they may also be found on the superior surface of the folds as well as subglottally. In the latter case, there may be little or no alteration in the voice. They may also involve almost the entire length of the vocal fold (Fig. 4.3).

Perceptual Signs and Symptoms

Typical perceptual signs of a polyp include hoarseness, roughness, or breathiness. In addition, the patient may report the sensation of something in the throat.

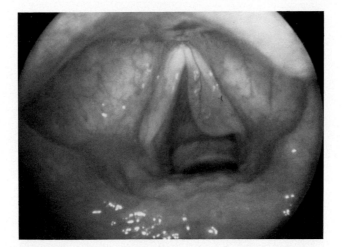

Figure 4.3. Large sessile polyp, involving the entire length of the vocal fold. (Color photograph on page xiii by Eiji Yanagisawa, M.D.)

Acoustic Signs

The acoustic features created by a polyp are very similar to those of a nodule. Increased jitter and shimmer would be expected (depending on the location of the polyp). Davis (1981) reported a PPQ of 0.60% and an APQ of 11.68% for his one patient with a polyp. Normal PPQ is 0.42% and APQ is 6.14%. Reduced phonational and dynamic ranges as well as increased spectral noise, would also be anticipated acoustic characteristics. Unfortunately, data to support these expectations about the magnitude of phonational ranges and spectral noise in patients with polyps are not available.

Physiological Signs

Increased airflow may be present if the polyp interferes with complete glottal closure. In one report, 18 patients with polyps had an average airflow rate of 162 ml/sec (Iwata et al., 1972), whereas in another report (Iwata et al., 1976) an average airflow rate of 253 ml/ sec was reported for 29 male patients and 247 ml/sec for 19 female patients with unilateral polyps. Patients with bilateral polyps had airflow rates of 256 ml/sec (8 males) and 359 ml/ sec (8 females). For their 7 patients with polyps, Tanaka and Gould (1985) reported a mean flow rate of 223.71 ml/sec. Woo et al. (1987) reported a mean flow rate of 265 ml/ sec for their combined polyp and nodule group, collapsed across 14 male and 18 female subjects. In their study, normal speakers produced a mean flow rate of 144 ml/sec. Subglottal or lung pressure also appears to show an increase due to attempts to produce phonation in the presence of a leaky glottis (Tanaka and Gould, 1985). We have observed that patients with polyps tend to have greater than normal vibratory flows. Electroglottograms tend to show decreased closing times of the vocal folds and irregular patterns. Muscle action potentials would be expected to be normal, unless the patient showed excessive laryngeal tension.

Stroboscopic Signs

Stroboscopically, asymmetry of motion of the vocal folds and increased aperiodicity are noted. Polyps tend to show distinct phase differences between the two folds, especially if the lesions are grossly different in size. The amplitude of the vocal folds is reduced, and

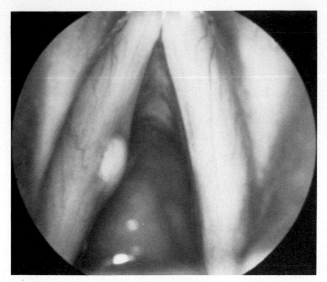

Figure 4.4.   Intracordal cyst. (Color photograph on page xiii by Eiji Yanagisawa, M.D.)

mucosal waves, expecially in the vicinity of the polyp, will be either decreased or absent. Glottal closure may also be affected (Hirano, Feder, and Bless, 1983; Kitzing, 1985).

Pathophysiology

A polyp will increase the mass of the cover of the vocal folds. If the polyp is soft, edematous, and pliable, the stiffness of the cover will be decreased (Hirano, 1981b). However, if bleeding, hyaline degeneration, or other histological changes are present, stiffness of the cover may be increased (see Chapter 3). The mechanical properties of the transition layers and the muscle will not be affected. As described in the case of the nodule, the mechanical properties of the cover will determine the vibratory characteristics of the vocal folds. The extra mass at the midpoint of the vibrating vocal folds results in increased aperiodicity of vibration, greater frequency perturbation, and greater hoarseness. However, if the polyp is pedunculated (attached only by a slim stalk), there will probably be little effect on vibration because the mass of the polyp does not affect the cover directly. Depending on the size of the polyp, glottal closure may be affected. If sufficient air can escape through the closed glottis, breathiness will be perceived.

Intracordal Cysts

Primary Voice Symptom

The primary voice symptom is hoarseness.

Description and Etiology

Intracordal cysts appear as small spheres on the margins of the vocal folds (Fig. 4.4). They may be mistaken for nodules because small nodule-like growths may appear on one cord but not the other. Cysts may also occur in association with vocal nodules (Monday, Cornut, Bouchayer, and Roch, 1983).

Intracordal cysts may be caused by blockage of a glandular duct in which there is retention of mucus (Monday et al., 1983). Because there is no way for the mucus to escape, a cyst may, with time, grow larger. Another type of cyst, usually smaller than a retention cyst, is the epidermoid cyst. Epidermoid cysts of the vocal folds have a strong similarity to epidermal cysts of the skin.

Most patients with intracordal cysts are young adult women (Monday et al., 1983; Bouchayer, Cornut, Witzig, Loire, Roch, and Bastian, 1985). Cysts often occur in professional voice users.

Perceptual Signs and Symptoms

Typical signs of a cyst include hoarseness and a lowered pitch. The patient may report a "tired" voice.

Acoustic Signs

Data are not available on the acoustic characteristics of the voices of patients with cysts. We might expect data similar to those for nodules, since the effect on the vocal folds appears to be similar.

Physiological Signs

Again, there are few physiological data available on patients with cysts. However, higher than normal average airflows might be expected as a result of elevated offset flows and higher than normal peak flows. The closing phase of the vocal folds, as seen in an electroglottogram, may also be slower than normal.

Laryngoscopic Signs

Identification of a cyst can be very difficult. Bouchayer et al. (1985) report that in only 10% of their cases was a cyst obvious on initial examination. However, the appearance of fullness of the vocal fold and dilated capillaries raised the suspicion of a cyst in 55% of cases.

Stroboscopic Signs

Stroboscopy has been found to be very helpful in the diagnosis of a cyst because there is an absence of mucosal wave in the area over the cyst. Other signs include greater aperiodicity and reduced glottal closure (Kitzing, 1985). We have found that the vibration of the two folds is asymmetrical, especially over the area of the cyst.

Pathophysiology

A cyst originates in the superficial layer of the lamina propria (Hirano, 1981b). As it grows, it increases the distance between the cover and the lamina propria but usually does not extend into the layers. A cyst increases the mass and stiffness of the cover, whereas the transition layers and the body are unaffected.

Edema

Primary Voice Symptom

The primary voice symptom is hoarseness.

Description and Etiology

Edema refers to the buildup of fluid somewhere in the vocal fold. It may occur deep in the vocal fold or in more superfical layers. When it occurs in the first layer of the lamina propria, it is referred to as Reinke's edema since Reinke's space occurs in this layer (Fig. 4.5). Other names used to refer to this problem are diffuse polyposis or polypoid degenera-

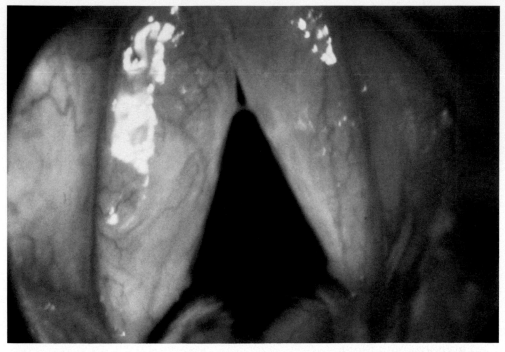

Figure 4.5.   Reinke's edema. (Color photograph on page xiii by Eiji Yanagisawa, M.D.)

tion. Some apparent swelling of the vocal folds, especially when localized, may also be a sign of a cyst.

Edema is a natural reaction of tissue to trauma and misuse. In addition to vocal abuse, chronic Reinke's edema is most often associated with smoking. It appears to occur more frequently in females, especially if they are long-term smokers (Bastian, 1986; Nielsen, Hojslet, and Karlsmose, 1986).

Perceptual Signs and Symptoms

Typical symptoms of edema include a lower than normal pitch level and hoarseness. If the condition is particularly severe, the patient may complain of shortness of breath because the edematous vocal folds may partially block the airway.

Acoustic Signs

The fundamental frequency of phonation is lower than that expected for the sex and age of the patient. Bennett, Bishop, and Lumpkin (1987) reported a mean fundamental frequency of 108 Hz for their group of 29 females with Reinke's edema, and 91 Hz for their 6 male patients. There may be increased frequency and amplitude perturbation, as well as the presence of spectral noise due to the hoarseness. There are, however, few experimental data available to support these hypotheses.

Physiological Signs

Unless there is incomplete closure of the vocal folds, airflow and air pressures may be within normal limits. Electromyographic recordings may also show no abnormalities. Vibratory airflow measurements may show the aperiodicity of phonation with greater than normal peak airflows.

Laryngoscopic Signs

The vocal folds, when visualized, appear full of fluid and boggy. The edema usually involves the full length of the vocal folds bilaterally. In some respects, Reinke's edema gives the appearance of a broad-based polyp occupying the full length of the vocal fold.

Stroboscopic Signs

The major stroboscopic features appear to be greater than normal movements of the mucosal wave and a more complete glottal closure. The former may be due to the fluid-filled vocal folds' having greater inertia to movement, and the latter due to the fluid filled folds' meeting much more firmly. We have found that the vibration of the two folds is often symmetrical.

Pathophysiology

Edema affects the superficial layer of the lamina propria. The mass of the cover is increased, whereas its stiffness is decreased. Bennett et al. (1987) suggested that Reinke's edema disturbs the elasticity of the cover, resulting in decreased stiffness. Such a reduction in stiffness would allow for greater amplitudes of vibration. The transition layers and body are not affected in Reinke's edema. The increase in bulk and reduction of stiffness would contribute to a lowered fundamental frequency of vibration.

Laryngitis

Primary Voice Symptom

The primary voice symptom is hoarseness.

Description and Etiology

Laryngitis is an inflammation of the vocal folds and larynx. It may result from exposure to noxious agents (tobacco, alcohol, drugs), environmental agents (allergens, dust, etc.) or vocal abuse. Laryngitis may also be the result of upper respiratory infections, which have a generalized effect on the mucosa of the respiratory tract, including the larynx (Fig. 4.6). The problem may be acute or chronic. Acute laryngitis resulting from bacterial infection is not directly related to vocal abuse. However, it does affect voice production and indirectly may be aggravated by abuse, as will be described later. Chronic abuse will lead to persistent inflammation and perhaps result in a thickening of the vocal folds. It may also lead to permanent changes, such as nodules, polyps, or hypertrophy of the laryngeal epithelium.

Perceptual Signs and Symptoms

The symptoms of laryngitis include marked roughness or hoarseness in the voice with accompanying discomfort and dryness in the throat. When secondary to infection, the hoarseness may persist for some time after the infection has been controlled. Continued heavy use of the voice during this time may contribute to the laryngitis and the continued hoarseness. The pitch levels of the voice may appear to be higher than normal, and it will be difficult to speak in a loud voice.

Acoustic Signs

Greater than normal frequency and amplitude perturbation would be expected. Takahashi and Koike (1975) found a mean RAP of 0.0069 and 0.0078 in their two female patients with chronic laryngitis. Their nine normal subjects had a mean RAP of 0.00582.

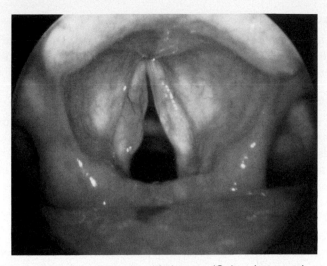

Figure 4.6. Chronic laryngitis, with polypoid change. (Color photograph on page xiii by Eiji Yanagisawa, M.D.)

Takahashi and Koike (1985) reported a mean fundamental frequency level of 103 Hz for one of their female patients with chronic laryngitis, and 284 Hz for the other. Thus, it appears that fundamental frequency may be either elevated or reduced. This may be related to the severity of the chordal involvement. One would also expect that phonational range would be reduced (Shipp and Huntington, 1965). Maximum sustainable intensities may be much lower than normal. Finally, there should be greater than normal spectral noise in the voice.

Physiological Signs

When laryngitis is present, airflow and air pressures may be elevated, especially if there is incomplete glottal closure. However, average airflows appear to be within normal limits (see Table 3.4 in Hirano, 1981b). Based on our experience, vibratory airflows show increased variability from one cycle to the next, and there may be greater than normal offset and peak airflows. Woo et al. (1987) reported a mean flow rate of 222 ml/sec for their combined acute, chronic, and radiation laryngitis group, collapsed across 7 male and 11 female subjects. In their study, normal speakers produced a mean flow rate of 144 ml/sec. The electroglottographic signal may show marked variability from one cycle to the next, although closure times may be normal. Electromyographic levels would be expected to be normal or slightly elevated.

Laryngoscopic Signs

Laryngitic larynges show a marked redness, and small, dilated blood vessels may be visible on the inflamed folds.

Stroboscopic Signs

The vocal folds may show greater asymmetry and aperiodicity, with reduced mucosal waves and incomplete vibratory closure, if there is a posterior chink. The propagation of the mucosal wave is diminished. We have noted a jerk-like movement of the mucosal wave, in which the wave appears to travel along part of the surface at one speed, then changes its speed for the remainder of its travel. The movement may also be called biphasic (Woo, personal communication, 1988).

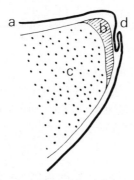

Figure 4.7.   Schematic of a coronal cross-section of the vocal fold with a sulcus vocalis. *a*, the mucosal cover; *b*, the vocal ligament; *c*, muscle; *d*, sulcus entrance. (From Bouchayer, Cornut, Witzig, Loire, Roch, and Bastian, 1985.)

Pathophysiology

Laryngitis affects the cover of the vocal folds by increasing its stiffness, with little effect on the mass of the vocal folds.

Other Comments

Chronic laryngitis, if allowed to continue untreated, may result in serious complications, including laryngitis sicca, which is characterized by marked atrophy of the mucosa of the larynx. The major abnormality is the lack of vocal fold lubrication due to the reduction or absence of glandular secretions. The vocal folds will become dry and sticky, and a chronic cough may be present as the system attempts to remove the thick secretions on the vocal folds. On occasion, laryngeal crusting may result, requiring surgical removal.

Other forms of laryngitis include diptheria, tuberculous, and syphilitic, all of which are extremely rare. Another special form of laryngitis is acute epiglottitis, in which the inflammatory changes affect the mucosa of the epiglottis. Epiglottitis may be life threatening if the epiglottis becomes sufficiently enlarged to result in airway obstruction. Emergency treatment may be required. Antibotics may be used to control the infection or steroids may be used to reduce the inflammation (Sataloff, 1987a).

Sulcus Vocalis

Primary Voice Symptom

The primary voice symptom is hoarseness.

Description and Etiology

Sulcus vocalis refers to a condition in which a furrow along the upper medial edge of the vocal folds is observed. Bastian (1986) describes it as an "epithelial-lined furrow or pocket whose lips parallel the free edge of the cords" (p. 1974). In a cross-section of the vocal folds, the furrow appears as a pocketed ledge on the medial surface of the vocal folds (Fig. 4.7). The longitudinal extent of the furrow is variable, as is its depth. If very deep, it seems to divide the cord in half. According to Arnold (1980), sulcus vocalis may be associated with other laryngeal or oral asymmetries.

The etiology of sulcus vocalis is uncertain, although Bastian (1986) attributes it to vocal misuse and abuse. Luchsinger and Arnold (1965) in their review of the literature summarized the possible etiological factors as being congenital, developmental, or traumatic. Bouchayer et al. (1985) argued for a congenital etiology. The disorder is rather rare, at least in Europe and the United States (Luchsinger and Arnold, 1965); it may be more prevalent in Japan (Hirano, 1981b).

Perceptual Signs and Symptoms

Symptoms include a breathy, hoarse voice quality that apparently is due to incomplete closure of the vocal folds. The pitch of the voice may be lower than normal, and the patient may have reduced loudness.

Acoustic Signs

Phonational and intensity ranges would be expected to be reduced, although there are no data available to support this expectation. There may be elevated levels of spectral noise in the voice. We might also find greater than normal frequency and amplitude perturbation, although of small magnitude.

Physiological Signs

Airflows may be slightly elevated (Shigemori, 1977). We would expect vibratory flows to show greater than normal perturbation and slightly greater than normal airflow leakage (offset flow). Electroglottographic recordings should show increased perturbation with the possibility of short closed times.

Laryngoscopic Signs

Laryngoscopically, a sulcus will be seen as a depression or line along the upper medial edge of the vocal fold. The depression may extend the entire length of the vocal fold and may vary in depth from shallow to very deep.

Stroboscopic Signs

We have found diminished amplitudes of vocal fold movement with little continuity of the mucosal wave across the sulcus. A mucosal wave can usually be seen across the uninvolved superior surface of the vocal fold.

Pathophysiology

The sulcus is located in the superficial layer of the lamina propria, which decreases the mass of the cover but may increase its stiffness. The body and the transition layers are normal.

Contact Ulcer

Primary Voice Symptom

The primary voice symptom is hoarseness.

Description and Etiology

A contact ulcer is a small ulceration that develops on the medial surface of the vocal processes of the arytenoid cartilages. The ulceration may be unilateral or bilateral and may present a "cup and saucer" appearance, with a protuberance on one cord and a crater or concavity on the other. Continued irritation in the presence of bacteria results in an ulceration on one side and the production of granulation tissue on the other.

Although many have reported that contact ulcers are the result of vocal abuse, there is uncertainty about this. The condition is relatively uncommon. The traditional view has been that contact ulcers occur predominantly in adult males with an average age of 50 years (Peacher, 1947) who engage in a great deal of forceful, aggressive speaking. However, there has been a paucity of experimental data to support this hypothesis, and even less to document the efficacy of a voice therapy approach. Contact ulcers have been removed surgically but have shown a propensity to recur following such treatment.

Von Leden and Moore (1960) described some of the anatomical and physiological variations of phonation that may contribute to the formation of a contact ulcer. They pointed out that at low pitches the arytenoids oscillate vigorously, in a rocking-type motion. Thus, at low pitches it is more likely that the arytenoids would be subjected to greater trauma. They also observed that at low pitches there is greater vocal fold approximation, the approximation is prolonged, and it tends to persist beyond the vibratory phase of the vocal folds. Greater loudness will also increase the degree of approximation as well as its duration. Harsh, gutteral sounds will increase the force of approximation of the vocal folds, as will other nonphonatory acts (throat clearing, etc.).

In a study relating gastric reflux to contact ulcer, Cherry and Margulies (1968) studied three patients who showed evidence of peptic ulcer. All were treated with antacids, reduced food intake at night, the elevation of the head during sleep, and all experienced resolution of the ulcer. Delahunty and Cherry (1968) demonstrated that continued exposure of the arytenoid vocal processes to stomach acids would create ulcers and granulation tissue in dogs in about a month's time. Histologically, these lesions exhibited epithelial necrosis with an organized fibrous exudate beneath. Submucosal edema and nonspecific inflammation were also described. In a control condition, saliva was applied to the arytenoids over the same time period, with no development of granulation tissue. It is apparent that a proportion of contact ulcers are produced by gastric reflux emanating from the stomach and irritating the vocal folds. Ward, Zwitman, Hanson, and Berci (1980) reported that contact ulcers result from constant throat clearing that is secondary to irritation of the mucosa due to gastroesophageal reflux (regurgitation of peptic acids at night), and with less frequency to irritation from nasal secretions (postnasal drip). They further reported that of 28 cases, only 2 failed to respond to medical treatment. Feder and Michell (1984) divided ulcers into two groups, hyperfunctional and hyperacidic. Watterson, Hensen-Magorian, and McFarlane (1988) reported that 51% of their patients with a contact ulcer also exhibited a hiatal hernia. Thus, it would appear that the etiology of contact ulcers is at least twofold: (a) hyperfunctional vocal abuse and (b) reflux, or bathing of the arytenoids by stomach secretions or secretions from the nose (Ward et al., 1980).

Benjamin and Croxson (1985) reported clinical and histological similarities between contact ulcers and granulomas. They studied 16 patients, of whom 7 had postintubation granulomas and the remainder contact ulcers. The most common symptom of all patients was hoarseness. They concluded that contact ulcer was not a precursor to granulomas since the history of the problems was different and the patient with a granuloma did not present the profile of a patient with a contact ulcer.

Perceptual Signs and Symptoms

The primary perceptual symptoms of a contact ulcer are constant throat clearing and vocal fatigue. There may be a breathy voice with some hoarseness, accompanied by discomfort or even severe, stabbing pain. The pain is usually unilateral and located in the area of the greater horn of the thyroid. The pain may radiate to the ear. There is usually the constant feeling of something in the throat, which accounts for the continual throat clearing.

Acoustic Signs

Depending on the severity of the voice symptoms, some increased frequency perturbation and spectral noise may be present in the voice.

Physiological Signs

Isshiki and von Leden (1964) reported a mean flow of 144 ml/sec for their group of patients with contact ulcers. This value is not much higher than would be expected in normal speakers. Increased air pressures might be expected due to the tendency to use higher than normal forces when speaking. Muscle activity levels should be within normal limits.

Laryngoscopic Signs

Laryngoscopically, a contact ulcer will be visible as a buildup of pink or pinkish-white tissue on one of the vocal processes of the arytenoids. This usually occurs at the tip of the process, but it is possible to find such an outgrowth elsewhere on the vocal process or on the lower base of the arytenoid. On the contralateral process, there may be injection of the mucosa or a depression. This has been described as the "cup and saucer" appearance because the two processes fit together in that way. Slight pinkness may be seen in the area of the arytenoids. In the early stages of contact ulcer development, even prior to tissue outgrowth, a strand of mucus may be seen between the two processes. This is referred to as a contact ulcer diathesis.

Stroboscopic Signs

Unless there are abnormal voice symptoms, normal stroboscopic features would be anticipated.

Pathophysiology

Since the contact ulcer does not involve the membranous vocal fold, there will be little change in the mass or stiffness of the cover, transition layers, or body.

Summary

Misuse and abuse of the voice have been defined, and the specific ways in which they occur have been discussed. The goal of this chapter is to sensitize the practitioner to the many forms that misuse and abuse of the phonatory mechanism may take. The primary misuses of the voice include hard glottal attack, elevated laryngeal posture, anteroposterior squeezing, and inappropriate pitch level. Abusive behaviors include excessive coughing and throat clearing, yelling, shouting, cheerleading, and prolonged loud talking. Abusive behaviors result in mechanical trauma to the vocal folds or vocal processes. Continued trauma may result in tissue change that will alter the vibratory characteristics of the vocal folds, which in turn results in hoarseness or roughness in the voice. In some cases, the tissue alteration will prevent complete glottal closure and result in the production of breathy phonation. An understanding of these behaviors will allow the clinician to help patients make a thorough inventory of their own behaviors.

The goal of this chapter's section on drugs is to increase awareness of the potential phonatory effect of a vast array of pharmaceuticals, many of which are frequently considered to be quite benign, especially if they are of the over-the-counter variety. There are certainly many overriding reasons why drugs must be used in the treatment of various conditions, even if some degree of voice change may occur. However, the practitioner

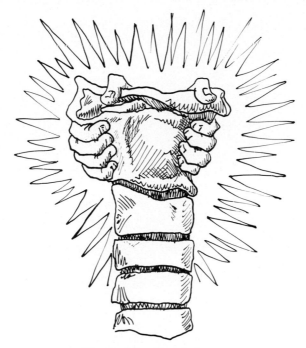

Figure 4.8.   Vocal abuse.

who works with the voice patient must be aware of the different drugs' possible effects on voice and/or on mucosal tissues. This can be critical for the professional voice user.

In the last section, a variety of specific tissue changes associated with vocal misuse and abuse have been reviewed, including vocal nodules, polyps, cysts, edema, laryngitis, sulcus vocalis, contact ulcer, keratosis, and granulomas. Although some of these conditions may be caused by infection, viral agents, external trauma, or disease, the primary etiology is most often considered to be vocal abuse. Recognition of the contribution of abusive behaviors to these conditions is necessary in order to arrive at a treatment protocol that will be effective in reducing and/or eliminating these vocal problems, with the least trauma and expense to the patient (Fig. 4.8).

5

Voice Problems Associated with Nervous System Involvement

Role of the Nervous System

The nervous system is that portion of the body concerned with the control of other body functions. Viewed as a unit, it is responsible for the total control of all systems in the body, even self-regulating systems that are capable of carrying out their own functions. The smaller units of the body's organizational system (cells, tissues, and organs) function only within their own little world and in an environment that must be controlled. It is the responsibility of the nervous system to create this environment by regulating systems that provide for the proper nourishment, temperature regulation, gas exchange, and by-product disposal necessary for all the component parts to work effectively.

Coordination of function is another aspect of the control exerted by the nervous system. One system must work at the proper time if another system is to function properly. Within a system, the various parts must perform their tasks at the proper times for the final output of the system to be meaningful and productive. The necessity for coordination is even more apparent in the production of skilled motor acts involving the various striated muscles of the body. Simple walking is an example of a highly skilled motor act involving the proper contraction and relaxation of different muscles for its action.

The nervous system is divided into two major parts: the central nervous system and the peripheral nervous system. The central nervous system (CNS) is that portion residing within the cranial cavity or skull. The peripheral nervous system (PNS) resides throughout the body outside of the cranium. The central nervous system is responsible for the initiation and coordination of function, whereas the peripheral nervous system carries the instructions of the central nervous system to the various organs and muscles of the body.

The nervous system may also be divided into two components, according to whether information is conducted to the central nervous system (afferent) or from the central nervous system (efferent). Indeed, information from muscles, organs, and tissues is needed by the central nervous system for proper control to be maintained. Information from the outside world via the several senses is also used by the central nervous system to make it possible for the body to exist in the hostile world. Without the nervous system, the body cannot live, much less function effectively in its environment.

General Characteristics of Nervous System Dysfunction

The nervous system may malfunction due to disease, abnormal growths, accidents, or trauma. The nature of the malfunction will depend on where the problem occurs. In some cases there will be difficulty in initiating an action or activity, while in others the activity will begin without difficulty but control of it may be impaired. In still other cases, incoming information will be distorted or nonexistent, so that the nervous system will not have the proper information for the control of motor or organ activity appropriate for the task at hand.

The central nervous system is responsible for initiating skilled motor acts that involve the starting and stopping of motor activity. Walking is a good example of an activity that must be initiated and terminated. Most internal body functions are ongoing; that is, once started, they continue or else the body will to cease to function (e.g., blood flow, respiration, temperature regulation). Other internal body functions are episodic and may be stopped and started (e.g., digestion, hormone production). Speech itself is a very good example of an act that is constantly started and stopped even during its execution. There are centers and cells within the central nervous system that have this function of starting an act. If damaged, the initiation of the act will never take place.

As mentioned previously, the central nervous system effects coordination of function. There are many examples of the need for coordination of body systems, the act of walking being just one. Speech is also a highly coordinated event involving coordination within bodily systems (e.g., phonation, respiration, articulation) and among these systems. Damage to the central nervous system may affect this form of control.

Lower brain centers, including the spinal cord, maintain a measure of control, albeit local, on muscles and systems. For example, muscles must be maintained in a state of readiness for action. This is manifested by the steady level of electrical activity in muscles even when they are not being used for a motor act. This state of readiness is maintained by these lower neuron systems. However, the central nervous system exerts its involvement through inhibition of the activity of these lower centers, so that they do not get out of control. Damage to the central nervous system can result in the disruption of this inhibition and the production of unnecessary or unwanted movements.

Finally, incoming sensory information is critical for the control process. The central nervous system must know when the right foot has touched the floor in order to command the left leg to rise and move the left foot forward. The central nervous system relies on visual information in order to properly control the hand and arm in reaching for the glass of water on the kitchen table. Deprived of sensory information, the organism will not know about the environment and its potential effects. Incoming sensory information need not be entirely external. Internal sensory information is also critical for neural control. Kinesthetic feedback from joints and muscles must be available if skilled movements are to be possible. The job of the central nervous system is to receive and integrate information and prepare a proper plan for dealing with it.

Role of the Nervous System in Phonation and Speech

Speech is a complex, fine motor act that involves several diverse systems or parts of systems for its execution. The respiratory system, basically designed for the exchange of gases for use by the tissues of the body, is also used for speech, with contributions from the digestive system, primarily the mouth, jaw, and teeth. Speech requires the use of the respiratory system mechanically, that is, for the generation and control of the airflows and pressures needed for speaking. Thus, the control of the respiratory system for life support and the control of the respiratory system for speaking are quite different. The nervous system must provide the control appropriate to the task at hand. Furthermore, during speech, there must be a high level of coordination among the chest wall/abdomen mechanical system, the larynx and pharynx, and the lips, tongue, teeth, and mandible so that all function at the correct time and for the length of time necessary for the production of the individual sounds. During the act of speaking, the system receives information about the state of its structures and muscles via both kinesthetic and acoustic feedback. Thus, the auditory system is yet another important system that must enter into the control exercised by the nervous system.

Disease, malformation, or injury will affect the control capabilities of the nervous system. The manifestation of nervous system damage will vary depending on where the lesion occurs. If the lesion occurs at the cortex, many components of speech may be affected, including the ability to use language, to initiate speech, to produce muscle movements necessary to produce intelligible speech or control muscle movements, or to receive information from the body systems about where they are and what they have done. The symptoms and signs that the patient presents are critical to the proper diagnosis of the problem and identification of the source of the problem.

In this book, we are interested in the effects of nervous system damage on the control of phonation. Although the system remains complex, there is a finite set of brain sites and pathways that have been shown to be important for the control of phonation. Lesions will produce specific symptoms that will help the diagnostician identify the site of lesion. Some of the possible problems affecting phonation and their possible locations in the nervous system are discussed by Barlow, Netsell, and Hunker (1986). They note that in the lateral precentral cortex, there appears to be a convergence of pathways from other parts of the brain that may be the site of the final common pathway through the brain to the periphery. Lesions at this site would be expected to result in complete loss of phonation because input from the higher control centers will have been lost. Furthermore, lesions in this area and other adjacent areas would also be expected to produce loss of function in other muscles concerned with speech. Consequently, such lesions will be expected to produce aphonia or dysphonia, dysarthria, and perhaps even aphasia. Lesions in the anterior cingulate cortex are also reported to produce akinetic mutism in humans (Barlow et al., 1986). In monkeys this area seems to be critical for the control of conditional, learned vocalization. Lesions in other areas of the brain (e.g., basal ganglia, periaqueductal gray) produce a disruption in phonation characterized by breathiness, roughness, tremor, or complete disruption of vocalization. Lesions in the cerebellum result in ataxic dysarthria and changes in the velocity of lip and jaw movements and would presumably affect the speed of movements of structures in the larynx. Larson, Sutton, and Lindeman (1978) concluded that the cerebellum is very important in the control of pitch and loudness of phonation but is not required for the initiation of phonation.

An effective and convenient organizational scheme for the consideration of the neurological problems that affect phonation would recognize the levels of organization within the nervous system, as discussed above. The following is such a scheme, proposed by Ward, Hanson, and Berci (1981). It is both simple and effective as an aid in understanding how a specific lesion or syndrome may affect phonation.

1. Afferent sensory, autonomic
2. Efferent motor
    Upper motor neuron (cortex and pyramidal tracts)
    Extrapyramidal (reticular substance)
    Cerebellar
    Nuclear (lower motor neurons)

We have adopted this scheme, with slight modifications, as the organizational framework for consideration of neurological problems that affect voice. It is most effective in emphasizing the role of a specific area of the nervous system in the control of phonation and in the ultimate determination of the pathophysiology of a voice problem.

Organization of the Nervous System and Voice Pathology

The following section is a brief review of the major systems involved in phonation. More complete information about the nervous system can be found in Chapter 12. Ward et al. (1981) discuss the role of the afferent or sensory system in the control of phonation. Our discussion here will concentrate on the efferent or motor system involved in the control of phonation (Fig. 5.1).

In the cortex, area 4 of the precentral gyrus is very important in the control of vocalization. Neurons from this and other areas of the cortex converge to form the corticobulbar tracts. These tracts pass through the internal capsule and cerebral peduncle and eventually comprise what is known as the pyramidal tracts. At the upper part of the medulla, many fibers cross over (decussate) to the opposite side and continue down to the nucleus ambiguus in the brainstem. As discussed in Chapter 12, the nucleus ambiguus houses the motor nuclei for the 9th, 10th, and 11th cranial nerves. Thus, lesions anywhere along this pathway may involve the precentral cortex, the corticobulbar tracts, the internal capsule or the cerebral peduncles, the medulla, the brainstem, or the nucleus ambiguus itself, causing differential effects on phonation.

The extrapyramidal system consists of the reticular substance, corpus striatum (with the caudate and lenticular nuclei), and the basal ganglia (specifically the globus pallidus and the substantia nigra) (Ward et al., 1981). Lesions here will affect the coordination of laryngeal function. Athetoid movements are characteristic of patients with lesions in these areas. Degeneration of the basal ganglia and the reticular substance produce the symptoms typical of parkinsonism (see ''Parkinsonism,'' below, for a more complete discussion of this disease). The Shy-Drager syndrome, in which there is progressive abductor paralysis of the larynx, is thought to be a disease affecting the extrapyramidal system, as well as the motor nuclei of the vagus (see ''Shy-Drager Syndrome,'' below, for a more complete discussion of this disease).

Lesions in the cerebellum affect the coordination of motor function and result in slurred speech and problems with coordination of the various speech systems, as well as nonspeech symptoms, such as ataxia, nystagmus, and gait problems. The voice may exhibit a breathy quality, or it may exhibit spastic behavior. In the Arnold-Chiari syndrome,

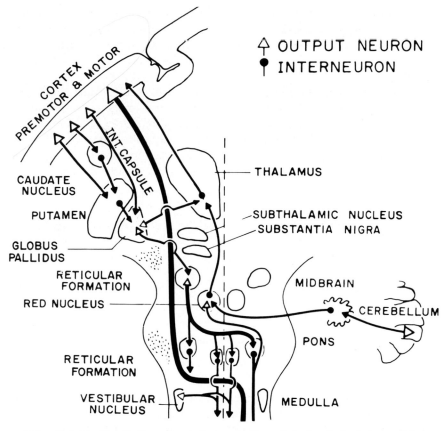

Figure 5.1. Schematic of the direct (pyramidal) and indirect (extrapyramidal) motor pathways. The direct reaches the neurons in the spinal cord without an intervening synapse (shown by heavy black line). The indirect has many synapses on its way to the lower motor neurons, with stops in the basal ganglia and reticular formation. Not shown are collaterals from the pyramidal system to the tegmentum of the pons and the midbrain, where they can interact with the extrapyramidal system. (From Darley, Aronson, and Brown, 1975.)

for example, the vocal folds may typically demonstrate involuntary abduction (see "Arnold-Chiari Malformation," below, for a more complete discussion).

Lower motor neuron problems occur in the brainstem and medulla. There are many syndromes that result from lesions in the medulla and in which voice will be affected, as will the functioning of the palate, pharynx, tongue, face, and other body parts. Lesions in the nucleus ambiguus may produce classic symptoms of a combined paralysis of the superior and recurrent laryngeal nerves, resulting in flaccid vocal folds. Such lesions, depending on their extent, may also affect the palate and pharynx.

Finally, there can be an interruption of control in the peripheral nerves supplying the larynx itself. Such disturbance can result from lesions or injury to the superior laryngeal nerve or the recurrent laryngeal nerve or both. Furthermore, the lesions may be either unilateral or bilateral. Again, the specific symptoms presented by the patient will help to determine the proper diagnosis and locus of the problem.

There are voice problems in which neurological involvement is suspected but cannot be determined with certainty. Some of these problems may involve diffuse areas of the brain, and no specific single site of lesion can be determined. In other instances, the etiology is unknown or described as idiopathic in nature. However, unknown or idiopathic is a nondiagnosis. It should signify a temporary condition during which further data are gathered in the search for the diagnosis. A more precise diagnosis may result from additional testing, but occasionally the simple passage of time reveals additional symptoms that help to refine the diagnosis; in some cases, a more specific diagnosis may remain undetermined or unknown.

In the following discussion about specific neurological problems that affect the voice, a primary vocal symptom will be stated. In most cases, this refers to the most frequently reported symptom for that disease, as reported by Aronson, Brown, Litin, and Pearson (1968a). In some cases, other studies were used to identify the primary vocal symptom. There will usually be additional voice symptoms associated with each neurological problem. These will be discussed for each disease in the section entitled ''Perceptual Voice Signs and Symptoms.''

Upper Motor Neuron Disorders (Cortical and Pyramidal)

Supra- or Pseudobulbar Palsy

Primary Voice Symptom

The primary voice symptom is hoarseness/harshness.

Description and Etiology

Two major pathway systems converge on the lower motor neurons for control of muscles that affect voice and speech. These are the pyramidal and extrapyramidal tracts. Selected damage to the extrapyramidal or indirect pathway usually results in spasticity and increased muscle reflexes. Selected damage to the direct or pyramidal pathway results in a loss of function, especially for skilled movements. The pyramidal system is said to be the newer system, phylogenetically. Lesions in these pathways would affect voluntary movement in four ways: spasticity, weakness, limitation of range, and a slowing of movement. The disease known as pseudobulbar palsy results when lesions affect these two systems.

Pseudobulbar palsy is actually a misnomer. The symptoms of the problem are in some instances very similar to those of bulbar disease (muscle weakness), and yet the evidence for bulbar lesions is equivocal. Langworthy and Hesser (1940) recommended the term ''supranuclear bulbar paralysis.'' Aring (1965) agreed, believing that the term had an anatomical basis, locating the lesions rostral to the appropriate cranial motor nerve nuclei. However, the term ''pseudobulbar palsy'' has remained in use.

Pseudobulbar palsy results from progressive lesions that occur bilaterally in the corticobulbar tracts. These lesions occur most frequently in the internal capsules (Langworthy and Hesser, 1940; Aring, 1965), although there may be pontine or midbrain lesions. These lesions are usually the result of a stroke, although other reported causes have been cerebral palsy, brain injuries, multiple sclerosis, and arteriosclerosis (Langworthy and Hesser, 1940; Darley, Aronson, and Brown, 1975). The chief symptoms are difficulties with speech and swallowing, plus emotional lability. The latter presents a unique feature of this problem. Patients may show bursts of laughter or crying in the presence of very mild stimuli or no stimuli at all. It is as if the patient's higher centers have released their control of these responses, and they appear uncontrolled. Kreindler and Pruskauer-Apostol (1971) documented these unusual behaviors, and Aronson (1985) emphasized that reduced thresholds for crying and laughter are critical cues in the diagnosis of this disorder.

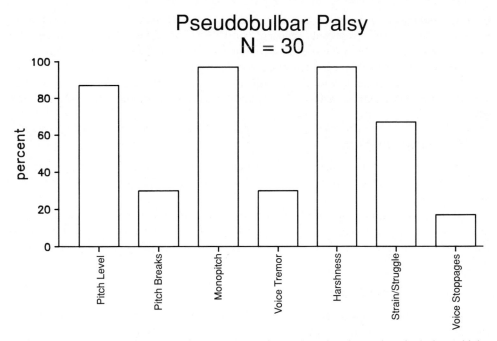

Figure 5.2. Percent of patients with pseudobulbar palsy showing voice deviations. Voice tremor was rated during contextual speech. (Drawn from data of Aronson, Brown, Litin, and Pearson, 1968b.)

Perceptual Voice Signs and Symptoms

A major sign of pseudobulbar palsy is the dysarthria of speech, as documented by Darley et al. (1969a, 1969b, 1975). They grouped perceptual signs into clusters of the dysarthric symptoms that best characterize a particular type of neurological dysfunction. The important perceptual signs in pseudobulbar palsy are reported to be (using Darley, Aronson, and Brown's terminology) (*a*) prosodic excess (relates to rate and stress characteristics of speech), (*b*) prosodic insufficiency (monopitch, monoloudness, reduced stress, short phrases), (*c*) articulatory-resonatory incompetence (imprecise consonants, distorted vowels, hypernasality), and (*d*) phonatory stenosis (harsh voice, strain/struggle, pitch breaks).

Aronson et al. (1968b) rated the voice characteristics of 30 patients with pseudobulbar palsy (same as Darley et al., 1969a, 1969b) and found that 97% of the patients were considered to have monopitch and harsh voices, 87% had a too-low pitch level, 67% demonstrated considerable strain and struggle in phonation, and 30% exhibited pitch breaks and voice tremor. (These voice signs of pseudobulbar palsy are shown in Fig. 5.2.) Aring (1965) commented that the speech of a patient with pseudobulbar palsy is nasal, monotonic, and of soft intensity and rapid rate, making it difficult to understand.

Acoustic Signs

There have been few data reported on the acoustic characteristics of patients with pseudobulbar palsy, other than a study by Kammermeier (1969), who reported a mean fundamental frequency of 124.1 Hz in male subjects with a mean age of 61.7 years. When compared to the mean fundamental frequency (F_o) values reported for normal adult male speakers by Mysak (1959; mean F_o 124.3 Hz, mean age 73.3 years) and Hollien and Shipp (1972; mean F_o 112 Hz, mean age 64.6 years), the pseudobulbar subjects are seen to produce fundamental frequencies that are equal to or slightly higher than normal speakers. Kammermeier (1969) reported reduced variability of fundamental frequency in pseudobulbar patients, as well as reduced intensity variation. These findings may be related to the perception of monopitch and monoloudness.

It appears that patients with pseudobulbar palsy exhibit normal or near-normal average fundamental frequency, reduced fundamental frequency variation, and reduced intensity variation.

Physiological Signs

We know of no data on the physiological characteristics of the speech of patients with pseudobulbar palsy. Higher than normal subglottal pressures might be expected because of the hypertonicity and strain/struggle characteristics of the voice. If breathy, the patient would probably exhibit greater than normal airflows. If the range and force of movement of the vocal folds are affected, this might be reflected in slow opening and closing times of the vocal folds and perhaps a short closed phase due to the inability to maintain sufficient muscle forces.

Laryngoscopic Signs

According to Darley et al. (1975), no laryngeal abnormalities have been reported. However, it is possible that vocal fold hyperadduction as well as hypofunction of other laryngeal structures might be observable, utilizing the improved instruments available today for laryngoscopic examination. Further study of these characteristics is needed.

Stroboscopic Signs

Again, there appear to be no reports on stroboscopic signs in patients with pseudobulbar palsy. When vocal fold hypertonicity is present, typical findings, according to Kitzing (1985), would include reduced vocal fold amplitudes, diminished mucosal waves, and excessive glottal closure. However, if the muscles have reduced force and movement, glottal closure may not be complete, and there may be asymmetry and aperiodicity of vocal fold movement.

Pathophysiology

Pseudobulbar palsy results in a loss of muscle coordination and a release of inhibition of the lower centers. The latter condition results in hyperactivity of the muscle reflexes and spasticity. In speech, pseudobulbar palsy patients will show a reduction in the force and range of the muscle movement (Darley et al., 1969a). In addition, the release of the lower motor centers results in hypertonicity of the vocal folds. Pseudobulbar palsy seems to be a condition in which both muscle weakness and muscle hyperactivity coexist, with differential effects on the motor act being performed. Hypertonicity would be consistent with the perception of harshness in the voice, as well as the strain and struggle to speak. It is not necessarily consistent with the perception of a low pitch level or the findings that the fundamental frequency of these patients is within the normal range. These findings might be understood by hypothesizing that the cricothyroid is minimally affected in pseudobulbar palsy but that the other adductors or abductors of the larynx are affected differentially. Breathiness (noted in 14 out of 30 patients with pseudobulbar palsy studied by Darley et al., 1969a) would be produced by excessive opening of the vocal folds or perhaps by hypertonicity of the abductor muscle of the larynx (posterior cricothyroid). Hyperactivity in the adductors would have an effect similar to hypertonicity and would be consistent with strain/struggle quality, as well as excessive hoarseness/harshness. The specific voice signs (perceptual, acoustic, or physiological) noted in a patient with pseudobulbar palsy may reflect lesions at different locations along the long pathway from the brain to the ultimate motor neurons controlling the muscles of the larynx.

Extrapyramidal Disorders

Parkinsonism

Primary Voice Symptom

The primary voice symptom is monopitch.

Description and Etiology

Parkinsonism is a central nervous system disease that results in rigidity, tremor, and reduced range of movement in the limbs, neck, and head. The general characteristic of parkinsonism is a slowness of movement or hypokinesia. All movements may be affected. Facial appearance is sometimes mask-like, with a flat, unemotional appearance. It is important to realize that the muscles are not paralyzed but rather lack the dynamic aspects of movement.

Parkinsonism is a disease of the basal ganglia, specifically the substantia nigra. Some cases of parkinsonism have been traced to an influenza epidemic in the early decades of this century. Other causes include some kind of slow-growing virus, head trauma, toxic buildup, or carbon monoxide poisoning (Darley et al., 1975).

Perceptual Voice Signs and Symptoms

The most frequently rated voice dimensions, as reported by Aronson et al. (1968) (Fig. 5.3), were monopitch, excessively low pitch, and harshness. According to Darley et al. (1969b), variability of loudness is reduced, but rate of speech is highly variable, sometimes with fast bursts and at other times a slow rate. Speech production is also affected by slurring and phoneme misarticulations.

In a study of 200 patients with Parkinson's disease, Logemann, Fisher, Boches, and Blonsky (1978) found that 87% showed some laryngeal dysfunction and that 45% had laryngeal dysfunction as the only symptom. The specific voice signs these authors reported were breathiness (15%), roughness (29%), hoarseness (45%), and tremulousness (13.5%).

Acoustic Signs

Canter (1963) reported a rather extensive study on the acoustic characteristics of intensity, pitch, and duration of patients with Parkinson's disease. He found no differences between a group of 11 Parkinson's patients and 17 control subjects on average intensity in a reading passage. Furthermore, the range of SPLs in the passage for the two groups was very similar. Parkinson's patients were found to have a higher mean fundamental frequency (129 Hz) as compared to the control group (106 Hz), and frequency variability in the Parkinson's group was found to be much less than for the control group (0.5 octave versus 0.86 octave). There were no differences between the two groups on vowel duration, number of pauses, mean pause length, mean phrase length, or mean syllable length. There was a tendency for the ranges of these measures to be higher in the parkinsonism patients.

There is a discrepancy between the Aronson et al. (1968a) study and the Canter (1963) study with respect to pitch and fundamental frequency. Aronson et al. reported a very low pitch level, but Canter reported a higher than normal fundamental frequency

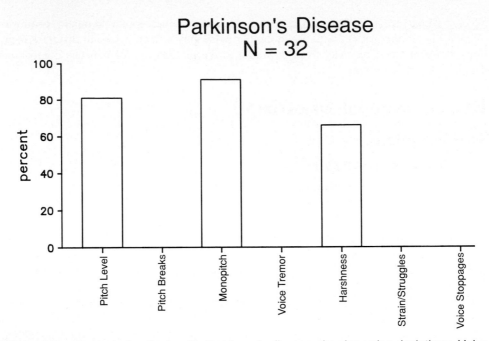

Figure 5.3. Percent of patients with Parkinson's disease showing voice deviations. Voice tremor was rated during contextual speech. (Drawn from data of Aronson, Brown, Litin, & Pearson, 1968b.)

level. Pitch and fundamental frequency are not synonymous, although they are related. During speech, judgments of pitch can be influenced by other characteristics of the signal, including degrees of roughness and breathiness. Apparently, in patients with Parkinson's disease the pitch of the voice is perceived to be very low, although the actual fundamental frequency is slightly higher than normal.

In a later study, Canter (1965) measured minimum and maximum intensity levels, pitch range, and maximum phonation time in 17 parkinsonism patients. The patients showed a higher SPL at their minimum intensity level ("quiet") and a lower maximum intensity level ("shouted") than the control group. The parkinsonism patients had a higher low fundamental frequency (100 Hz versus 80 Hz for controls) and a lowered maximum fundamental frequency level (200 Hz versus 260 Hz for controls). Finally, the parkinsonism patients had a much shorter maximum phonation time (9.5 seconds) compared to the control subjects (20.6 seconds). Thus, all ranges of function were reduced.

Logemann et al. (1978) reported that of all symptoms affecting the speech of Parkinson's patients, voice symptoms were reported most frequently, with articulation errors being the next most often cited symptom. Consonants (stops, fricatives, and affricatives) are most often affected by errors in place and manner. The severity of the disease appeared to be related to the speech errors exhibited. Although a severity-to-voice-symptom relationship might be expected to be present, data are not available to document it.

Physiological Signs

Patients with parkinsonism appear to produce higher resting and background activity in the interarytenoid and posterior cricoarytenoid muscles (Guidi, Bannister, Gibson, and Payne, 1981). Lip muscles also show greater resting and background activity levels, and the degree of activity seems to be related to the side of the body most affected by the disease (Leanderson, Meyerson, and Persson, 1972).

Laryngoscopic Signs

Cisler (1927) reported diminshed vocal fold movement, and Schilling (1925) described a rigor of the vocal folds. Darley et al. (1969a) reported no abnormal laryngoscopic signs.

The most extensive description of laryngoscopic signs in parkinsonism patients was reported by Hanson, Gerratt, and Ward (1984). They studied 32 patients, of whom 30 had abnormal laryngoscopic signs. The most prominent sign was bowed vocal folds, and the vocal folds appeared to vibrate with greater amplitude. In 26 patients, varying degrees of laryngeal asymmetry were observed. Many patients showed a characteristic pattern consisting of a more posterior position of the vocal process, a more posterior and lateral position of the apex of the arytenoid, and a more contracted ventricular fold than seen in normal speakers. These signs were associated with the side of the body affected by the disease.

Many patients also showed overclosure of the vocal folds, and 5 of the 32 exhibited an extreme degree of supraglottal constriction. In these cases, the ventricular folds seemed to squeeze the midportion of the vocal folds.

Stroboscopic Signs

Data on the stroboscopic signs associated with Parkinson's disease are unavailable.

Pathophysiology

Muscle rigidity and squeezing of structures within the larynx may produce a symptom of strain/struggle in the voice. Unequal tensions in the vocal folds, as noted by Hanson et al. (1984), would be expected to produce greater aperiodicity in the voice, resulting in greater hoarseness or roughness in the voice. Some patients have been reported to have associated voice tremor (although Aronson et al. [1968b] did not report any perceptual signs of tremor in their parkinsonism patients).

Shy-Drager Syndrome

Primary Voice Symptom

The primary voice symptom is hoarseness.

Description and Etiology

Shy-Drager syndrome is a progressive disease of the central nervous system that affects the autonomic and the motor nervous systems. It is a disease of later middle age and affects males more often than females. The initial symptoms are postural hypotension (decrease of blood pressure when the patient stands), impotence, and sphincter problems. In their study of 12 patients with Shy-Drager syndrome, Hanson, Ludlow, and Bassich (1983) reported symptoms of weakness of the accessory muscles of respiration, respiratory obstruction, limited movement of the soft palate, and dysphagia. They suggest that these symptoms are indicative of extrapyramidal, pyramidal, and bulbar involvement.

Shy-Drager syndrome was first described by Shy and Drager (1960), who described two cases. In one case, they were able to examine the brain and reported changes in the spinal cord, autonomic ganglia, and medulla (i.e., marked changes in the inferior olives) and a reduced number of Purkinje cells in the cerebellum, as well as extensive changes in the substantia nigra and the caudate nucleus of the basal ganglia.

Williams, Hanson, and Calne (1979) reported on 12 cases of Shy-Drager syndrome in which 8 had moderate to severe bilateral abductor paresis or paralysis of the vocal folds.

Two patients, upon initial examination, showed a unilateral paresis, but these patients eventually developed bilateral paralysis as the disease progressed. They concluded that the combination of vocal fold paralysis and respiratory difficulties in some of their patients may be consistent with a lesion in the nucleus ambiguus and the retrofacial nucleus.

Linebaugh (1979) reviewed 35 patients with Shy-Drager syndrome who presented with a dysarthria. He identified three major types of dysarthria: ataxic, hypokinetic, and mixed. Fifteen of the 35 presented with ataxic dysarthria, which involves the cerebellum and affects the accuracy, force, range, and timing of speech movements; 11 exhibited a hypokinetic dysarthria in which the extrapyramidal system was affected, resulting in muscular rigidity; and nine showed a mixed dysarthria involving combinations of the extrapyramidal, cerebellar, and pyramidal systems. Linebaugh presented examples of patients with these various types and commented on how careful listening can help to distinguish among them.

Perceptual Voice Signs and Symptoms

The most complete description and study of the speech signs and symptoms of Shy-Drager syndrome was presented by Hanson, Ludlow, and Bassich (1983). They rated the speech of 12 Shy-Drager syndrome patients, using scales reported previously by Darley et al. (1969a). Shy-Drager syndrome patients were rated most severe on scales of rate of speaking (variable rate and rate). The mean ratings on four voice scales are shown in Figure 5.4. The format of this figure is different from that of the first two figures in this chapter. Hanson, Ludlow, and Bassich (1983) did not report the proportion of patients with aberrant ratings on the scales used, probably because of the small number of patients. Rather, the mean ratings were reported using a seven-point scale on which 1 means normal and 7 means very severe. Other speech scales on which these patients were rated severely affected included intensity (this scale may relate to the overall level of voice), imprecise consonants, reduced stress, monopitch, and monoloudness. These authors performed a discriminant analysis of these ratings to determine if they could separate groups of Shy-Drager syndrome patients from parkinsonism patients who exhibit some of the same symptoms and from a group of normal subjects. Three scales did a very good job of distinguishing among these groups and included strain/struggle, glottal fry (a low-pitch, popping sound), and monopitch. Thus, it would appear that perceptual speech scales can be useful in distinguishing Shy-Drager syndrome from parkinsonism and both from normal speakers.

Acoustic Signs

There have been no data reported on the acoustic signs of patients with Shy-Drager syndrome. Acoustic signs similar to those manifested by patients with parkinsonism might be anticipated.

Physiological Signs

In a study of activity in the laryngeal muscles, Guidi et al. (1981) reported that all five of their Shy-Drager patients showed denervation of the posterior cricoarytenoid muscle, and two of the five showed fibrillation potentials in the interarytenoid muscle. These electromyographic characteristics were very different from the muscle activity recorded in patients with parkinsonism.

Laryngoscopic Signs

The primary laryngoscopic sign seen in Shy-Drager syndrome is bilateral abductor vocal fold paresis. Hanson, Ludlow, and Bassich (1983) reported that 11 of their 12 pa-

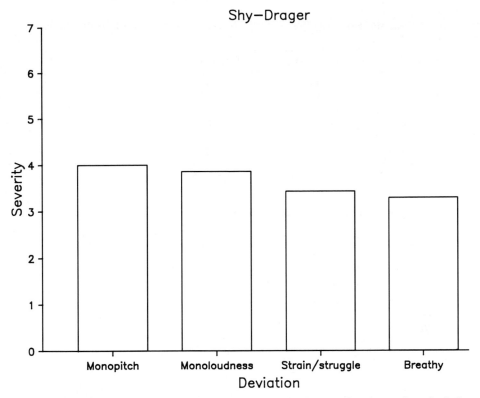

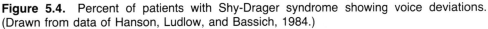

Figure 5.4. Percent of patients with Shy-Drager syndrome showing voice deviations. (Drawn from data of Hanson, Ludlow, and Bassich, 1984.)

tients presented moderate to severe abductor paresis. Longridge (1987) reported a case of Shy-Drager with bilateral vocal fold paralysis but did not specify whether it was of the adductor or abductor type.

Stroboscopic Signs

We know of no studies in which the stroboscopic signs of patients with Shy-Drager syndrome have been reported.

Pathophysiology

Shy-Drager syndrome is a disease involving the pyramidal, extrapyramidal, and cerebellar systems. It affects the control and coordination of speech and voice. Lesions that affect the upper motor neurons will result in the loss of muscle coordination. Lesions in the cerebellum will also affect muscle coordination, whereas lesions in the medulla and brainstem will affect the motor nuclei of the muscles serving the larynx, producing problems of muscle tone and function. Interestingly, the disease affects the neurons that control abductory function and not adductory function. The hyperadduction that results in strain/struggle in speech is produced by lesions higher in the brain. In many respects the disease is similar to parkinsonism, but with its own unique features. The outlook for patients with Shy-Drager syndrome is bleak, with few surviving more than 5 years (Thomas and Schirger, 1970). The course of the disease is a steady increase in neuromuscular impairment that will eventually affect the respiratory muscles and compromise respiratory function.

Table 5.1.
Percent of Patients with ALS Presenting Physical Abnormalities in the Head and Neck Region[a]

Area	Weakness	Fasciculations
Tongue	66	54
Extremities	66	30
Neck	41	10
Face	23	8
Palate and pharynx	23	2
Masseter muscle	8	2

[a]Adapted from Carpenter, McDonald, and Howard, 1978.

Amyotrophic Lateral Sclerosis

Primary Voice Symptom

The primary voice symptom is hoarseness/harshness.

Description and Etiology

Amyotrophic lateral sclerosis (ALS) is a progressive, degenerative disease of the central nervous system that involves both upper and lower motor neurons. As a result, the patient with amyotrophic lateral sclerosis may have symptoms such as spasticity (upper motor neuron symptom) along with muscle weakness (a symptom of lower motor neuron lesions). The lower motor neuron lesions usually affect the ventral horn cells (Janzen, Rae, and Hudson, 1988). The incidence of amyotrophic lateral sclerosis is about 0.4 to 1.8 per 100,000 people (Janzen et al., 1988). The initial manifestation is muscle weakness, cramps, and fasciculation (Carpenter, McDonald, and Howard, 1978). The disease usually affects people later in life.

In the study by Carpenter et al. (1978), 28% of the amyotrophic lateral sclerosis patients presented symptoms in the head, neck, larynx, or voice (123 patients). The mean age of these patients was 61, and the ratio between males and females was about equal. Of the 123 patients, 68% exhibited slurred speech, 14% hoarseness, and 13% dysphagia as the presenting ENT symptom. On physical exam, the patients presented muscle weakness and fasciculation in various areas, as shown in Table 5.1. In many patients, excessive drooling may exist and presents unique problems for management.

Speech symptoms in amyotrophic lateral sclerosis include flaccid dysarthria or spastic dysarthria or both. A more detailed list of speech symptoms in amyotrophic lateral sclerosis is presented in Table 5.2. There are many possible etiologies of this condition. Aronson (1985) listed infection, malignancy, and genetic defects. Janzen et al. (1988) added toxins, autoimmunity problems, and metabolic deficiencies. There is no effective treatment, although certain drugs have been used to ease the symptoms.

Perceptual Voice Signs and Symptoms

The primary symptom is hoarseness/harshness, with slurred speech as an additional symptom. In their classic study of the perceptual characteristicsof dysarthria, Darley et al. (1969b) listed imprecise consonants, hypernasality, harsh voice, slow rate, and monopitch as the prominant speech characteristics in their group of 30 subjects with amyotrophic lateral sclerosis. Figure 5.5 presents a summary of the voice symptoms found in a group of patients with amyotrophic lateral sclerosis patients, as reported by Aronson et al. (1968a).

Table 5.2.
Frequency of Speech Deviations in Patients with ALS[a]

Deviation	Percent
Harsh voice	79.75
Hypernasality	74.68
Breathy voice	64.56
Voice tremor	63.29
Strained/strangled voice	59.49
Imprecise consonants	56.96
Reduced intelligibility	46.84
Slow rate	46.84
Phonemes prolonged	45.57
Audible inspiration	40.51
Continuous phonation	37.97
High pitch	37.97
Phrases short	36.71
Inappropriate silences	32.91
Nasal emission	30.28
Vowels distorted	24.05
Low pitch	7.59
Fast rate	2.53

[a]Adapted from Carrow, Rivera, Mauldin, and Shamblin, 1974.

Similar speech and voice symptoms were reported by Carrow, Rivera, Mauldin, and Shamblin (1974).

Acoustic Signs

Caruso and Burton (1987) reported that the stop gaps in stop consonant syllables and vowel duration were much longer in the speech of patients with amyotrophic lateral sclerosis than in normal speakers. Voice onset time in the two groups was very similar. These authors suggest that laryngeal structures may move more slowly in amyotrophic lateral sclerosis. They point out that because the nucleus ambiguus is often affected, the neural control of adduction/abduction by the vocal folds may be impaired. Data on other acoustic variables in these patients are not available.

Physiological Signs

There have been no data reported on the physiologic characteristics of the speech of amyotrophic lateral sclerosis patients. However, electromyographic studies have been reported on nonlaryngeal muscles and reveal sporadic action potentials, a reduction in the number of potentials, and fibrillation (Carpenter et al., 1978). Similar findings might be expected in the laryngeal muscles.

Laryngoscopic Signs

The larynx in amyotrophic lateral sclerosis usually presents a normal appearance (Aronson, 1985). However, it is possible to observe hyperadduction if the major component in the disease is spastic, and less than normal speed of vocal fold movement if the major component is of the flaccid type.

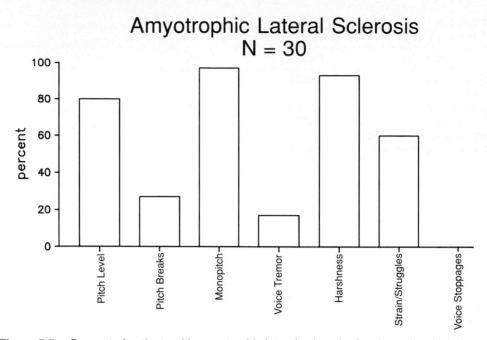

Figure 5.5.   Percent of patients with amyotrophic lateral sclerosis showing voice deviations. Voice tremor was rated during contextual speech. (Drawn from data of Aronson, Brown, Litin, and Pearson, 1968b.)

Stroboscopic Signs

There have been no data reported on stroboscopic signs specifically in amyotrophic lateral sclerosis patients. However, signs typical of flaccid paralysis (no mucosal wave, incomplete closure) or those associated with problems affecting the upper motor neurons (spastic characteristics) would be consistent with the nature of the effects of the disease.

Pathophysiology

Amyotrophic lateral sclerosis impairs central nervous system control of the muscles of the larynx. Furthermore, if the lower motor neurons are affected, muscle tone and strength are affected.

Huntington's Chorea

Primary Voice Symptom

The primary voice symptom is hoarseness/harshness.

Description and Etiology

Chorea refers to a hyperkinetic disorder in which there are abrupt, jerky movements of the head, neck, or limbs. In children it is many times called Sydenham's chorea, whereas in adults it is referred to as Huntington's chorea.

Chorea is a disease of the basal ganglia with an incidence of 4 to 7 per 100,000 (Merritt, 1979). It has a genetic basis, and 50% of an affected person's offspring have a good chance of developing the disease. It usually appears in the 3rd through 5th decades of life, although it has been reported to appear as early as age 5 and as late as age 70 (Merritt, 1979). The basic symptoms are choreiform movements (abrupt, jerky, purposeless) and

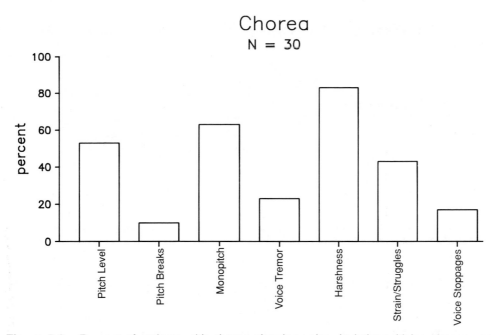

Figure 5.6. Percent of patients with chorea showing voice deviations. Voice tremor was rated during contextual speech. (Drawn from data of Aronson, Brown, Litin, and Pearson, 1968b.)

progressive mental deterioration. The abnormal movements appear to increase with heightened emotional levels, are dramatically reduced during sleep, and, of course, will superimpose themselves on any voluntary movements, thereby affecting them. Mentally, a patient with Huntington's chorea experiences a progressive loss of memory and intellectual capacity.

Ramig (1986) reasoned that generalized instability of muscle contraction (involuntary contractions, variable tone or tremor) would be expected to affect the muscles of the larynx. Therefore, disorders of phonation associated with Huntington's chorea would be likely.

Perceptual Voice Signs and Symptoms

The most prominent perceptual voice sign is harshness, followed by monopitch and strain/struggle voice quality (Aronson et al., 1968b; Aronson, 1985). Figure 5.6 presents the percentage of patients exhibiting the various voice signs rated by Darley et al. (1969b).

Acoustic Signs

Jarema, Kennedy, and Shoulson (1985) studied some acoustic characteristics in 12 adults with Huntington's chorea. There were 7 females with a mean age of 44 years and 5 males with a mean age of 42 years. These authors measured habitual (mean) fundamental frequency and intensity during sustained vowel production and obtained estimates of phonational range and maximum phonation time. Their data on fundamental frequency and vocal intensity are summarized in Table 5.3. The habitual fundamental frequency is defined as that fundamental frequency at a patient's most comfortable effort level, whereas the low and high fundamental frequencies represent the extremes of the patient's phonational range. The authors also collected these data for a normal-speaking group. There is no statistically significant difference between the two groups on habitual fundamental fre-

Table 5.3.
Fundamental Frequency and Intensity Characteristics of the Speech of Huntington's Chorea[a]

	Female		Male	
	Patient	Normal	Patient	Normal
Fundamental frequency (Hz)				
Habitual	166	182	106	103
Low	155	143	92	83
High	592	716	390	422
Intensity (dB SPL)				
Habitual	71	71	74	72
Soft	68	66	71	66
Loud	100	108	104	106

[a]Adapted from Jarema, Kennedy, and Shoulson, 1988.

quency. Although there were some restrictions at both ends of the patients' phonational and dynamic ranges, the differences were not statistically significant. The male patients in the study were found to produce shorter maximum phonation times (15 seconds) than the normal male speakers (23 seconds), but this difference was not significant. However, the female patient phonation times (14 seconds versus 23 seconds) were significantly shorter than those for the normal group.

Ramig (1986) also measured some acoustic features in the speech of eight patients, four males and four females. She noted frequent abrupt low frequency segments during a sustained vowel (sudden drop of fundamental frequency, then a return to almost the same fundamental frequency), voice arrests, and reduced duration of the sustained vowels /ah/, /ee/, and /oo/. Voice arrests (370 to 510 msec in mean duration) occurred in six of the eight patients. Mean vowel durations for the patients ranged from 0.50 to 9.75 seconds, whereas mean normal vowel durations on the same task were 14.61 seconds.

Physiological Signs

Few physiological data have been reported on voice in chorea. Jarema et al. (1985) measured airflow rates during sustained vowel production for their 12 adults with Huntington's chorea and found much higher flow rates (220 ml/sec for females, 320 ml/sec for males) than for their normal control subjects (178 ml/sec for females, 254 ml/sec for males). These data would suggest increased breathiness in patients with Huntington's chorea.

Ramig (1986) suggested that the previously noted voice arrests had to be associated with sudden adductory or abductory movements of the vocal folds, as they occurred much too fast to be produced by articulatory movements. This could be seen as indirect evidence of either hyper- or hypotense vocal folds.

Laryngoscopic Signs

Usually, the larynges of patients with Huntington's chorea appear normal (Aronson, 1985). However, close observation may reveal short periods of adductory or abductory movement, especially in patients exhibiting voice arrests. Sudden shifts of fundamental frequency (usually downward) may be accompanied by jerky movements of the vocal folds. Further research is needed on the laryngoscopic signs of Huntington's chorea.

Stroboscopic Signs

No data have been reported on the strobosopic signs in Huntington's chorea. Because the movements in Huntington's chorea are very jerky and irregular, visualization of the larynx with stroboscopy might be difficult.

Pathophysiology

The jerky, sudden, and abrupt movements of Huntington's chorea would seriously interfere with the production of smooth, controlled sound. Sudden adduction of the vocal folds may result in intensity bursts or voice arrests. Sudden abductory bursts would be accompanied by excessive airflow and breathiness or aphonic episodes. It is possible for a patient to exhibit both conditions, although one or the other characteristic will probably be the most prominent.

Cerebellar Disorders

Ataxic Dysphonia

Primary Voice Symptom

The primary voice symptom is hoarseness/harshness.

Description and Etiology

Ataxic dysphonia (or the more general term, ataxic dysarthria) is a disorder of the cerebellum. A lesion in the cerebellum results in a loss of muscle coordination and movement. Fulton and Dow (1937) considered two kinds of defects in cerebellar lesions: (a) errors in the rate, range, direction, and force of movements and (b) hypotonia. Kent, Netsell, and Abbs (1979) presented some acoustic evidence for scanning speech and suggested that it may be the result of the cerebellum's failing to properly integrate movements, or it may be due to an alteration in the motor programming plan of the cerebellum. In their study of ataxic speech, Brown, Darley, and Aronson (1970) concluded that excess and equal stress plus irregular articulatory breakdown were the speech scales most suggestive of ataxic dysarthria.

The etiology of dysphonia in ataxic dysarthria is varied. In their study, Brown et al. (1970) reported that 3 patients had a neoplasm, 1 had experienced trauma, 1 had an infarct, 1 was thought to have multiple sclerosis, and 24 were diagnosed with cerebellar degeneration. They suggested that the important areas of the cerebellum serving speech were the vermis and the adjacent paravermis. Lechtenberg and Gilman (1978) implicate the left cerebellar hemisphere as important for the control of speech. Based on that implication, Kent et al. (1979) hypothesized that the right cerebral hemisphere must send its informationto the left cerebellar hemisphere, making both hemispheres responsible for the control of speech prosody. If true, one might expect patients with ataxic dysarthria to have greater difficulty in the control of the suprasegmental features of speech (i.e., stress and intonation) both of which involve the vocal folds.

Perceptual Voice Signs and Symptoms

In their rating study of the speech of patients with various kinds of neuromuscular diseases, Aronson et al. (1969b) noted the voice features of harshness, monopitch, too-low pitch, strain/struggle, and pitch breaks as prevalent in ataxic dysarthria. The percentage of patients showing these perceptual signs of the voice is shown in Figure 5.7.

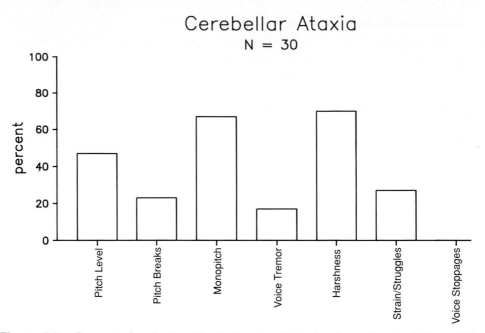

Figure 5.7. Percent of patients with ataxic dysarthria showing voice deviations. Voice tremor was rated during contextual speech. (Drawn from data of Aronson, Brown, Litin, and Pearson, 1968b.)

Aronson (1985) noted that some ataxics may exhibit normal voice quality but that many will show harshness, monopitch, and monoloudness as characteristic features.

Acoustic Signs

There are very few data on the acoustic characteristics of the voice of ataxic dysphonia. Kent et al. (1979) reported a study on the acoustic characteristics of the speech of five ataxic patients. They found abnormally long vowel and segment durations and strongly suggested that there were aberrations in the control of fundamental frequency. In an earlier study, Kent and Netsell (1975) reported on the speech characteristics of a female ataxic patient. Among other variables, they examined fundamental frequency contours during the production of words and sentences. They noted that many fundamental frequency contours had a monotone appearance, while others had marked variability of fundamental frequency. They suggested that ataxics may have more difficulty controlling fundamental frequency during speech than they have in articulating the phonemes. They also noted spectrographic evidence of harshness and/or vocal fry.

Physiological Signs

There appear to be no data available in the literature concerning the physiological characteristics of the voice of ataxic patients. In their single-subject analysis, Kent and Netsell (1975) reported that cineradiographic analysis of the oral cavity during speech revealed abnormal but small anteroposterior lingual adjustments. Furthermore, they found that the patient's articulatory movements were longer in duration than normal movements. Thus, valving movements of the vocal folds might show abnormally long durations and perhaps vibratory movements as well.

Brown et al. (1970) reported that electromyographic recordings were made on 6 of their 30 patients with ataxic dysarthria but failed to specify which muscles were studied. They reported normal electromyographic patterns in 2 patients, evidence of a motor lesion in 1 patient, and evidence of a peripheral neuropathy in 3 patients. Similar abnormalities might be found in the laryngeal muscles, although not in all patients.

Laryngoscopic Signs

Aronson (1985) expects to find a normal-appearing larynx in patients with ataxic dysphonia. Evidence of reduced speed of adduction/abduction during valving and movements of the vocal folds might be observed on careful study.

Stroboscopic Signs

There are no reported data on the stroboscopic signs in patients with ataxic dysphonia.

Pathophysiology

Ataxic dysphonia/dysarthria seems to be characterized by hypotonia and an incoordination of muscles. Hypotonia manifests itself as a delay in the generation of a force, a reduced rate of muscular contraction, and a reduced range of movement (Brown et al., 1970; Kent and Netsell, 1975; Kent et al., 1979). Reduced muscle activity may account for the reduced fundamental frequency range during conversational speech, since in order to increase vocal pitch, cricothyroid muscle activity must be increased. Reduced muscle tone may also account for hoarseness in ataxic voices because of tension differences between the two vocal folds. Hypotonicity will have a similar effect on the control of intensity, although few data have been reported on this acoustic variable. Incoordination of phonation may be manifested by difficulty in controlling the magnitude and extent of laryngeal movements as well as the control of the magnitude and extent of articulatory movements.

Arnold-Chiari Malformation

The Arnold-Chiari malformation is a congenital anomaly of the hindbrain where the brainstem and cerebellum are squeezed into the cervical portion of the spinal column, causing injury to the cerebellum, medulla, and lower cranial nerves (Merritt, 1979, pp. 437–440). It was first described by Arnold (1894) and later by Chiari (1896). In some cases, this malformation can result in vocal fold paralysis (Rullan, 1956) in which voice symptoms will appear that are similar to cerebellar ataxia (see "Ataxic Dysphonia," above) or to lesions affecting the medulla or the peripheral nerves as they leave the cranium and causing flaccid paralysis. In the latter case, perceptual, acoustic, physiological, laryngoscopic, and stroboscopic signs as seen in recurrent nerve paralysis would be expected (see "Peripheral Nerve Lesions" for a more complete discussion.)

Lower Motor Neuron Disorders (Brainstem and Medulla)

Spastic Dysphonia

Primary Voice Symptom

The primary voice symptom is strain/struggle.

Description and Etiology

Spastic dysphonia is a problem affecting vocalization and speech that has received much attention over the past 15 to 20 years, perhaps out of proportion to its incidence. It is a relatively rare voice disorder, although the many recent reports of patients with the problem make it appear that their numbers have increased. This may appear to be so due to the fairly recent availability of methods to provide some form of symptom relief. Spastic dysphonia seems to occur equally in men and women (Aronson et al., 1968a), with onset most frequently in middle age, although we have seen patients as young as 20 years with a history of onset in the teens.

The nature of the onset of spastic dysphonia is variable. In some patients, onset is associated with a major upper respiratory infection (Aronson et al., 1968a), in others a traumatic emotional event is identified (Brodnitz, 1976; Aronson, 1985), and in still other patientsthe onset is insidious, beginning as a mild hoarseness and progressing to interrupted, strained phonation. The progression of symptoms may be rapid or may take place over a number of years.

The etiology of spastic dysphonia is unclear (Salamy and Sessions, 1980; Aronson, 1985). Some authors have advocated a psychological origin (Arnold, 1959; Heaver, 1959; Bloch, 1965; Brodnitz, 1976; Henschen and Burton, 1978), whereas others have implicated a neurological origin (Robe, Brumlik, and Moore, 1960; Aronson et al., 1968a, 1968b; Aminoff, Dedo, and Izdebski, 1978; Schaefer, 1983).

One rationale for the psychological etiology is that patients often report a traumatic emotional event closely associated with the awareness of the onset of symptoms. Brodnitz (1976) described the case of a woman whose symptoms appeared after her husband tried to kill her. Other patients have reported severe marital crises, an accident, the death of a loved one, or the threat of loss of a job preceeding the onset of the symptoms. Another rationale suggests that the population of patients with this disorder tends to be tense and high strung individuals with many personal problems. Advocates of the psychological etiology theory point to some success in therapy (voice or psychiatric) or to relief of symptoms with the use of tranquilizing or neuroleptic drugs (e.g., amobarbital [Amytal], Brodnitz, 1976) as positive evidence of the correctness of the theory.

Advocates of the neurological etiology of spastic dysphonia point to the sizable body of evidence of associated neurological signs in these patients (Aronson et al., 1968a) and to the documented existence of abnormal findings in various tests of brain function (Robe, Brumlik, and Moore, 1960; Dordain and Dordain, 1972; Sharbrough, Stockard, and Aronson, 1975; Aminoff et al., 1978; Finitzo-Hieber, Freeman, Gerling, Dobson, and Schaefer, 1982; Schaefer, 1983). Many of these authors also point out that there has been little actual documentation of symptom relief as a result of voice therapy or in response to psychiatric treatment. Reports of successful treatment have been anecdotal (Cooper and Cooper, 1977), and moreover, the lack of success of these treatment protocols for patients with spastic dysphonia has been extensively noted (Aronson, 1985). On the other hand, there have been reports of symptom relief in patients with spastic dysphonia who have undergone a recurrent nerve section (Dedo, 1976; Izdebski, Dedo, and Shipp, 1981; Dedo and Izdebski, 1981, 1983).

Blitzer, Lovelace, Brin, Fahn, and Fink (1985) have suggested that spastic dysphonia should be considered a focal dystonia. In their electromyographic study of 16 patients with spastic dysphonia, they found normal spontaneous activity but increased activity on phonation. They claim that in spastic diseases, there is usually an irregularity and dyssynchrony of muscle action potentials. These abnormalities were not observed in the patients with spastic dysphonia. Furthermore, they report the presence of other forms of dystonia (not spasticity) in some of their subjects, onset typically in the adult years, causing excessive activity when purposeful activity is attempted and an inability to control the spasms, which increased when the patient was under stress. Based on this evidence, the authors conclude that spastic dysphonia is a type of dystonia specific to the larynx.

Aronson (1985) believes that spastic dysphonia should be considered a disorder that may have either a neurological or a psychological etiology. In cases thought to be neurogenic, the site of the lesion appears to be somewhere in the brainstem (Sharbrough et al. 1975; Finitzio-Hieber et al., 1982; Schaefer, 1983), although more recent evidence may implicate other areas of the brain (Schaefer, Freeman, Finitzo, Close, Cannito, Ross, Reisch, and Maravilla, 1985; Finitzo, Pool, Freeman, Cannito, Schaefer, 1987; Schaefer and Freeman, 1987). In some cases, the etiology may be in doubt or referred to as idiopathic.

Another distinction that should be made concerning this problem is whether the symptoms are indicative of an adductor (closing) type of disorder or an abductor (opening) type of disorder. The specific symptoms of each form are quite different (see below, "Perceptual Voice Symptoms and Signs"). Presumably, the underlying pathophysiology will also differ, and the form of treatment should differ. Some authors (Shipp, Mueller, and Zwitman, 1980; Hartman and Aronson, 1981) have even suggested that abductor spastic dysphonia is so dissimilar to the adductor type that it should be given a name more indicative of its pathophysiology. Hartman and Aronson (1981) have suggested the term "intermittent breathy dysphonia," whereas Shipp et al. (1980) advocate the term "intermittent abductory dysphonia."

Another consideration is whether or not the use of the term "spastic" is appropriate. "Spastic" implies lesions in the corticobulbar or corticospinal (pyramidal) systems. That does not seem to be the case in this disorder. Current evidence suggests that the underlying disease state in spastic dysphonia affects structures in the extrapyramidal system (see below). Aronson et al. (1968a) suggested that the term "spasmodic" would be more appropriate. Unfortunately, the name "spastic dysphonia" has become so commonplace that there has been much resistance to adoption of the more accurate terminology, "spasmodic dysphonia."

Perceptual Voice Signs and Symptoms

Adductor Spastic Dysphonia.   The most characteristic symptom (and sign) is the struggle and strain to talk, in association with intermittent stoppages of voice (Aronson et al., 1968a; Brodnitz, 1976; Aronson, 1985). Associated symptoms may include hoarseness, harshness, and tremor (Fig. 5.8). Other patients present with a creaking, choked, tense, or squeezed voice with extreme tension noted in the entire speech production system. Perceptual signs include strain/struggle, sudden interruption of voicing, tension, loudness and pitch variations, pitch breaks, and stoppages of phonation.

Abductor Spastic Dysphonia.   In the abductor type of spastic dysphonia, there are intermittent episodes of breathy dysphonia, drops in pitch, and vowel prolongations (Zwitman, 1979; Merson and Ginsberg, 1979; Hartman and Aronson, 1981). In many respects it is the mirror image of adductor spastic dysphonia (Aronson, 1973, 1985).

Acoustic Signs

There have been considerable data reported in the literature about the various acoustic signs accompanying spastic dysphonia.

Fundamental Frequency Signs. *Adductor Spastic Dysphonia.*   Davis, Boone, Carroll, Davenzia, and Harrison (1988) reported the average fundamental frequencies during a reading passage for 16 female and 7 male patients with adductor spastic dysphonia and compared these data to those of a set of control subjects. The female patients had a mean fundamental frequency of 162 Hz compared to a mean fundamental frequency of 175 Hz for the 17 female control subjects. The male patients had a mean fundamental fre-

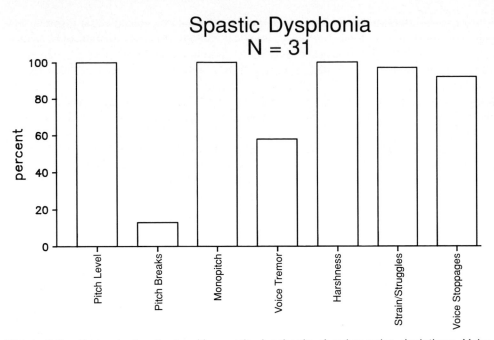

Figure 5.8. Percent of patients with spastic dysphonia showing voice deviations. Voice tremor was rated during contextual speech. (Drawn from data of Aronson, Brown, Litin, and Pearson, 1968b.)

quency of 134 Hz compared to a mean fundamental frequency of 106 Hz for 7 male controls. These authors also reported that the spastic dysphonia patients had a much greater variation of fundamental frequency during the passage than the controls (21.8 [females] and 14.7 [males] semitones compared to 12.2 [females] and 11.8 [males] semitones for the control group).

Fritzell, Feuer, Haglund, Knutsson, and Schiratski (1982) analyzed the distribution of fundamental frequency in the voices of four patients (three males and one female) reading a short passage. Mean fundamental frequency ranged from 111 to 238. The distribution of fundamental frequency was bimodal, with a major peak centered above 200 Hz and a minor peak centered around 150 Hz. These patients underwent section of the recurrent laryngeal nerve for relief of symptoms (see Chapter 8). Postsurgically, the fundamental frequency distribution was much lower (mean fundamental frequencies ranged from 125 to 171 Hz) and unimodal.

Abductor Spastic Dysphonia. Merson and Ginsberg (1979) reported mean fundamental frequencies of 161.3 Hz and 203.8 Hz for two female patients with abductor spastic dysphonia reading a sentence.

Vocal Intensity Signs. Hartman and Aronson (1981) reported the amplitude variations observed in the speech of 17 abductor-type spastic dysphonia patients. They found a steady but random variation of amplitude in some patients, rhythmic variation in other patients, and evidence of moments of breathiness in still other patients. We know of no data on vocal intensity in the adductor type of spastic dysphonia. It has been our experience, however, that some of these patients use much-reduced intensity levels in conversation, even to the point of aphonic whisper. This is perhaps a compensatory behavior adopted in order to avoid voice stoppages.

Spectral Signs. Izdebski (1984) measured the long-term average spectrum (LTAS, a spectrum computed over a sentence or paragraph) in 23 patients with adductor spastic

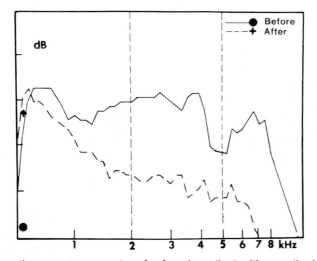

Figure 5.9. Long-time average spectra of a female patient with spastic dysphonia before (——) and after (— —) recurrent nerve section. (From Izdebski, 1984.)

dysphonia. Figure 5.9 illustrates his results. The solid line shows the spectrum of a female speaker before surgery (recurrent nerve section), and the dotted line shows the same patient after surgery. Note the high levels of high frequency energy in the speech before surgery, but the dramatic decrease of high frequency energy after surgery.

Fritzell et al. (1982) analyzed the LTAS in the voices of four patients reading a short passage. They reported only a slight difference of spectral shape and levels after surgery. Because there was no control group, it is not known whether the levels of energy at the higher frequencies were greater than normal. Informal comparisons of the data presented by Fritzell et al. (1982) to those presented by Hammarberg, Fritzell, Gauffin,and Sundberg (1986) for normal speakers suggests that the patient group exhibited greater than normal energy levels in the high frequencies.

Hartman, Abbs, and Vishwanat (1988) observed pronounced peaks between 4 and 7 Hz in the spectrum of sustained /ah/s produced by four patients with adductor spastic dysphonia. These peaks may be indicative of vocal tremor. The finding of low frequency tremor in the frequency spectrum of these patients is of interest. Wolfe and Bacon (1976), using spectrographic analysis of a patient with adductor spastic dysphonia, showed a breakdown in the harmonic structure of vowels, dark areas on the spectrogram (indicating greater loudness), and sudden changes of gray levels on the spectrogram, indicating the irregular variation of voicing present in adductor spastic dysphonia (Fig. 5.10). They also reported spectrographic findings for a patient with what appears to be abductor spastic dysphonia, in which there is evidence of interruptions of voicing (probably due to the sudden blowing apart of the vocal folds), as well as irregularly spaced vertical striations indicating a variation of voicing associated with the strain and struggle to speak. Zwitman (1979) reported similar findings for two patients with abductor spastic dysphonia. He also reported that voiceless stops seem to be distinguished from voiced stops by a sustained frication during the voiceless stops. Some of the spectrographic features of abductor spastic dysphonia can be seen in Figure 5.10.

Physiological Signs

Several studies have reported airflows and air pressures for spastic dysphonia patients. Hirano, Koike, and von Leden (1968) reported flows within the normal range for

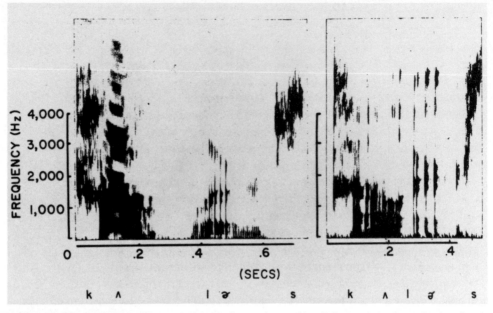

Figure 5.10. Broad band spectrogram of a patient with abductor-type spastic dysphonia (left panel) and adductor-type spastic dysphonia (right panel). The utterance was the word "colors." (From Wolfe and Bacon, 1976.)

their 8 spastic dysphonia patients, whereas other studies have reported low (Davis et al., 1988, 14 female patients: 90.5 ml/sec; 6 male patients: 77.2 ml/sec) to very low flows (Briant, Blair, Cole, and Singer, 1983, 9 patients: 29.3 ml/sec). In adductor spastic dysphonia, patients may exhibit strain during voicing, which may produce small glottal apertures through which air can flow. Low flows would be expected in this situation. On the other hand, in abductor spastic dysphonia, high flows would be expected as a result of the sudden opening of the vocal folds, releasing large quantities of airflow. Merson and Ginsberg (1979) reported such large flows in two patients with abductor spastic dysphonia (e.g., 321 ml/sec on a sustained /ah/ vowel, 400 ml/sec and 435 ml/sec during sentence for two patients).

Shipp, Izdebski, Schutte, and Morrissey (1988) studied subglottal air pressure magnitudes in two patients with adductor spastic dysphonia. They reported much higher pressures (13 to 14 cm/H_2O) than normal (about 6 cm/H_2O). These very high pressures are consistent with patients' reports of the increased effort required to speak. The elevated pressures in combination with the low flows suggest increased glottal resistance during voicing for patients with adductor spastic dysphonia.

Laryngoscopic Signs

Anatomically, the larynx appears essentially normal. However, during phonation it is possible to observe the hyperadduction of the adductor type of spastic dysphonia or the sudden opening of the vocal folds in the abductor variety. Hartman and Aronson (1981) reported the appearance of bowed vocal folds in 2 of 17 patients with otherwise normal-looking vocal folds. Hartman et al. (1988) reported the observations of quick adductory movements of the true vocal folds, the ventricular folds, and much of the supraglottal structures in one patient; small, irregular movements of the true vocal folds in another patient; and, in a third patient, periodic laryngospasms. In the study reported by Davis et al. (1988), most patients had normal laryngoscopic exams, but interruption of voicing was reported to occur in seven patients due to action of the true vocal folds, in two patients tremor seemed to cause the interruption, and in four other patients the ventricular folds appeared to cause the voice stoppage.

Stroboscopic Signs

Few data have been reported on the vibratory characteristics of patients with spastic dysphonia as seen via stroboscopy. Fritzell et al. (1982) report that stroboscopy was carried out prior to recurrent nerve section, but no data were presented. Postsurgically, two patients showed symmetrical vocal fold vibrations, indicating a return of function to the muscle. Because patients with spastic dysphonia have difficulty in sustaining phonation, stroboscopic visualization of the vocal folds might be unproductive. The presence of tremor will also reduce the possibility of obtaining an adequate stroboscopic examination.

Pathophysiology

The spasm activity of the vocal folds, be it adductory or abductory, will have a pronounced effect on the production of sound. Excessive adductory forces will require greater than normal pressures to force the vocal folds apart during phonation. Greater air pressures will be associated with greater sound pressure levels and a more rapid opening and closing phase of the vocal folds. Rapid closing phases are associated with the production of greater energy in the higher frequencies and high energy, high frequency spectra. The intermittent nature of the problem will produce wide variations of spectrum and fundamental frequency unless some compensatory mechanism is employed in the attempt to maintain a steady, smooth flow of speech. In abductory spastic dysphonia, the sudden spasm results in a sudden increase of flow and relatively short closed times. The combination of rapid airflows and short closed time would be expected to produce much less energy in the higher frequencies of the spectrum. The voice will be perceived as breathy and weak. Again, there are periods of normal vocal fold vibration, but it is the sudden, unexpected stoppages (or openings) that create havoc in the production of voice and speech.

Other Considerations

In many patients with spastic dysphonia, other neurological signs will appear, including voice tremor, jaw or facial jerks, hand or limb tremor, hyperreflexia, sucking reflex, torticollis, or asymmetries in the face or palate (Aronson et al., 1968a; Davis et al., 1988). The high incidence of tremor in spastic dysphonia patients (58%, Aronson et al., 1968b) suggests that perhaps a proportion of patients diagnosed with spastic dysphonia are in fact patients with essential tremor (Aronson et al., 1968b). On the other hand, it is possible that in some cases spastic dysphonia is another manifestation of essential tremor (Aronson and Hartman, 1981). At the very least, the frequency of occurrence of additional neurological signs suggests that spastic dysphonia may have as one etiology a neurological substrate somewhere in the brain, probably in the extrapyramidal system (Critichley, 1949).

Sharbrough et al. (1975) reported brainstem abnormalities in 7 of their 18 spastic dysphonia patients. They concluded that spastic dysphonia is "a symptom due to organic CNS disease which, in some cases, incidentally produces asymptomatic slowing of conduction within the brainstem auditory pathway" (p. 200).

Finitzo-Hieber et al. (1982) reported that five of their six spastic dysphonia patients had abnormal auditory brainstem responses. They also concluded that the capacity of the brainstem to conduct impulses is impaired in patients with spastic dysphonia.

Essential Tremor

Primary Voice Symptom

The primary voice symptom is tremor.

Description and Etiology

Essential tremor is a disorder of the central nervous system that may result in tremor in the head, limbs, tongue, palate, and larynx. It tends to start in the hands and then progress to the arms, head, neck, face, and so on (Brown and Simonson, 1963). Although the larynx may not be involved, in some patients voice tremor may be the primary or sole characteristic. In others, the tremor may not be observable when the affected body part is at rest, but it becomes obvious when some kind of movement is attempted, including speech.

In the Brown and Simonson study (1963), only 6 of 31 essential tremor patients exhibited isolated voice tremor, while the remaining 25 had, in addition to voice tremor, tremor in the head or extremities or both. In a vast majority of cases, the onset was gradual, and many had family members with some kind of tremor. Associated neurological signs, including a positive sucking reflex, spasmodic torticollis, bilateral facial spasms, incoordination, and adiadochokinesis, were present in 17 of the patients.

Larsson and Sjogren (1960) reported that essential tremor occurred more frequently in males, with a mean age of onset of 48 years. Aronson and Hartman (1981) reported the mean age of onset at 57 years. They also found extralaryngeal tremor in 93% of their patients.

Thus, essential tremor seems to be associated with aging, although the reasons for this are unclear. Heredity may affect the development of the tremor. In those cases where the onset was sudden, Brown and Simonson (1963) suggested that some kind of arterial disease may have been responsible.

It is difficult to determine the locus of the central nervous system lesion that results in essential tremor. Critchley (1949) suggested that the extrapyramidal system is involved, but it is possible that other structures might be affected.

Perceptual Voice Signs and Symptoms

The most prominent voice symptom and sign is tremor that is most noticeable during prolonged production of a vowel and is also apparent during contextual speech. In 100% of their patients with essential tremor, Aronson et al. (1968b) reported tremor on a sustained /ah/ vowel, (not shown is Figure 5.11) as well as harshness and strain/struggle. Figure 5.11 presents a summary of the voice symptoms in essential tremor as reported in the Aronson et al. (1968b) study.

In general, the voice of essential tremor patients may be described as sounding quavery and tremulous. Most patients will have a relatively constant and noticeable tremor during speech. Some may have such severe tremor that stoppage of voice occurs, as reported by Ardran, Kinsbourne, and Rushworth (1966).

Acoustic Signs

There are few data on many of the acoustic signs of voice in essential tremor. Most studies have concentrated on the variation of amplitude during sustained vowel production. Brown and Simonson (1963) measured the rate of tremor from oscillograms of 23 patients. Tremor frequencies of 5 to 6 Hz were measured in 16 of the 23 patients. Ardran et al. (1966) reported spectrographic evidence of low amplitude noise during the production of monosyllabic words by a single patient. This noise, they suggested, gave evidence of

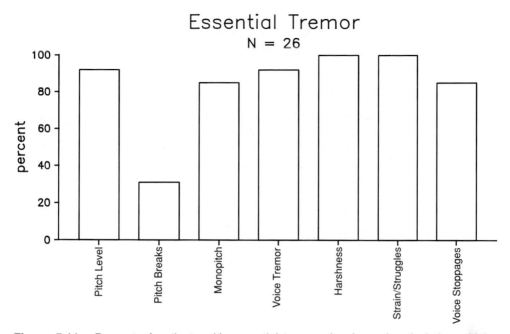

Figure 5.11. Percent of patients with essential tremor showing voice deviations. Voice tremor was rated during contextual speech. (Drawn from data of Aronson, Brown, Litin, and Pearson, 1968b.)

breathiness in the patients' speech. Aronson and Hartman (1981) analyzed the tremor in oscillograms of 14 patients with essential tremor and reported a mean tremor frequency of 5.7 Hz.

Laryngoscopic Signs

By and large, the larynges of patients with essential tremor will show normal structure and movement. Rhythmic movement of one or more structures may sometimes be observed during phonation and at rest. Brown and Simonson (1963) reported normal-appearing larynges in 13 of their essential tremor patients and vocal fold bowing in 1 patient. However, 17 of their patients were not examined laryngoscopically.

Physiological Signs

There have been few data reported on the physiological characteristics of patients with essential tremor. Ardran et al. (1966) performed electromyograms on the cricothyroid and hyoglossus muscles of a 72-year-old female patient. They showed that at rest, both muscles had regular variation in activity at about a rate of 5 to 6 Hz. They comment that this was low level activity that did not result in movement of the structures. This variation in muscle activity was not entirely regular and disappeared occasionally. Furthermore, the variation of activity between the hyoglossus and the cricothyroid muscle was not synchronized. Ardran et al. (1966) also reported finding resting tremor in the electromyogram of the pectoralis major and external intercostal muscles in this patient. However, these disappeared when the patient contracted these muscles.

Stroboscopic Signs

We know of no data on the stroboscopic signs in essential tremor. We would expect that obtaining good stroboscopic recordings would be very difficult since the variation of amplitude level and fundamental frequency would make tracking of the fundamental frequency difficult. In patients we have observed with tremor, it has not been possible to obtain good stroboscopic pictures that would permit reliable observation of the significant stroboscopic signs.

Pathophysiology

The rhythmically changing activity in the muscles of the larynx would create varying degrees of tension in the vocal folds and lead to a rhythmic change in fundamental frequency. Furthermore, the degree of adduction would systematically vary in synchrony with the variation of muscle activity, creating a rhythmic change in the force of adduction. This would result in variations of subglottal air pressure and thus of vocal intensity. If the tremor is severe, the adductory force could become large enough to completely stop voice production. Voice stoppages are also characteristic of spastic dysphonia. Aronson and Hartman (1981) have suggested that some forms of spastic dysphonia may have essential tremor as their etiology. If so, perhaps some of the treatment modalities attempted for the relief of essential tremor would be effective in the treatment of spastic dysphonia. Only time will tell.

Miscellaneous Syndromes

Lesions in the upper neck or the medulla result in various syndromes that have paralysis of the vocal folds as one characteristic. There is involvement of the recurrent and superior laryngeal nerves, with a characteristic combined paralysis of the vocal folds. Other cranial nerves are usually also affected in these syndromes. Table 5.4 presents a summary of syndromes as discussed by Ballenger (1985). Note how often these syndromes include some effect on the pharynx, palate, and tongue, as well as the larynx. In Table 5.5, syndromes with a vocal fold component that result from lesions in the neck are presented.

Generalized Central Nervous System Damage or Unknown Locations

Gilles de la Tourette Syndrome

Gilles de la Tourette syndrome develops in early childhood, usually between 2 and 13 years. It is characterized by twitching and grimacing, with tics of the face and eyes being the most common symptom (Merritt, 1979; Golden, 1977). The tics may later spread to the limbs. The speech of these individuals is characterized by unusual noises, explosive outbursts, and the unexpected utterance of profanities. Contrary to most belief, coprolalia (foul explicatives) and echolalia are not frequently heard in childhood. The disease increases in severity during childhood, but the symptoms may diminish in adulthood. The disease can usually be controlled by the use of the drug haloperidol, although there have been reports of unwanted side effects in some patients. Lang and Marsden (1983) reported a case in which spastic dysphonia developed during the use of haloperidol and persisted after removal of the drug.

Gilles de la Tourette syndrome, although interesting and unusual, does not present any unique challenges for the speech pathologist insofar as the voice is concerned. The symptoms are not under voluntary control and cannot be altered or controlled through a behavioral approach. It would appear that pharmacologic treatment can be effective in reducing or eliminating the symptoms.

Table 5.4.
Miscellaneous Medulla Syndromes Affecting the Vocal Folds[a]

Name	Effect	Etiology
Wallenberg's	Paralysis of half of larynx, pharynx, palate; loss of sensation to the face, vestibular dysfunction, ataxia, Horner's syndrome	Infarction of posterior inferior cerebellar artery
Babinski-Nageotte	Similar to Wallenberg's, including paralysis of tongue, loss of position and vibratory sense	Similar to Wallenberg, plus involvement of medial bulbar area
Cestan-Chenais	Similar to Babinski-Nageotte, except little or no involvement proximal to nucleus ambiguus	Infarction of vertebral artery below the posterior inferior cerebellar artery
Avellis's	Causes laryngeal, pharyngeal, and palatal paralysis with dysphonia and dysphagia	Vascular or inflammatory lesion in medulla; lesion in nucleus ambiguus of vagus, plus cranial part of spinal accessory
Hughlings-Jackson	Results in ipsilateral paralysis of the soft palate, pharynx, larynx, tongue, and sternocleidomastoid muscles	Intramedullary lesion or a lesion high in the lateral pharyngeal space; affects vagus, spinal accessory, and hypoglossal nerves
Schmidt's	Ipsilateral paralysis of soft palate, pharynx, larynx, sternomastoid, and trapezius muscles	Vascular lesion in caudal part of medulla
Mackenzie	Unilateral paralysis of soft palate, pharynx, larynx, and tongue	Vascular lesion in medulla
Bonnier's	General weakness	Lesion in Deiters's nucleus or associated vestibular tracts

[a]Adapted from Ballenger, 1985.

Multiple Sclerosis

Primary Voice Symptoms

The primary voice symptoms are impaired loudness control and hoarseness/harshness.

Description and Etiology

Multiple sclerosis was first described by Charcot (1881), who referred to it as disseminated sclerosis. It is a disease characterized by multiple scarring (sclerosis) of the white matter in the brain, brainstem, and spinal cord. The initial symptoms of the disease may be very mild. As it progresses, the severity of the symptoms may increase, yet intermittently there may be long periods of remission or latency during which the person may seem well,

Table 5.5.
Miscellaneous Peripheral Syndromes Resulting in Laryngeal Paralysis[a]

Name	Effect	Etiology
Collet-Sicard	Last four cranial nerves	Tumor, meningitis, or trauma to posterior cranial fossa
Vernet's	Nerves 9,10,11; dysphagia and dysphonia	Lesion in jugular fossa
Villarets	Like Vernet's, including sympathetic paralysis and Horner's syndrome	Lesion in retroparotid or lateral pharyngeal space
Tapia's	Ipsilateral paralysis of tongue and larynx	Neoplasm where hypoglossal crosses vagus and internal carotid
Gard-Gignoux	Paralysis of vocal folds, weakness of trapezius and sternomastoid muscles	11th and vagus below nodose ganglion
Klinkert	Paralysis of recurrent and phrenic nerves	Lesion in root of neck or mediastinum

[a]Adapted from Ballenger, 1985.

but then the symptoms return. In the United States, the incidence of multiple sclerosis is about 50 per 100,000. It is much more common in the temperate regions of the northern and southern hemispheres, with the incidence dropping markedly close to the equator. The male/female ratio is unclear. The disease frequently develops in young adulthood, although it has been suggested that the onset of the very slowly progressing symptoms occurs in childhood but only becomes apparent in the adult (Millar, 1971).

Approximately 50% of patients with multiple sclerosis initially seek medical attention because of ENT symptoms, including vertigo (25%), nystagmus (40% to 70%), and dysarthria (20%) or dysphagia (10% to 15%) (Ward, Cannon, and Lindsay, 1965; Garfinkle and Kimmelman, 1982). Bilateral abductor paralysis of the vocal folds may also occur. Noffsinger, Olsen, Carhart, Hart, and Sahgal (1972) documented many of the auditory and vestibular system dysfunctions in multiple sclerosis patients. Of course, a patient may present more than one of these symptoms.

The reported loci of central nervous system involvement are not consistent. In a study of 234 multiple sclerosis patients, 85% were reported to have pyramidal involvement, followed by cerebellar involvement in 77% and brainstem in 73% (Kurtzke, Beebe, Nagler, Auth, Kurland, and Nefzger,1972). Multiple system involvement was also noted by Garfinkle and Kimmelman (1982). Patients with multiple sclerosis present a variety of neurologic signs. Some of these are summarized in Table 5.6, based on the data presented by Darley, Brown, and Goldstein (1972).

It has been stated that the cardinal signs of multiple sclerosis are scanning speech, nystagmus, and intention tremor (Ivers and Goldstein, 1963). However, available data suggest that speech/voice problems, although sometimes present, are not pervasive. Darley et al. (1972) found that 59% of their 168 patients presented normal speech patterns, and another 29% had minimal speech impairment. Table 5.7 presents a summary of the speech and voice symptoms in their patients. These authors also noted that the severity of speech difficulty increased with an increase in the severity of the neurologic deficit. They

Table 5.6.
Neurologic Signs in Multiple Sclerosis[a]

Neurologic Sign	Percent
Finger to finger/toe to finger tests	82%
Dysdiadochokinesis	71%
Impairment of posterior column sense	60%
Pyramidal signs (sucking reflex, Hoffman's sign, Babinski's sign, increased muscle-stretch reflexes)	92%
Muscular weakness	9%

[a]Adapted from Darley, Brown, and Goldstein, 1972.

concluded that dysarthria was not characteristic of multiple sclerosis speech, nor was scanning speech. Kurtzke et al. (1972) reported that scanning speech was present in only 18.9% of their 525 male patients with multiple sclerosis.

Perceptual Voice Signs and Symptoms

The primary voice symptoms associated with multiple sclerosis are impaired loudness control and harshness (Farmakides and Boone, 1960; Darley et al., 1972). Hypernasality is also prominent (Farmakides and Boone, 1960), while impaired pitch control, inappropriate pitch level, and breathiness can occur less frequently. Speech characteristics include a slowing of speech rate, defective articulation (Jensen, 1960; Darley et al., 1972), impaired emphasis (scanning speech), and occasionally poor respiratory control.

Acoustic Signs

The range of fundamental frequencies produced by patients with multiple sclerosis appears to be very similar to that of normal speakers, with the possible exception of a slightly greater fundamental frequency range and larger variability of fundamental frequency (Zemlin, 1962).

Table 5.7.
Speech Deviations in Multiple Sclerosis[a]

	Percent	
Normal speech performance		59%
Defective speech performance		41%
Impaired loudness control	77%	
Harshness	72%	
Defective articulation	46%	
Impaired emphasis	39%	
Impaired pitch control	37%	
Hypernasality	24%	
Inappropriate pitch level	24%	
Breathiness	22%	

[a]Adapted from Darley, Brown, and Goldstein, 1972.

Physiological Signs

We know of no data on the phonatory physiological characteristics of patients with multiple sclerosis. If harshness is present, suggestive of vocal fold hypertonicity, low flows and high subglottal pressures might be expected. The vibratory cycle of the vocal folds is probably highly variable because of the harshness and impaired muscle control.

Laryngoscopic Signs

In most patients, the larynx would be expected to appear normal. In patients with abductor paralysis, vocal fold opening should be impaired, and the patient may present problems related to air intake. There may be reduced range of motion of the vocal folds and momentary stoppages of vocal fold motion.

Stroboscopic Signs

We know of no data on the stroboscopic signs in multiple sclerosis. We might expect to find good closure of the vocal folds (unless the patient is very breathy), but there may be a reduction of the amplitude of vibration and perhaps poor phase symmetry.

Pathophysiology

Multiple sclerosis is characterized by increasing incoordination, spasticity, and weakness of the muscles in the body. When the laryngeal musculature is affected, these same characteristics might be evidenced by impaired phonatory coordination and control and by reduced range and force of movement. Spasticity and muscle weakness will affect the ability of the vocal folds to adduct smoothly and to maintain the proper adductory forces needed for phonation. Weakness of vocal fold adduction may mean an inability to produce the proper subglottal pressures needed for speech. This will manifest itself in reduced vocal loudness. The spastic characteristic of multiple sclerosis may impair the ability to maintain control over vocal fold adduction and therefore may result in uneven vocal loudness. Poor coordination of the vocal folds may produce aperiodicity of vibration and lead to greater perceived hoarseness/harshness. The rate of movement of the vocal folds may also be impaired similarly to the impaired rate of speaking (Jensen, 1960).

Disorders of Muscle and Myoneural Junction

Myasthenia Gravis

Primary Voice Symptom

The primary voice symptom is breathiness.

Description and Etiology

Patients with myasthenia gravis show a characteristic weakening of the striated muscles and a prolonged return of function after activation. Muscles innervated by cranial nerves seem most susceptible to this disease. The disease is relatively rare, with an incidence between 2 to 10 per 100,000 (Garfinkle and Kimmelman, 1982). It tends to affect the sexes differentially in terms of incidence and age of onset. It occurs twice as often in females, and much earlier than in males. Onset for females is reported in the 3rd decade of life, while in males it is during the 6th decade (Garfinkle and Kimmelman, 1982).

Patients with myasthenia gravis tend to show bulbar symptoms, with the earliest and most common being ptosis or drooping of the eyelids (Grob, 1961). Other symptoms include diplopia, weakness of the legs, fatigue, dysphagia, dysphonia, and blurred vision. All patients will not exhibit all symptoms. Furthermore, these symptoms are not unique to myasthenia gravis but are encountered in other disease states. The symptom of diplopia, for example, can be associated with infection, glioma of the brainstem, multiple sclerosis, toxicity, aneurysms, tumors, and trauma (Baker, 1958). Paralysis or muscle weakness can also be a sign of poliomyelitis or brainstem glioma in children. In adults, paralysis can be a sign of poliomyelitis, Guillain-Barré syndrome, brainstem glioma, cerebellopontine angle tumor, cerebral artery occlusion, amyotrophic lateral sclerosis, and pseudobulbar palsy or tumor (Baker, 1958; Stuart, 1965). Carpenter et al. (1978) emphasized the differential diagnosis of myasthenia gravis, amyotrophic lateral sclerosis, and multiple sclerosis. The unique features of myasthenia gravis are fatigability, fluctuation of function, and restoration of function after rest. These features do not occur, for example, in amyotrophic lateral sclerosis or multiple sclerosis. The voice symptoms of myasthenia gravis, because of their variability, have been been mistaken for hysterical aphonia (Ball and Lloyd, 1971).

Some myasthenia gravis patients may present with voice or speech dysfunction as their initial symptom. Wolski (1967) reported a case of myasthenia gravis in which nasality was the initial presenting symptom. Colton and Brewer (1985) and Levine, Hatlali, and Zaggy (1985) each reported a case diagnosed as myasthenia gravis who presented unusual fiberoptic laryngoscopic findings.

Myasthenia gravis seems to be a disease of the myoneural junction. It may result from inadequate release of acetylcholine or other aberrant chemical activity at the myoneural junction (Osserman, 1958).

Perceptual Voice Signs and Symptoms

The primary symptom of myasthenia gravis is the general fatigability of muscle functions in the head, neck, tongue, pharynx, and larynx. Voice signs include hoarseness, breathy voice, and vocal weakness (Carpenter et al. 1978). In one study, 60% of myasthenia gravis patients presented voice symptoms (Rontal, Rontal, Leuchter, and Rolnick, 1978). The following voice characteristics were reported in ratings of 11 patients with myasthenia gravis: hypernasality, nasal emission, inspiratory voice, dysphonia, intermittent aphonia, and aspirate voice (Maxwell and Locke, 1969). Interestingly, these symptoms were completely eliminated with pharmacologic treatment.

Acoustic Signs

Few studies have been reported about the acoustic characteristics of patients with myasthenia gravis. In a study of 11 females and 1 male with myasthenia gravis, average fundamental frequency of speech was found to be very similar to normal expectations in both medicated and unmedicated states (Maxwell and Locke, 1969).

Rontal et al. (1978) presented spectrographic evidence of aperiodicity and high frequency noise in the speech of patients with myasthenia gravis.

Physiological Signs

Electromyographic studies have shown a characteristic decrement of activity with repetitive stimulation (Warren, Gutmann, and Cody, 1977). We have studied the airflow and electroglottogram characteristics of a patient with myasthenia gravis. The data are shown in Figure 5.12. Note the extremely long opening phase of the airflow waveform

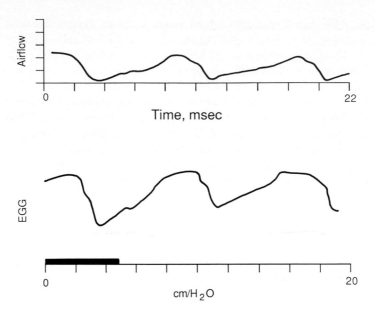

Figure 5.12. Inverse filtered and electroglottogram waveforms for a 65-year-old female with myasthenia gravis. Note the extremely long opening phase of the vocal folds and the slow closing phase. The electroglottogram waveform mirrors these slow variations of vibration. Lung pressure was within normal limits. (From Colton and Brewer, 1985.)

cycles, with a rather slow (but faster than the opening phase) closing phase. The electroglottogram waveform seems to mirror these slow opening and closing phases of the vocal folds. The airflow/slope ratio (ratio of the closing slope to the opening slope) and the electroglottogram closing time were significantly greater than the normal subjects.

Laryngoscopic Signs

The characteristic sign seen in laryngoscopic evaluations is sluggishness of vocal fold abduction. Continued phonation by a patient with myasthenia gravis over a period of time may show increasing weakness of arytenoid and vocal fold motion. Normal movement will return, however, with sufficient rest.

Stroboscopic Signs

There have been no data reported on the stroboscopic signs associated with myasthenia gravis. Normal mucosal waves but reduced amplitude of motion might be expected.

Pathophysiology

Muscle weakness will be expected to affect the patient's ability to raise the vocal pitch and produce loud voice. However, these changes may occur only when the mechanism has fatigued following phonation over a period of time. The inability to maintain the proper tension in the vocal folds will result in increased aperiodicity and the inability to maintain good glottal closure. These conditions will produce roughness or hoarseness and breathiness in the voice.

Lesions of the Peripheral Nerves

Primary Voice Symptom

The primary voice symptom is breathiness.

Description and Etiology

Lesions that affect the vagus nerve somewhere along its course from the base of the skull to the larynx will result in a paresis (weakness) or paralysis of muscles in the larynx. These peripheral lesions of the vagus are the most common cause of vocal fold paralysis. The intrinsic laryngeal muscles affected will depend on the exact location of the lesion. Recall that the superior laryngeal nerve (SLN) of the vagus controls the cricothyroid muscles, whereas the recurrent laryngeal nerve (RLN) controls the remaining muscles of the larynx. The SLN branches off from the vagus high in the neck. The RLN branches off somewhat below the SLN. A paralysis of all the muscles suggests that the lesion is high in the neck or higher still, in the brainstem itself. Lesions affecting only the RLN will be much lower in the neck or as far down as the thorax.

Lesions of the SLN or RLN may affect the position of the vocal folds. In RLN paralysis, the lesion may be unilateral or bilateral and may be of the adductor or abductor type, depending on the muscles affected. In the instance of a unilateral adductor paralysis, the affected vocal fold will not be actively moved toward the midline when phonation commences. When the glottis cannot be completely closed, the quality of the voice produced will be weak and breathy. In bilateral adductor paralysis, neither vocal fold will be capable of moving to the midline, thus making phonation impossible. The position of the paralyzed vocal folds, that is, how far apart they are, will depend partly on whether or not the SLN is affected. The SLN innervates the cricothryoid muscle, which when contracted tends to contribute to adduction of the vocal folds, in addition to tensing them to create a rise of vocal pitch. Paralysis of this muscle in addition to the RLN will further reduce the adductory forces on the vocal folds, thereby increasing their distance from each other over what it might be with an RLN lesion alone. Other factors, such as degree of fibrosis of the affected fold, tension of the conus elasticus, and freedom of joint movement may also affect the final position of the vocal folds after paralysis of the RLN or SLN (Ballenger, 1985).

Lesions may also affect the abductory function of the vocal folds, which opens the airway for inspiration. Such lesions may produce unilateral or bilateral abductory paralysis. Bilateral abductor paralysis in which the vocal folds remain in an adducted posture causes serious respiratory problems (dyspnea), for which most patients will require a tracheotomy.

The etiology of vocal fold paralysis is varied and, as mentioned previously, can include lesions in the brainstem itself. These high vagal lesions (from the nodose ganglion up) will affect all laryngeal muscles, as well as muscles supplied by other cranial nerves. The lesions include tumors at the base of the skull, carcinoma of the nasopharynx, or trauma. A listing of some of the lesions in this area that could affect the larynx is shown in Table 5.5.

The possible etiologies of low vagal lesions are even more numerous. Neuritis is a frequent cause and occurs with upper respiratory infection, infectious mononucleosis, sarcoidosis, and infections of the parapharyngeal spaces (Ballenger, 1985). Neoplasms in the neck, bronchi, and chest may invade and affect the nerve. Mechanical stretching or compression of the nerve may also result in paralysis of the laryngeal musculature. Among the most common etiologies are acute external trauma to the neck, surgery, and idiopathic etiologies (Tucker, 1980; Ballenger, 1985). A summary of the etiologies of laryngeal paralysis for adult patients as reported by Tucker (1980) is presented in Figure 5.13. Note that thyroidectomy is a relatively rare cause of a unilateral paralysis, but the major cause of bilateral paralysis.

Cohen, Geller, Birns, and Thompson (1982) reported on the causes of laryngeal nerve paralysis in children, the symptoms of which will usually be observed shortly after birth. In some cases, however, the symptoms may be so minor that a vocal fold paralysis may not be recognized until many years later. Such was the case of K. B. reported in Chapter 2. The major cause of vocal fold paralysis in children is birth trauma (19%), with central nervous system disease the next most common etiology. The other causes of paralysis in children are shown in Figure 5.14. Also shown in this figure are the presenting ENT signs. Interestingly, 65% of infants with laryngeal paralysis had a normal delivery, and 38% had unilateral paralysis, whereas 62% had bilateral abductor paralysis.

Perceptual Voice Signs and Symptoms

The most common perceptual symptoms of unilateral paralysis are breathiness and hoarseness. Occasionally diplophonia may be present. Bilateral paralysis of the adductor type will cause severe breathiness or aphonia, but near-normal voice may be present in the abductor type. An additional perceptual sign of bilateral abductor paralysis is inspiratory stridor that results from the passage of ingressive air over approximated vocal folds that are incapable of opening.

Acoustic Signs

Acoustically, increased aperiodicity (jitter and shimmer), a reduced pitch range, reduced variability of pitch, higher noise levels, and a reduced vocal intensity range would all be expected to be present.

Murry (1978) reported the fundamental frequency characteristics of 20 patients with unilateral paralysis of the vocal folds as they read a standard reading passage. The patient group had a mean fundamental frequency of 127 Hz, whereas a group of 20 normal speakers had a mean fundamental frequency of 121.9 Hz. This difference was not statistically significant. The variability of fundamental frequency (pitch sigma) between the two groups of subjects was also not significant.

Davis (1981) reported pitch perturbation quotient (PPQ), or jitter, and amplitude perturbation quotient (APQ), or shimmer, values for 2 patients with unilateral paralysis of the vocal folds. The average PPQ was 9.165% for the patients versus 0.42% for a group of 10 normal speakers. The APQ was 12.96% for the patient group and 6.14% for the 10 normal speakers. It is difficult to generalize about these findings based on only 2 subjects, but they appear to be in the direction hypothesized. That is, patients with unilateral paralysis will show greater frequency and amplitude perturbation than speakers with normal-functioning vocal folds.

Kim, Kakita, and Hirano (1982) carried out spectrographic analysis of some acoustic characteristics of the voices of 10 persons with unilateral RLN paralysis. They were unable to obtain fundamental frequency measures, suggesting that these subjects' voices exhibited a large amount of aperiodicity. The only difference between the patient and the normal group on amplitude variation and extent (a rough analog of shimmer) occurred between males. Other differences measured in these spectrograms included higher harmonic energy in the patient group, as well as greater noise energy. These latter features may correlate with the greater breathiness and noise levels that are present in many patients with unilateral recurrent nerve paralysis.

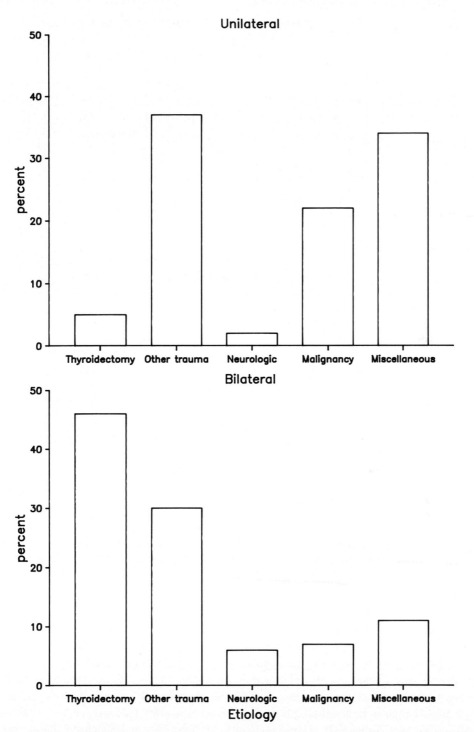

Figure 5.13. Etiology of unilateral and bilateral adductor vocal fold paralysis in adults. Shown is the percent of patients with the etiologies listed, as reported by Tucker, (1980.)

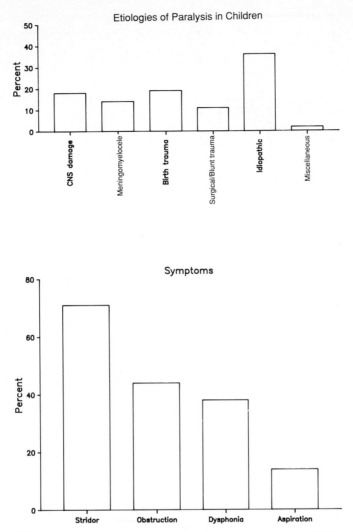

Figure 5.14. Etiology and symptoms of peripheral nerve paralysis in children. There were 50 male and 41 female children in this sample. In the top panel is shown the percent of patients with the specific etiology. In the bottom panel is shown the percent of patients with ENT symptoms. (Drawn from data of Cohen, Geller, Birns, and Thompson, 1982.)

Physiological Signs

There have been several investigations concerned with the measurement of average airflow during the speech of patients with vocal fold paralysis. Hirano (1981a) summarized several of these studies, noting that the mean flow rates in paralysis are much higher than normal, although they range from a low of 35 ml/sec to a high of 1150 ml/sec (see Table 3.3, p. 30, in Hirano, 1981a). Normal-speaking males produce rates of about 110 ml/sec, females about 94 ml/sec (Koike and Hirano, 1968). Yanagihara and von Leden (1967) reported a mean flow rate of 442.2 ml/sec for their 10 patients with unilateral paralysis, whereas Iwata et al. (1972) reported a mean flow of 353 ml/sec for their group of 19 unilateral paralysis patients. Hirano et al. (1968) reported a mean flow rate of 312.8 ml/sec for their 10 patients with bilateral paraly-

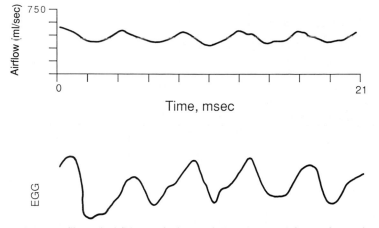

Figure 5.15. Inverse filtered airflow and electroglottogram waveforms for patient K. B., a female with a congenital unilateral vocal fold paralysis. Note the large airflow offset, indicative of a large leak through the vocal folds. The electroglottogram also exhibits unusual waveforms with marked change from one cycle to the next. Due to technical problems, we were unable to record the lung pressure used with this phonation. (From Casper, Colton, and Brewer, 1985.)

sis. Thus, it would appear that higher mean flow rates occur in unilateral paralysis than in bilateral paralysis.

We have recorded the inverse filtered flow characteristics and electroglottograms of several patients with unilateral paralysis. One patient is shown in Figure 5.15. This is the same female (K. B.) whose case was presented in Chapter 2. Note the high levels of offset flow (from baseline to lowest point on the airflow waveform), which were much greater than for the normal subjects. The airflow waveform is variable, perhaps indicative of the greater aperiodicity of the vocal folds. This increased aperiodicity is also evident in the electroglottographic trace shown below the airflow trace.

Kuroki (1969) studied the subglottal pressures produced by patients with unilateral and bilateral recurrent nerve paralysis. Most patients with unilateral paralysis produced higher than normal subglottal pressures (normal, about 6 to 8 cm/H_2O), and two bilateral paralysis patients showed much higher than normal subglottal pressures. This might be expected in view of the air loss during phonation and the natural tendency for the speaker to attempt to compensate for this loss with greater driving pressures below the vocal folds. On the other hand, patients with vocal fold paralysis may produce greater pressures (and therefore greater flows) because of their inability to achieve glottal closure during the vibratory cycle.

Laryngoscopic Signs

The typical laryngoscopic view in unilateral paralysis is that of one relatively immobile vocal fold that does not adduct during phonation, while the unaffected fold moves to the midline. There may be some apparent movement of the affected vocal fold caused by movements of other structures, or by contraction of the cricothyroid (assuming an intact SLN), which will tend to exert some adductory force on the vocal folds (as described earlier), or perhaps the affected fold is driven by air pressure. Movement in the pyriform sinus on the affected side may be reduced or absent (Brewer and Gould, 1974) in patients with unilateral vocal fold paralysis. It may be possible to see differences in the horizontal level of the two vocal folds. There seems to be a lack of agreement, however, as to

Table 5.8.
Stroboscopic Signs in Laryngeal Paralysis[a]

1. Abnormal vibration with predominant vertical movements
2. Large irregular amplitudes
3. Poor vocal fold closure
4. Asymmetrical vibration
5. Affected fold seems to flutter
6. Absence of edge deflections (upward, on affected fold)

[a]Adapted from Hirano, Feder, and Bless, 1983.

whether the affected fold assumes a higher or lower position relative to the normal fold (Adran, Demp, and Marland, 1954; Lee, 1973; Ballantyne and Groves, 1978; Casper, Colton, and Brewer, 1985).

Stroboscopic Signs

Hirano, Feder, and Bless (1983) discussed some of the stroboscopic signs seen in patients with peripheral nerve paralysis. These signs will vary depending on the severity of involvement and the type of problem, that is, superior or recurrent nerve involvement, or both. A summary of the important signs they report for unilateral adductor paralysis is presented in Table 5.8.

Kitzing (1985) reported that stroboscopic signs in vocal fold paresis include vocal fold asymmetry and aperiodicity, greater than normal vibratory amplitudes, absence of a mucosal wave, and incomplete glottal closure. These signs are consistent with the nature of the disease and the perceptual, acoustic, physiological, and laryngoscopic signs discussed earlier.

Pathophysiology

A paralyzed vocal fold may be unable to move to (adduct) or away from (abduct) the midline. Voice problems are most commonly associated with unilateral adductorparalysis. In bilateral adductor paralysis, the voice problem is great but the patient's primary and potentially life-threatening problem, in need of urgent attention, will be loss of protection of the airway and the attending risk of aspiration. The incidence of unilateral laryngeal paralysis is much greater than that of bilateral paralysis. Patients with bilateral abductor paralysis may present with acceptable voices but severe airway problems and may suffer significant air hunger. This life-threatening situation takes precedence over any vocal concerns.

In unilateral paralysis, the affected fold cannot move to the midline and assist in closure of the glottis. Because of this incomplete closure, greater than normal airflows and a weak voice will be produced. The affected fold may also exhibit muscle tensions vastly different from the unaffected cord, resulting in asymmetrical tension and the exhibition of greater aperiodicity in the voice. This will be perceived as greater roughness or hoarseness. A difference in level between the two folds may also contribute to the increased aperiodicity and excessive airflow, although its precise effect remains unknown.

Summary

Vocal fold vibration depends on an intact neurological system in order to maintain the proper tension in the vocal folds, produce the proper airflow and air pressures needed for voicing, and adduct or abduct the vocal folds in accord with the requirements of the speaking act. Disruption of this control will affect the normal vibration of the vocal folds. This disruption may occur either in the central or the peripheral nervous system. When lesions occur in the peripheral nervous system, the phonatory system will show signs of denervation and flaccidity. The muscles controlled by the nerves will fail to receive the proper innervation and will not contract.

When lesions occur within the central nervous system, the phonatory system may show signs of flaccidity or hyperfunction depending on the site of the lesion(s). Lesions high in the central nervous system but not in the cortex affecting the pyramidal or extrapyramidal systems will produce hypertonia and exaggerated reflexes. Lesions in the cerebellum will produce deficits in the control of muscles, especially groups of muscles needed for the complex motor act of speech. The signs and symptoms of phonatory difficulty that develop will depend on the site of lesion. A good working knowledge of the appropriate physical signs and symptoms as well as the voice signs and symptoms is needed before the clinician can properly diagnose and/or understand the nature of the difficulty presented by a patient. In this chapter we have presented an overview of many different neurological problems in which voice may be affected, including parkinsonism, myasthenia gravis, amyotrophic lateral sclerosis, Shy-Drager syndrome, multiple sclerosis, cerebellar ataxia, spastic dysphonia, essential tremor, and many of the problems that may affect the recurrent and superior laryngeal nerves when they exit the central nervous system or as they travel in the neck and thorax to their ultimate destinations.

6

Voice Problems Associated with Organic Disease and Trauma

The conditions discussed in this chapter represent various organic disease states that have an effect on phonation. The etiology of these conditions is unrelated to ways in which the voice has been used, and their treatment is primarily medical and/or surgical. It is important for clinicians to be familiar with these conditions and their effect on phonatory physiology, and to be prepared to offer the appropriate level of service as the need for it becomes timely. The conditions include keratosis, granulomas, pachydermia laryngis, ankylosis of the cricoarytenoid joint, papillomas, carcinoma and other malignancies, blunt or penetrating trauma, and chemical or heat trauma.

Benign Lesions

Keratosis

Primary Voice Symptom

The primary voice symptom is hoarseness.

Description and Etiology

Keratosis refers to epithelial lesions in which there is abnormal tissue growth on the vocal folds (Fig. 6.1). Other terms may be used to describe this condition, including leukoplakia, hyperkeratosis, keratosis with cellular atypia, and dyskeratosis. Two kinds of lesions may be seen: flat, white, plaque-like lesions (leukoplakia) or irregular growth of epithelium that results in a warty lesion (papillary keratosis). There is a full spectrum of

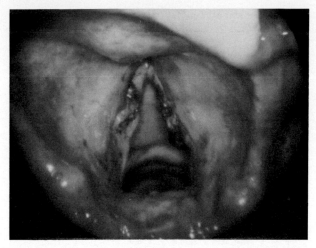

Figure 6.1. Hyperkeratosis of the vocal folds. (Color photograph on page xiii by Eiji Yanagisawa, M.D.)

premalignant laryngeal tissue changes observed in smokers that are not seen in non-smokers (U.S. Dept. of Health and Human Services, 1982). These lesions must be carefully monitored.

Smoking, environmental pollutants, and other factors have been implicated in the development of keratotic epithelium on the vocal folds. These lesions tend to occur more often in males than females.

Perceptual Signs and Symptoms

The primary symptom is hoarseness or roughness in the voice.

Acoustic Signs

There are few data available on the acoustic characteristics of patients with keratosis of the vocal folds. Due to the growths on the vocal folds, greater than normal frequency and amplitude perturbation as well as greater than normal spectral noise would be expected.

Physiological Signs

Minimal physiological data exist on patients with keratosis of the vocal folds. Iwata, von Leden, and Williams (1972) reported a mean airflow rate of 227 ml/sec for patients with leukoplakia of the vocal folds. Lesions that might have a similar effect (papilloma, epitheial hyperplasia) also show greater than normal airflows (see Table 3.6 in Hirano, 1981b).

Laryngoscopic Signs

In patients with leukoplakia, there will be whitish plaque-like lesions on the mucosal surface of the vocal folds. These may be limited in extent or may cover almost the entire vocal fold. Ballenger (1985) reports that another form of this lesion, papillary keratosis, may show a piling up of small, reddish epithelium or an irregular mucosa covered by keratin.

Stroboscopic Signs

There are few data on the stroboscopic signs in hyperkeratosis. In extensive lesions, diminished amplitude of vibration and limited mucosal waves, especially over the sites occupied by the lesion, would be expected. With superficial hyperkeratosis, we have seen a normal mucosal wave. If fact, this stroboscopic feature may be important in distinguishing keratosis from cancer, because in carcinoma there is usually little or no mucosal wave over the site of the lesion.

Pathophysiology

Keratotic-type lesions, for the most part, affect the cover, increasing its mass and stiffness.

Granulomas

Primary Voice Symptom

The primary symptom is hoarseness.

Description and Etiology

Granulomas most commonly are a complication of intubation (Fig. 6.2). It may be an early complication occurring at some point between intubation and extubation, or a late complication, the morbid sequelae of extubation (Balestrieri and Watson, 1982). The passing of an intubation tube between the vocal processes may be necessary in order to provide access to the airway for purposes of delivering anesthesia and maintaining appropiate oxygenation during a surgical procedure. Intubation may also be necessary in nonsurgical situations to maintain adequate oxygen supply for persons in need of respiratory assistance. Contact between the tube and the vocal processes may occur at the time of intubation or with the tube in situ. During such contact the mucoperichondrium of the vocal processes may be traumatized, causing a small ulcer to appear on the vocal process. The bare process will eventually be covered by granulation tissue, which will become epithelialized and present as a granuloma. The condition is surprisingly uncommon in light of the frequency with which intubation is required, and spontaneous resolution occurs within a few weeks in most cases. The incidence of granuloma is dependent on factors such as duration of intubation, the method of intubation, the patient's age and general condition, nursing techniques, and other factors. All reported cases have occurred in patients 15 years or older, and women are more prone to develop an intubation granuloma because of small laryngeal size and a thinner mucosal layer covering the vocal processes (Snow, Marano, and Balogh, 1966).

Endotracheal intubation is being accepted for longer and longer periods of time. Although it is not a benign procedure, mortality and morbidity rates, when compared to the option of tracheotomy, are much lower. Weymuller (1988) presents a thorough review of the pertinent factors relating to endotracheal injury, its nature, the biomechanical factors of the tube itself, and the efforts made to prevent injury from the procedure. A prototype endotracheal tube using a foam cuff is described, and initial results of its use in animals have shown an absence of the typical injury expected even after a 2-week period of intubation. If adopted, it appears that the tube's use could substantially reduce the injurious effects of endotracheal intubation and reduce trauma to the vocal folds and larynx.

Perceptual Signs and Symptoms

The symptoms of granuloma are breathiness and hoarseness.

Acoustic Signs

There are no data on the acoustic characteristics of patients with granulomas. Greater than normal frequency and amplitude perturbation would be expected, and depending on the severity of the hoarseness, greater than normal spectral noise could be present.

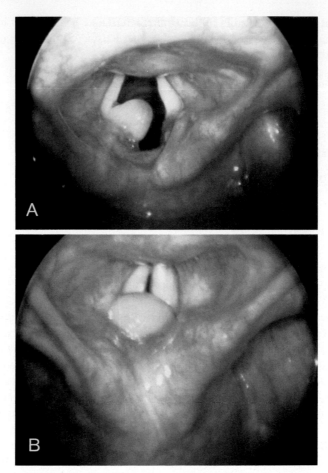

Figure 6.2.   Granuloma involving the posterior part of the glottis. **A,** The granuloma during respiration. **B,** During phonation. (Color photographs on pages xiii and xiv by Eiji Yanagisawa, M.D.)

Physiological Signs

Normal airflow rates have been reported in patients with contact granulomas (see Table 3.7 in Hirano, 1981a). Few other physiological data are available on the physiological characteristics associated with granulomas of the vocal folds.

Laryngoscopic Signs

Granulomas manifest themselves laryngoscopically as irregularly shaped masses of tissue either at the site of the vocal processes of the arytenoids (if an intubation granuloma) or elsewhere on the vocal folds or larynx (Friedman, 1973).

Stroboscopic Signs

The vocal folds will show normal stroboscopic signs unless the granuloma appears on the vocal fold margins, which may affect the mucosal wave and closure.

Pathophysiology

Intubation granulomas affect the mucosa of the vocal processes of the arytenoids.

Pachydermia Laryngis

Primary Vocal Symptom

The primary vocal symptom is hoarseness.

Description and Etiology

This is a relatively rare problem whose etiology is unknown. Some suspect smoking and other irritants to be the major cause. Pachydermia laryngis is characterized by a thickening of the epithelium with acanthosis and keratosis (Ballenger, 1985). Clinically it appears as a whitish mass of tissue in the interarytenoid space. The membranous vocal folds may also be injected and thickened. Conservative treatment although minimally effective, usually consists of voice rest and cessation of smoking and alcohol use. Surgical removal may be necessary.

Perceptual Signs and Symptoms

Hoarseness will be a primary perceptual sign of this disease.

Acoustic Signs

There are few data on the acoustic signs for this vocal problem. A lower fundamental frequency may be expected if the vocal folds are thickened sufficiently.

Physiological Signs

We have no knowledge of physiological data on this vocal problem. One might expect that if the lesion interfered with glottal closure, excessive airflows would result.

Laryngoscopic Signs

On direct or indirect laryngoscopy, the vocal folds may look thickened and rough, and there is an excess of rough, uneven tissue present in the interarytenoid space.

Stroboscopic Signs

We know of no data concerning the stroboscopic signs associated with pachydermia laryngis. Glottal closure may be compromised, and there may be abnormal mucosal waves due to the thickened mucosa.

Papilloma

Primary Voice Symptom

The primary vocal symptom is hoarseness.

Description and Etiology

Papilloma is a rather common benign tumor that affects the epithelium and is thought to be caused by a virus, probably of the papovavirus group. It occurs in both children and adults. In children it is referred to as juvenile papilloma, and it is very resistant to eradication. Surgical excision is required, as papillomas tend to proliferate and can obstruct the airway. It is not uncommon for children with this problem to require multiple surgical excisions before the condition runs its course. If juvenile papilloma persists or begins in adulthood, it continues to be a condition that is highly resistant to treatment. The papilloma may occur in various parts of the larynx: subglottally, at the level of the vocal folds, and supraglottally. It is sometimes necessary for children with aggressive papilloma

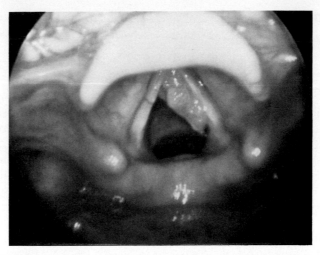

Figure 6.3. Papilloma of the vocal folds. (Color photograph on page xiv by Eiji Yanagisawa, M.D.)

growth to undergo tracheotomy. When the papillomas have ceased recurring, or perhaps between episodes of recurrence, voice therapy may be appropriate in order to maintain or restore the best possible voice production. The prognosis will depend largely on the state of the vocal fold mucosa.

Perceptual Signs and Symptoms

Hoarseness is the primary symptom and sign of the voice disorder caused by this condition. Because of the sometimes extensive involvement of the true vocal folds, a low pitch level might also be evident, although there are no data to support this hypothesis.

Physiological Signs

We know of no physiological data reported for individuals with papillomas of the vocal folds.

Laryngoscopic Signs

A papilloma will typically present as a whitish cluster of tissue, somewhat comparable in texture to a raspberry. An example of the laryngoscopic appearance of a papilloma is shown in Figure 6.3. In Figure 6.4 multiple papillomas are evident, illustrating the potentially extensive nature of the disease.

Stroboscopic Signs

We know of no data on the stroboscopic signs of papillomas. One might expect to find little mucosal wave and perhaps poor glottal closure. When multiple surgical excisions have been required for vocal fold papilloma, the membranous cover of the vocal folds may have been sufficiently damaged so that there may be a reduced or absent mucosal wave.

Pathophysiology

Papillomas affect vocal fold vibration by increasing the mass of the vocal folds and altering the biomechanical characteristics of the mucosa. Although they can be removed surgically, preferably with a CO_2 laser, the lesions tend to recur, especially in children

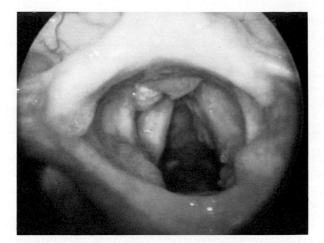

Figure 6.4. Multiple papillomas of the vocal folds. (Color photograph on page xiv by Eiji Yanagisawa, M.D.)

(Bastian, 1986). Treatment with interferon has been tried but with inconclusive results (Benjamin, Gatenby, Kitchen, Harrison, Cameron, and Basten, 1988).

Ankylosis of the Cricoarytenoid Joint

Primary Voice Symptom

The primary vocal symptom is hoarseness.

Description and Etiology

Fixation of the cricoarytenoid joint may be due to several causes, including arthritis, trauma, or joint disease. Ankylosis of the cricoarytenoid joint is sometimes difficult to distinguish from paralysis of the vocal folds. Clinically they appear very similar (Cummings, 1986). However, pain may be a symptom of ankylosis due to arthritis and would usually not be a symptom of paralysis. An attempt to manipulate the joint under direct laryngoscopy may be necessary in order to distinguish between the two conditions. Treatment of ankylosis requires surgical arytenoidectomy or arytenoidopexy (Ballenger, 1985). Voice therapy is usually not helpful.

Perceptual Signs and Symptoms

The primary perceptual symptoms of unilateral arytenoid fixation are hoarseness and breathiness secondary to the anticipated inadequacy of posterior vocal fold closure. In the event that the condition is bilateral, stridor may be present, and the patient may display symptoms of dyspnea.

Acoustic Signs

We know of no experimental data concerning the acoustic characteristics of voice in the presence of cricoarytenoid ankylosis. In unilateral ankylosis, these might include increased frequency and amplitude perturbation (jitter and shimmer), reduced phonational and dynamic ranges, increased spectral noise, and reduced phonation time. Acoustic signs in bilateral ankylosis may be minimal.

Physiological Signs

Physiological signs of ankylosis are not documented. As with unilateral vocal fold paralysis, if the glottis is not fully adducted during phonation, we would expect increased airflows and an electroglottogram that would reveal the incomplete closure and reduced closed time. On the other hand, in the bilateral condition, airflows might be expected to be reduced, and the electrogram should reveal minimal vocal fold opening phase.

Laryngoscopic Signs

As noted previously, the laryngeal appearance of ankylosis might be difficult to distinguish from vocal fold paralysis. If unilateral, we would expect to observe lack of movement of the arytenoid and incomplete glottal closure. In bilateral ankylosis, the position of both arytenoids would be fixed and unmoving, resulting also in lack of either adduction or abduction of the folds. We have observed that in paralysis, movement in the opening to the pyriform sinuses may be absent, while in ankylosis such movement continues to be present. If the cause of ankylosis is an arthritic condition (usually rheumatoid arthritis), mucosal edema, inflammation, or both may be seen in the area of the cricoarytenoid joint.

Stroboscopic Signs

We know of no data on the stroboscopic signs of a fixed arytenoid. One might expect to see incomplete glottal closure, but minimal aberrations in the vibratory motion of the vocal folds.

Pathophysiology

The movement of the ankylosed arytenoid cartilage(s) is reduced or absent. The glottis may be incompletely adducted, or, in the case of bilateral ankylosis, it may be neither fully adducted nor abducted.

Blunt or Penetrating Trauma

A variety of traumatic injuries may affect the larynx. These may include attempted strangulation, a penetrating neck wound, blunt trauma resulting from a blow to the neck or from the body's being hurled with force, and the neck's striking an object. In severe trauma, the structures of the larynx may be fractured or severely damaged, compromising the airway and resulting in vocal difficulty. An example of the effects of trauma to the vocal folds is shown in Figure 6.5.

Most cases of blunt or penetrating trauma require medical/surgical treatment. The most urgent concern is management of the airway. Subsequently there will be an attempt to repair or reconstruct the damaged structures. Voice restoration, following the completion of the repair, may be very difficult. A speech pathologist may be asked to help the patient achieve the best possible voice. In these cases, the speech pathologist should ask for and expect to receive detailed information about the altered laryngeal anatomy, in order to understand the constraints upon the system and to be able to plan the treatment approach accordingly.

Inhalation and Thermal Trauma

There is a paucity of information in the literature about the long-term laryngeal and phonatory sequelae of the inhalation of gases, smoke, or steam. Inhalation injuries are usually referred to as chemical tracheobronchitis, a term that seems to exclude laryngeal

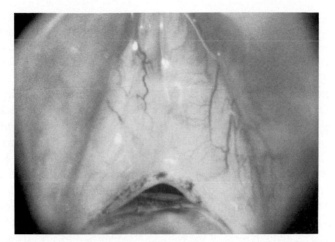

Figure 6.5. Trauma of the vocal folds. (Color photograph on page xiv by Eiji Yanagisawa, M.D.)

and supraglottal effects of such injury even though they occur as frequently and almost always with greater severity (Hunt, Agee, and Pruitt, 1975; Miller, Gray, Cotton, and Myer, 1988). Hot fumes cause reflex closure of the glottis, which, in combination with the cooling capacity of the upper respiratory tract, protects the trachea and lower tract (Miller et al., 1988). Acute airway obstruction can result from either supraglottal or laryngeal edema, or both. Hunt et al. (1975) point out that laryngeal and supraglottal structures tend to show massive amounts of edema in a short period of time due to the loose attachment of the surface mucosa to the underlying basal layers.

During the acute stage, those who suffer inhalation injury are frequently at risk for survival, making their medical condition and treatment of the utmost urgency. The severe edema of the respiratory tract may appear immediately or may develop within a matter of hours and can quickly lead to airway obstruction and to death (Crapo, 1981; Cudmore and Vivori, 1981). Intubation or tracheotomy may be required. A risk of intubation is the possibility of damage to the already compromised mucosal tissue. Symptoms of inhalation trauma include swelling, inflammation, burns, or soot around the nose and mouth and in the oropharynx (even with minimal body surface injury), respiratory distress, stridor, wheezing, and hoarseness (Crapo, 1981). The symptoms will depend on the severity of the trauma, the type of fumes or gases inhaled, and the stage of the body's response to the trauma. The trauma may result not only from heat but also from the particles and toxic chemicals released as the burning material breaks down, and from the reduction in oxygen. The heat capacity of steam is 4000 times greater than that of air; thus, steam inhalation can quickly produce thermal burns of the respiratory tract. Steam inhalation burns may occur with a scald injury in young children. According to Cudmore and Vivori (1981), inhalation of hot, dry gases causes damage primarily to the upper airway (including the larynx) because there is a rapid decrease in temperature of the gases as soon as they enter the airway. Chemical damage to the entire airway results from inhalation of smoke. Smoke from the combustion of polyurethane foams is reported to be especially damaging (Dyer and Esch, 1976). This fact is all the more disturbing in view of the increased numbers of house fires resulting in an increase in inhalation burns in children (Chisnall, 1977) and the increased use of plastics and polyurethane foam.

Voice can only become a concern after the patient has survived the acute stage of trauma and has completed the major portion of treatment for the injuries sustained. If there has been extensive body surface burn in addition to the inhalation injuries, treatment may be quite lengthy. Only when the patient is sufficiently recovered is it appropriate to focus on aspects of vocal recovery. However, during that recovery period, consultation by the speech/language pathologist may be helpful in establishing the most efficacious means of communication for patients whose ability to communicate has been significantly compromised.

As noted previously, there is little documentation of the long-term effects of laryngeal trauma. Close, Catlin, and Cohn (1980), reporting on the chronic effects of ammonia inhalation burns, cite one case in which breathy phonation was present and showed some improvement with voice therapy. In another instance, severe and progressive hoarseness noted in the early post-trauma stage, apparently resolved spontaneously. Recently 22 patients who had been treated in the regional burn unit at the SUNY Health Science Center over a 10-year period were examined for voice problems (Casper, Clark, and Kellman, unpublished data). Of these, 11 or 50% were judged by an experienced voice clinician to show some degree of voice abnormality that, according to patient reports, was not present prior to the trauma. Although most of the patients so identified had been either intubated or tracheotomized or both, some patients had not experienced either of these procedures. Thus, injury resulting from intubation or tracheotomy cannot fully account for the resulting voice abnormality.

In view of these findings, we would suspect that there are more residual voice problems in inhalation burn survivors than have previously been recognized. The pathophysiology is not well understood and may differ from patient to patient. There are many unanswered questions relative to phonatory function in this population, such as whether problems result from changes in laryngeal mucosa, peripheral nerve damage from the burn or from subsequent surgery, or central nervous system damage due to hypoxia.

Our experience in voice therapy with this population is very limited. Nevertheless, the case study of C. H. is instructive.

CASE STUDY   C. H. was a 17-year-old young man who had suffered extensive burns of the head, neck, face, hands, and upper body, following the crash of an ultralight plane that he had been flying alone. He also suffered inhalation injury. His treatment course included two periods of intubation, the first for a week and the second for 4 days, with a 2-day period between. He survived a long and painful course of treatment and surgeries. Although now he was being followed as an outpatient, he faced further surgery in the future. He was in constant physical pain and discomfort, and his emotional pain due to his grotesquely deformed appearance was perhaps even greater. He was essentially aphonic, as he had been throughout the entire posttrauma course. Ear, nose, and throat examination was reported to be negative, with no observable reason for the aphonia. The vocal folds were reported to show good movement, although they did not adduct completely during speaking.

C. H. responded minimally to questions, offered no information spontaneously, and did not make eye contact with the clinician. He generally kept his eyes downcast or looked out of the window. Several sessions were required to work through this resistance and to establish a relationship. As he began to open up, C. H. talked more about the crash, and also about his parents, who were divorced. He was living with his mother; he would have preferred to have been with his father, but the accident had occurred during a time spent with the father, who was apparently finding the guilt related to the event overwhelming. C. H. was supposed to be returning to school but had thus far been resisting that because he saw himself as a "monster" whom others saw as disgusting. As therapy progressed, C. H. was increasingly willing to attempt voicing. Indeed, he was able to produce voice, but with a hoarse and somewhat breathy quality. The sound of this voice was just one more abnormality that he could not deal with, and his response had been to be aphonic.

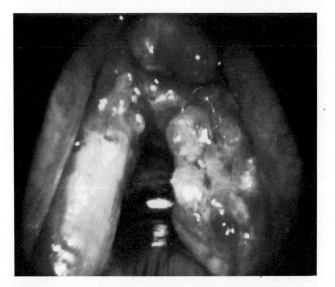

Figure 6.6. Carcinoma of the vocal folds. (Color photograph on page xiv by Eiji Yanagisawa, M.D.)

Work with C. H. continued for a period of time, during which he began to use voice routinely and with some improvement in quality. He was clearly in need of psychological counseling but had previously refused to consider such referral. Leading him to an acceptance of such counseling had been one of the goals of therapy, and indeed, after his experience with us he was able to accept the support that had been offered and to recognize his need for continuation of such support. Although his voice quality was not "normal," C. H. was using voice routinely and finding that communication was easier.

The reason for C. H.'s hoarse voice quality was never fully understood. However, more testing, given his initial level of resistance and the subsequent determination of his very vulnerable psychological state, was not entirely necessary and might result in his withdrawal from further therapy. He made sufficient progress so that his voice was entirely usable, and although still hoarse, was not severely so. The reason for his aphonic presentation appeared to be primarily psychological. This case highlights the need to be alert to more than a single problem being present at one time, especially when there may be an obvious cause that might explain the problem.

Carcinoma and Other Tumors

Carcinoma

Cancer is one of the diseases that may affect the structures of the oral cavity, pharynx, and larynx. If allowed to proceed unchecked, it is life threatening. The incidence of laryngeal cancer is reported to be between 2% and 5% of all malignancies. Persistent hoarseness is well known as one of the primary symptoms of cancer. If a malignant lesion affects one or both vocal folds directly, hoarseness will result. Figure 6.6 shows a cancer involving both vocal folds. Laryngeal lesions that do not affect the vibratory characteristics of the vocal folds will not necessarily result in a change in the voice.

There are many possible etiologies for cancer, including smoking, environmental irritants, chemicals and other contaminants, metabolic disturbances, and unknown causes.

Table 6.1.
Classification of Glottal Cancers[a,b]

T:	Location of primary tumor
	Tx—Cannot be staged
	T0—No evidence of tumor
	Tis—Carcinoma in situ
	T1—Confined to vocal folds
	T2—Supraglottal or subglottal extension, normal or impaired mobility
	T3—Confined to larynx but with fixed cord
	T4—Massive tumor
N:	Involvement of regional lymph nodes
	Nx—Cannot be assessed
	N0—No involvement
	N1—A single small node on one side
	N2—A single large or multiple small nodes on one side
	N3—Massive nodes on one or both sides
M:	Distant metastasis
	Mx—Cannot be assessed
	M0—No known metastasis
	M1—Metastasis present

[a]Adapted from Sasaki and Carlson, 1986.
[b]Based on the American Joint Committee for Cancer Staging and End Results Reporting System, 1983.

According to the Surgeon General's report (U.S. Department of Health and Human Services, 1982), "Cigarette smoking is a major cause of cancers of the lung, larynx, oral cavity and esophagus" (p. vi). Furthermore, 50% to 70% of oral and laryngeal cancer deaths are associated with smoking. The report also states that a synergistic effect is created by the use of alcohol in conjunction with smoking that greatly increases the risk of oral and laryngeal cancers. The ratio of men to women who develop these cancers was reported to be 5 to 1 in 1985 (Ballenger, 1985), but that ratio has been narrowing steadily for the past 20 years. The carcinogenic effects of cigar and pipe smoke are similar to those of cigarette smoke.

The severity of the malignancy is evaluated using the "TNM" system or its variants (American Joint Committee for Cancer Staging and End Results Reporting, 1983). The *T* refers to the site of the primary tumor, the *N* indicates the involvement of lymph nodes, and the *M* signifies spread of the lesion to other parts of the body (metastasis). Low numbers associated with each code indicate a lesser involvement; the numbers increase as severity or extent increase (Table 6.1). Thus, a patient described to have a T1N0M0 lesion has a locally confined tumor with neither node involvement nor any distant metastasis (Fig. 6.7).

The signs of cancer of the larynx may include (*a*) a lump in the neck, (*b*) a broadening of the larynx, detected on palpation; (*c*) tenderness in the neck; and (*d*) hoarseness. Other symptoms may include dysphagia, odynophagia, and dyspnea. Laryngoscopic examination may reveal anything from a small, well-defined tumor to a large and diffuse one involving any part of the larynx or vocal folds. Precise diagnosis of carcinoma usually requires biopsy and histological analysis.

There are several approaches to cancer treatment. These include surgery, radiation therapy, and chemotherapy. Their use depends on many factors and is determined on a case-by-case basis. Spector and Ogura (1985) have discussed some of the considerations in

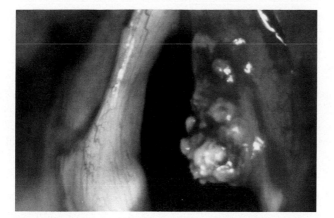
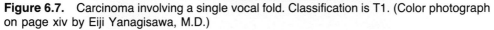

Figure 6.7.   Carcinoma involving a single vocal fold. Classification is T1. (Color photograph on page xiv by Eiji Yanagisawa, M.D.)

the diagnosis and treatment of carcinoma. Patients who undergo radiation therapy as the primary treatment mode may experience some alterations in voice during the course of the treatment (Colton, Sagerman, Chung, Young, and Reed, 1978). Depending on the extent of the lesion, a patient may still have a normal-sounding voice after radiation therapy. Voice therapy is usually not necessary or indicated.

There are a variety of surgical approaches in the treatment of laryngeal cancer, which may involve excision of the lesion, of up to half of the larynx, of supraglottal structures only, or of the entire larynx. The effect on voice production capability will depend on the extent and the nature of the surgery performed. In addition to concerns about voice, patients who have had extensive surgery may also have difficulty with swallowing. A full discussion of the problems of dysphagia and those associated with the total absence of the larynx is beyond the scope of this book. These topics are well covered in the literature.

The voice problems associated with partial laryngeal excisions will vary a great deal. Both voice problems and dysphagia will require the assistance of a speech pathologist. The role of the speech pathologist is to assist the patient in producing the best possible voice. In order to do so, the speech pathologist must be completely informed about the specifics of the surgical procedure. It is important to know what structures remain intact, how the anatomy is altered, and what functional skills remain relative to phonation.

Some patients with laryngeal cancer have extremely extensive disease that requires excision of not only the larynx but also of other structures essential to the production of speech, such as the tongue. The speech pathologist should also be involved with these patients in an effort to provide a means of communication.

Other Tumors

A variety of benign and malignant tumors may be found in the laryngeal or neck area in both children and adults. Such tumors may obstruct the airway directly, or they may occupy space and place pressure on the trachea or larynx, thereby creating airway problems indirectly. The effect on the voice will depend on the position of the tumor. These lesions require medical and/or surgical treatment. In many cases of small or benign tumors, surgery is a viable treatment option. In cases of extensive malignant tumors, radiation therapy or chemotherapy or a combined protocol may be possible treatment choices. Rarely is there need for speech therapy services unless the tumor (or surgery) has compromised vocal or speech function. Tumors that are frequent in children include cysts, hemangiomas, and lymphoangiomas; malignant neuroblastomas and lymphomas also occur. Many of these same tumors may also be found in adults.

Summary

In this chapter, some organic problems that may affect the voice have been reviewed. The etiology of these problems is not related to voice use. However, their effects can drastically alter voice production. A variety of medical and surgical approaches are the primary treatment modalities. Vocal rehabilitation may be helpful in establishing the best voice the patient is capable of producing.

7

The Voice History, Examination, and Testing

Voice History

The clinical skills of the practitioner are critical when working with a patient with a voice problem. The interview with the patient, the search for information, and the elicitation of the history require a combination of art and science. The art is the skill of the clinician with the interview process. The science is the knowledge base that guides the selection of questions and informs the interpretation of responses. The two are inseparable, and there is a constant interplay between them throughout the interview and the treatment. It is not enough to know what questions to ask, if there is no skill in the asking. It is not enough to know what questions to ask, if there is no understanding of their implications or of why it is important to ask. It is not enough to know what questions to ask, and to have skill in the asking, without adequate knowledge and understanding for interpretation of the responses.

Another way to distinguish between what we have referred to as art and science is to think of them as process and content (Reiser and Schroder, 1980). All communication between people involves a process level. It is at this level of communication that many unspoken associations, silent questions, and feelings are expressed by both the patient and the professional through both verbal and nonverbal means. The content level of the interview refers to information specific to the problem.

The Interview Process

Interviewing as a skill and communication with patients are woefully neglected topics in the training of most speech pathologists and physicians. Aronson (1985) states:

Any in-depth study of voice disorders forces us to conclude that so long as clinicians obtain privileged information from patients; so long as people have voice problems because of life stress and interpersonal conflict; so long as voice disorders produce anxiety, depression, embarrassment and self-consciousness; so long as patients need a sympathetic person with whom they can discuss their distress, will speech pathologists [and physicians (author's addition)] need to consider their training incomplete until they have learned the basic skills of psychologic interviewing and counselling. (p. 271)

Aronson presents further rationale for the need for good interviewing and counseling skills and also discusses the personal characteristics clinicians must bring to the process. Although Aronson targets his discussion on the interaction of the clinician with patients whose voice problems are largely of psychological etiology, we feel the concepts are pertinent to interactions with all voice patients.

During the past decade, the field of medicine has shown an increasing awareness of the emotional components of disease processes. Furthermore, there has been recognition of the fact that effective treatment of these components occurs when there is a positive relationship between the patient and the health professional (Bernstein and Bernstein, 1985). The initial interview, usually the history-taking session, establishes the patient-clinician relationship. It is the foundation on which the success of treatment may depend (Hersen and Turner, 1985; Bernstein and Bernstein, 1985).

An interpersonal relationship by definition involves the dynamic interaction of at least two people, each of whom brings emotions, expectations, experience, and knowledge to the process. How these two sets of baggage match up, or fail to do so, will determine how well the process unfolds. Indeed, some studies have indicated that the breakdown in this relationship may be a major cause of malpractice suits (Blum, 1960; Rosenthal, 1978).

The clinical interview is an interaction of a particular type. Its specific purpose is to explore the nature and history of the patient's presenting symptoms. Unfortunately, it occurs within set time limits and a busy office environment. Despite these limitations, the interaction need not and must not be allowed to become rigid with preset boundaries.

Before we become clinicians, we are people who have been socialized into avoiding certain topics of conversation, not asking overly personal questions of relative strangers, and not probing when a topic appears to make our conversational partner uncomfortable. As clinicians we must recognize that clinical interviews are different from social conversations. The professional has not only the right but indeed the obligation to ask personal questions and to probe gently when areas require further exploration. A patient's indication of discomfort or avoidance may be a very important sign to the skilled clinician who knows how to probe without shutting off the flow of information. A clinician can only do this successfully by reaching a level of self-comfort in discussing sensitive areas.

What the Patient Brings to the Process

The patient comes to an evaluation or examination with a heightened sense of anxiety. The patient brings a personal history not only of the current problem but also of previous problems, previous contacts with members of the health professions, relationships, education, social ease, personal needs, and culture. The patient's ethnic background may shape attitudes toward illness and affect interaction with professionals (Bernstein and Bernstein, 1985). The patient may also have need for support and guidance in understanding the current problem. All of these factors will fashion the patient's behavior and responses.

What the Professional Brings to the Process

The most obvious contribution of the professional is expertise with a body of knowledge concerned with voice production. But the professional also brings a history of encounters with many patients, relationships with peers as well as with family and friends, personal needs, and the pressures of time. In the current climate of frequent litigation, the practitioner may also bring a sense of anxiety or wariness to the process, perhaps generating a defensive posture toward the patient.

Bernstein and Bernstein (1985) identify the following as the responsibilities of the professional in the interview process:

1. Assume responsibility for the conduct of the interview.
2. Avoid control and rigidity that inhibits or intimidates the patient.
3. Keep the interview in focus.
4. Maintain flexibility.
5. Remain sensitive to the patient's feelings expressed both verbally and nonverbally.
6. Do not permit expression of subjective, personal feelings.
7. Remain open and accepting of the patient even when the patient is hostile or uncooperative.

To that list we would add that the professional must be able to speak in language tailored to the individual patient—language that the patient can understand and that is neither insulting to the patient's intelligence nor patronizing in manner.

Listening

Although we cannot fully explore all of the crucial aspects of interview skills in a single chapter, the art and skill of listening demands more discussion. A frequent request of beginning clinicians, or of those who have not developed a level of understanding of a particular area sufficient to allow them to be comfortable with it, is for a checklist of questions to ask. Indeed, forms providing such questions are readily available (see Appendix and Wilson and Rice, 1977; Darley and Spriestersbach, 1978; Wilson, 1979, 1987; Boone, 1983). They will, however, prove to be of little help to the inadequately trained clinician. For the trained and skilled practitioner, a form is a convenient way to organize the interview, as long as one recognizes that it is not meant to be adhered to strictly. The value of a form is directly dependent on the skill of the clinician in conducting the interview and extracting the relevant information.

Attentive and sensitive listening on the part of the professional, rather than extensive talking, is the key. Some argue that engaging in note taking during an interview is disruptive to the process of attentive listening. Furthermore, patients may be influenced to focus on specific areas if the clinician's note taking appears to indicate those as areas of importance. Others, however, feel that patients are made to feel confident about the importance of their reporting when they observe the practitioner taking notes. Whichever system is used by a given clinician, it is important that the taking of notes be done in such a way as to minimize interference with active and attentive listening.

Listening is more than hearing the spoken words. It involves observation of facial expressions, both as one's questions are heard and during the response. It involves observation of body language. It involves attention to the sound of the voice, the suprasegmentals of stress and inflection and prosody. And it involves hearing messages sometimes hidden behind the words, the well-known "listening with the third ear" (Reik, 1948), and utilizing the sixth sense of feelings or intuitions (Browne and Freeling, 1976). If the clinician is focused on self or the next question to be asked, all of this will be missed. Indeed, much information will never be elicited.

As a component of developing good listening skills, it is necessary to develop a tolerance for moments of silence. The beginning or nonconfident clinician tends to abhor silence, and the very busy and rushed clinician has no time for it. Moments of reflection, of allowing the patient to provide additional information or sometimes to raise a new point, can be exceedingly valuable. The silence must be a comfortable one, however, in which the clinician must nonverbally project a sense of ease and of understanding.

Listening well need not be a lengthy process. Good listening skills enable the clinician to shape and control the interview. A balance must be maintained between the patient's need to talk and the clinician's need to elicit pertinent information. The clinician learns to pick up the important cues, to follow them while always targeting the problem, to ask directed questions when indicated, and to refocus responses when necessary. Patients will usually provide all the information needed by the professional, if they can be helped to express it in their own way in an environment of understanding and acceptance.

It is difficult to learn the skill of interviewing by reading about it. Our intent here is not to exhaust the topic but rather to raise it and recognize its importance. It is so extremely important when dealing with voice patients because of the very close linkage between voice and personality and emotional states. There are readily available resources that provide skills training in listening and in interview skills. We would strongly urge that all academic courses in voice disorders incorporate such skills training as part of the curriculum. Suggested readings on interviewing may be found at the end of this chapter.

Before leaving this topic, we must not ignore the use of history questionnaires that can be completed by patients prior to their appointments. There is some value in the use of such questionnaires because they make it possible for patients to review personal medical records, to validate their impressions against those of other family members or friends, and to think about the issues raised by their answers. However, if questionnaires are taken at face value, they clearly eliminate the immensely important interview process and abort the establishment of a relationship between the patient and the clinician. If such forms are to be used, it is very important for their contents to be reviewed verbally, allowing the patient to elaborate and clarify and opening the door for further probing by the clinician.

Content of the Interview: The Case History

The Problem

After initial introductions and review of identifying and demographic data, it is usually appropriate to begin the interview by asking the nature of the problem that has brought the patient for the examination. Not only is this a natural place to begin the interview, but the patient's response may hold a vast amount of information. The clinician will begin to get an impression of how aware the patient is of the problem, how articulate the person is in providing descriptive information, and what the patient's level of concern or motivation is relative to the problem. It is important to recognize that these early impressions should be recognized as just that—impressions, which need to be verified or altered as the interview progresses. Indeed, what eventually results from the interview and subsequent examination may be quite different from the concerns voiced initially. Nevertheless, it is important to have this starting point.

Some patients will provide an almost nonstop narrative in response to the very first question, whereas others will have to be prodded and asked many questions. Either type of patient will require that the clinician manage the questioning skillfully so as to obtain all the important information without being either drowned by trivia or blinded by an absence of response. It is important to ask many open-ended questions in an attempt to elicit information without putting words into the patient's mouth. For example, the open-ended request "Tell me about the problem that brought you to see me today" may bring a more complete response than "I understand you are here because you have a polyp on your vocal folds."

In response to the question concerning the nature of the problem, it is helpful to obtain the patient's description of the sound of his voice and how it differs from other voices or from his own preproblem voice. We have found that patients often are accurate in describing the problem and that their statement of the primary symptom is an important one.

It is instructive to ask what patients believe may have caused the problem or what they have been told about the problem by others they have consulted. Patients frequently indicate a lack of understanding, or perhaps a misunderstanding, of information received from the physician. It is not unusual for a patient to say, "My doctor said I have polyps or something growing in my throat, but I don't know what that means or what it has to do with my being sent to you." Other patients, of course, can quote the dates of office visits, procedures that were done, and their outcome. Despite what they have been told, or in the absence of having been given any information, patients often have their own ideas about the cause of the problem. Frequently heard comments include "It's this postnasal drip," "It's probably my sinus condition," and "I think I'm allergic." It is important for the clinician to recognize that patients frequently have difficulty giving up such ideas, even when they are unsubstantiated, and that the inability to do so may compromise the treatment program. Therefore, it will be important for these issues to be raised at the appropriate time in the process, and for the patient to be provided with information that is understandable and acceptable. The nature of the clinician-patient relationship established during the initial contact will have an important impact on this subsequent interaction and the patient's acceptance of new ideas.

Effect of the Voice Problem

If the patient has not spontaneously provided comments concerning the effect of the voice problem on his life, it is important to ask about this as a follow-up question. Once again, this information will help the clinician to understand the degree of importance of the problem to the patient. Voice problems may exert profound effects on people, including depression, anxiety, withdrawal, embarrassment, and self-consciousness. Indeed, a voice problem may have a profound effect on the individual's total being. On the other hand, for some the voice problem may be a minor embarrassment or have little effect on lifestyle. The severity of this reaction is not always directly related to the severity of the voice problem. Equally as important is information as to what effect the problem has had on family members, on work-related activities, and on co-workers or superiors—that is, on all aspects of the person's life. Some patients may express denial of a problem and a lack of personal concern. Such statements must be fully explored before they are accepted as valid. Feelings expressed by the patient in this discussion must be listened to carefully. The clinician must use skill in helping the patient to discuss feelings openly without fear of being judged or humiliated.

Developmental History of the Problem

Very valuable information may be obtained from this section of the case history. It is important to learn as much as possible not only about the onset of the current episode but also about how it has developed. Information relative to previous episodes of voice difficulty and any prior treatment and outcome must be known. When patients suggest dissatisfaction with the outcome of previous treatment, it is well to inquire whether there is any litigation in progress or in planning. This information may sometimes be obtained in an oblique or indirect manner rather than by a direct, confrontational question. In some instances patients may have been referred by a lawyer specifically for a second opinion. This knowledge may have little impact on your assessment of the patient, but it is helpful to know it in advance, and it may have some impact on the degree to which the entire interaction is documented.

Onset

The onset of a voice problem may be gradual or precipitous. Why is this a critical piece of information? In understanding the natural history of the development of laryngeal pathologies, we know that it is most likely that certain problems will develop over a period of time, while others may have a very sudden onset. While some patients can provide only rather vague information about the onset of the problem, others will provide the date, time, and exactly what they were doing at the very moment that the problem began. Clues to the diagnosis may be contained in each of these types of responses, as well as in the host of responses that lie between these two extremes. Patients frequently date the onset of the symptoms of a problem to another stressful occurrence in their lives. This is a natural tendency that can sometimes be misleading if accepted without full and careful exploration. Another common report is the association of an episode of laryngitis or upper respiratory infection with the onset of the current problem. This event may indeed have some bearing on the problem, but it requires verification.

Most laryngeal lesions develop over time. An exception to that would be the apparently rapid development of a polyp coinciding with a specific episode of excessively strenuous voice use. Patients have reported the sensation of a sudden, sharp pain during shouting or loud, stressful singing, with the subsequent finding of a hemorrhagic polyp. We know that professional singers may show evidence of beginning nodules immediately after a performance; these usually resolve spontaneously if the voice is allowed to rest in a state of less strenuous use.

The majority of patients with laryngeal growths of various types that affect the vibratory behavior of the vocal folds and thus the sound of the voice report a gradual onset of voice symptoms over a period of weeks, months, or even years. Often they describe early episodes of voice change lasting only brief periods of time, with return to what they describe as normal voice. The episodes increase in frequency and in duration over time, and the normal voice does not return. By the time they seek medical attention, the problem may have become chronic and be worsening.

Voice changes that result from vocal misuse, including increased musculoskeletal tension, also tend to run a gradual course even though observable laryngeal pathology may not be present. Indeed, it is not uncommon for patients to be totally unaware of when or how a problem developed. Small,gradual changes tend not to be noticed, and persons unaware of these minor changes show little or no concern until a more obvious change is noticed either by themselves, a friend, or a family member.

Neurologically based voice problems may have either a sudden or a gradual onset. Progressive deteriorating neurological diseases that affect the voice tend to do so in a gradual manner, while the precipitous nature of a stroke or a head injury may have an equally precipitous effect on voice production. Recurrent laryngeal nerve paralysis is not an uncommon result of severing the nerve during thyroid surgery (Johns and Rood, 1987). Obviously, the resulting voice problem will be immediately noted postoperatively. However, the history provided by patients with idiopathic recurrent laryngeal nerve paralysis is not so clear. Some patients report a slight voice change at first, with worsening of the voice symptoms over a relatively short period of time. Others report a very sudden change that neither worsens nor improves.

The voice of the adolescent male that fails to lower in pitch despite normal laryngeal growth no longer sounds exactly like it did prior to laryngeal growth, but it usually takes months, or more likely years, for it to be recognized as unusual.

Sudden, marked vocal change that can be pinpointed as to date and time, in the absence of other symptoms suggestive of an organic etiology, is often the first clue of a psychogenic dysphonia. It is important to caution, once again, that the process of differential diagnosis involves the exploration of all facets of a problem and does not allow for premature conclusions. Clues such as this must be viewed as only one piece of a puzzle, and the clinician must be careful to maintain an open mind so as not to overlook important information that might not fit a preconceived notion.

Duration

When a voice problem has occurred in a sudden manner, its effect on the person is usually more disturbing than a gradual change, and as a result, consultation may be sought more quickly. Nevertheless, it has been our experience that a period of months has usually elapsed from the onset of the problem to the time the person is referred for a voice evaluation. The pattern usually involves a period of consultation and treatment with the family physician, pediatrician, or other practitioner, followed by referral to an otolaryngologist. Another period of treatment may ensue, and if the problem persists, referral is made to a voice management team, to an otolaryngologist who specializes in laryngeal problems, or to a speech pathologist.

As noted previously, many problems have a gradual onset or may have been tolerated at a low level of dysfunction for lengthy periods of time. It is often not possible to determine how long a condition has been present. The germane question, then, is, does it matter? And the answer is yes—and maybe. Obviously, if the patient's problem involves a malignant lesion, time is of the essence. The earlier a malignancy is identified, the more positive the prognosis and the less traumatic the treatment. Early identification of any organic condition is, of course, a desired goal. It is easier to obtain resolution of a small, soft, new nodule than one that has become increasingly fibrotic over time. It is also easier to change abusive habits that have not had a lengthy period to develop. Early identification of certain neurological disease processes may allow early treatment of symptoms, if possible, although such treatment may not change the course of the disease. Early diagnosis and treatment of psychogenic dysphonias may shorten the period of time during which the patient must be dysfunctional.

The clinician needs to obtain the best estimate possible of the duration of the problem. This information, put into context, will help the clinician plan a treatment protocol.

Variability Versus Consistency

The reporting of these characteristics of a voice problem is very important. It is unlikely, for example, for a person with paralysis of the recurrent laryngeal nerve to report much variability in voice production from hour to hour or day to day. (It is important to recognize, however, that return of nerve function and thus return of normal voice may occur in cases of idiopathic paralysis. This would not constitute variability of symptoms so much as a change or improvement of voice.) We would not expect a person with a mass lesion to experience periods of normal voice. Such a patient may report improved voice for periods of time, but if questioned carefully it will become apparent that improved does not mean a return to normal voice. Another caution here is that patients who have experienced months or years of disordered or changed voice may no longer have a very clear auditory memory of how they used to sound, nor be sensitive to minor variability.

Variability in voice production can be understood in the light of certain neurological disorders. For example, patients with myasthenia gravis may experience periods of entirely normal voice production but will report a gradual worsening of voice with prolonged speaking and increased fatigue. Patients with voice disorders of psychological origin frequently report much variability in voice production. This variability, usually unpredictable, may occur throughout the day, from day to day, or at other time intervals.

Some patients report that their voices are at their worst in the morning, for the first hour or two after arising. Such report should raise the suspicion of esophageal reflux problems associated with a hiatal hernia. Such reflux frequently occurs while the person is sleeping in the prone position, allowing acidic stomach contents to actually wash up over the posterior laryngeal areas, including the arytenoids.

Variability of voice production may be situation related, use related, or related to general physical well-being. Voice-disordered patients frequently report a worsening of vocal function when under stress and when physically fatigued. Both of those states have a tendency to exacerbate any existing condition, but the clinician must not assume psychological causation based on such reports. When patients report variability in symptoms, they should routinely be asked to describe those things that seem to make the problem better and those that make it worse.

Once again, it is important to emphasize that in order to understand the implications of information received, the clinician's knowledge base must include awareness of the ways in which phonation can be affected by pathology and use factors.

Associated Symptoms and Sensations

It is always important to ask patients about any other symptoms they may have experienced that they associate with the voice problem. These may include difficulty in swallowing, slurring of speech, loss of fluids through the nose, weight loss, excessive coughing, increased fatigue, heartburn, and the like. In addition, it is important to inquire about sensations in the neck, throat, and larynx, either accompanying phonation or at other times. Patients with patterns of vocal abuse and increased musculoskeletal tension frequently report the sensation of pain localized lateral to the larynx and a feeling of fatigue. It is not uncommon for a patient to say, "I just feel my throat is too tired to talk." Some patients with mass lesions or laryngeal irritation report the sensation of a constant lump in the throat and a need to strain to produce voice loud enough to be heard. A feeling of dryness in the mouth and throat is often reported. Reporting of many other sensations may be provided by the patient. Such reports may be helpful not only in the diagnostic process but also as useful indicators of change in response to treatment.

Patient History

Voice Use

Exploration of how much a person talks and of where and how the voice is used constitutes a crucial part of the total history. An individual's job and lifestyle may not give indication of excessive or abusive voice use until it is discovered that she is or was a cheerleader, or he is the soloist in a church choir, or she performs with an amateur theater group.

There are specific concerns relative to voice use and, indeed, the entire voice history, if the patient is a professional voice user, that is, a singer, actor, or public speaker. Of major importance is whether or not the person has had professional voice training. It has been our experience that among the most difficult patients to treat are singers who have had no vocal training but who have had a few years of success in singing with a small group or choir, or in amateur theatrical productions. They have not recognized their abusive vocal behavior, which now has "caught up with them," often resulting in laryngeal tissue changes. It is difficult for these patients to understand or accept the fact that what they have been doing is what constitutes the problem.

Vocal performers work in a variety of settings and environments and engage in many styles of performance. Some must sing above the sound of amplified music, while others perform in large areas without adequate amplification; some use a belting style, some sing rock, some perform in smoke-filled rooms, and some may be performing at night after rehearsing all day. The vocal demands of actors' scripts vary from job to job. All of these factors must be explored. Not to be forgotten, however, are the nonperformance vocal demands and voice habits of professional voice users. It is not at all uncommon for well-trained performers who have learned their art to use their voices well when singing or on stage but to show little transfer of those habits to everyday speaking behavior. In addition, professional voice users are not immune to vocal abuse when engaging in noisy postperformance parties, loud talking backstage, teaching, and during other strenuous uses of the speaking voice. Sataloff (1987a,1987b, 1987c) presents a thorough discussion of the voice history to be used with professional singers, as well as samples of case history forms.

Children constitute another group for whom the voice use history must be carefully investigated. Some children may use their voices at appropriate levels and in acceptable ways much of the time, but the voice of the playground may be excessively loud, or making "weird sounds" may be a hobby. There are, of course, children who use their voices loudly and aggressively much of the time.

The voice and the manner of voice usage demonstrated in the office situation during the initial visit may not be an accurate reflection of potentially abusive voice use on the job, at the playground, or in the home. It is necessary to explore all these areas thoroughly during the interview and perhaps pursue them further during the voice evaluation.

Health

Because the voice is such an integral part of the whole person, it serves to reflect not only emotional states and personality but also physical states. We recognize the weak voice of the very ill, the lifeless voice of the pharmacologically subdued, or the tired voice of the physically exhausted. It has been said that the whole person "is considered to be greater than the sum of its parts; each part can only be understood in the context of the whole; a change in any one part will affect every other part" (Papp, 1983). It is for these reasons that the voice history must explore a patient's health history. The vital importance of the proper functioning of all body systems for the professional singer has been described by Sataloff (1987a, 1987b, 1987c), who provides as one example the effect a broken leg may have in altering the singer's posture, thereby affecting abdominal support for singing.

It is most appropriate to inquire first about the patient's present health status. We are most interested in whether the patient has any neurological problems, respiratory problems, problems affecting the gastrointestinal tract, allergy-related problems, or psychiatric problems; suffers from any chronic conditions such as arthritis; has any congenital anomalies or hearing loss; or has any other current health problem. The past health history, which may be relevant to the present vocal difficulty, is also important, as is the patient's history of surgeries and hospitalizations. It is important to know the nature of surgical procedures that the patient has undergone, particularly those that may have some connection to the present difficulty, such as laryngeal, head and neck, thoracic, or cardiac surgery. For example, a history of appendectomy at 4 years of age may not be pertinent in the case of a 35-year-old patient. However, the history of cardiac surgery in that same patient should be explored to determine whether any sequelae of that surgery were directly related in time to the onset of the voice problem. What kind of sequelae may accompany such surgery? The most obvious might be hoarseness following intubation. However, recalling the course of the left recurrent laryngeal nerve, injury to that nerve might also be a possible sequelae of cardiac surgery.

When exploring the surgical and hospitalization histories of a patient, it is important to learn either from the patient or from medical records whether the patient was intubated and, if so, whether it was a difficult or traumatic intubation, the duration of the intubation, and whether there is a time relationship between the procedure and the present voice problem.

Another related area to be explored is whether or not the patient has experienced any trauma, the effects of which might have an impact on the structure of the larynx or the mucosa. Some possible categories of such trauma would be blows to the neck, knife or gun wounds, automobile or other vehicular accidents, chemical ingestion or inhalation, and body burns or thermal inhalation.

A thorough history of substance use is important and takes some skill to elicit truthfully and completely. Substance abuse, that is, excessive use of alcohol or illegal drugs, is often not readily admitted. Questions about these areas must be asked in the same manner as inquiries into all other areas. The clinician must, however, be prepared to pursue vague responses or to probe further if there is reason to believe that the patient may be withholding information. It is often necessary for patients to be reassured about the confidential nature of the interaction. But patients do not seem to be reticent in divulging a history of tobacco use even when it is quite excessive.

There is widespread use of over-the-counter and prescription drugs in the treatment of illness or various physical discomforts. Because drugs work systemically, they often have an effect on all mucosa or tissues, not just that which is being targeted. For example, diuretics are used in many conditions in which release of fluids from body tissues is desired. However, it must be recognized that the laryngeal mucosa is not exempt from the diuretic action. Whereas release of excess body fluid may be very helpful to a person with certain medical conditions, the associated drying of laryngeal mucosa may have a negative effect on phonation.

Because the effect of various drugs on the laryngeal mucosa and laryngeal motor control is such an important yet relatively unreported area, additional information on it was presented in Chapter 4.

Vocational

It is not sufficient to simply obtain a person's occupation. It is necessary to discuss the nature of the work done, the environment in which it is done, the need for an adequate voice to carry out the job requirements, interactions with co-workers and superiors, and the level of job satisfaction. In this area, as well as throughout the history taking, open-ended questions such as "Tell me about your job and the people with whom you work" may elicit more complete information than closed questions such as "Do you need to talk as part of your work?"

Social

The focus of questioning in this area is designed to obtain information about the patient's lifestyle, family constellation, and even living arrangements. Environmental factors such as lack of adequate humidification or the use of a wood stove may have adverse effects on laryngeal tissues. People often do not recognize vocally abusive behavior that may occur in the home when yelling to the children or pets who are out in a large backyard or upstairs in another part of a house. Perhaps a hard-of-hearing person is a member of the family, requiring louder than usual voice usage. Home life is replete with examples of the need to raise the intensity level of the voice: talking above the television or music, talking above the level of others' speech in order to gain their attention, arguments. If the lifestyle includes much entertaining of large groups or frequenting of bars where extremely loud music is a constant background noise, vocal abuse may well be involved in the voice problem. Relationships with family members or ''significant others'' may be a source of stress or anxiety, that may be reflected in a problem with the voice.

Recreational

Certain recreational activities may have implications for the voice. For example, the weightlifter who strains mightily while lifting, simultaneously producing harsh, grunting phonation, is placing considerable stress on the laryngeal tissues, and so, too, the golfer or tennis player who phonates with each swing of the club or racket. Forceful phonation accompanying strenuous exercise of any type may constitute abusive behavior.

Psychological

Placing this information at the end of this section should not suggest that it has the least importance. Indeed, psychological factors may be of utmost etiological importance. Furthermore, as stated previously, all disease processes carry components of emotional stress.

Throughout this chapter, and elsewhere in this book, frequent reference is made to the close link between voice and personality, voice and self-identity, voice and emotions. After our physical appearance, it is the voice that sets us apart from others and serves to identify us to others. It reports about our physical condition as well as our emotional state and well-being. How often during a phone conversation have you commented to a friend that she sounds tired or depressed or, perhaps, really happy? Because of this close linkage, the voice may also be the primary reflector of inner turmoil. The importance of recognizing stress-related voice usage and the need to explore the patient's social interactions and interpersonal relationships cannot be overstated. The skilled clinician will be alert to indications, both verbal and nonverbal, of psychological stress factors. A patient's history of previous or current involvement in counseling or psychotherapy is valuable information.

Examination of the Voice

Examination of the larynx and testing of its performance can be carried out through a variety of techniques. It is our bias that no one or two procedures are enough to provide the best and most complete information about a person's vocal functioning. Furthermore, each procedure adds to our understanding of normal voice production as well as of the deviations altering that normal state. We are well aware that many assessment techniques are not immediately available to many speech pathologists or voice coaches, nor to all practicing otolaryngologists (Feder, 1986). However, within the past decade there has been a mini-explosion of interest in the voice and a concommitant development of voice laboratories. These laboratories can often provide testing, examination and diagnosis by an interdisciplinary team of voice specialists. It is therefore highly likely that full information is obtainable from sources within the community or in close geographic proximity, if it is sought.

Examination Procedures

Indirect Laryngoscopy

Indirect laryngoscopy is the traditional means of examining the larynx through the use of a laryngeal mirror. This technique requires that the tongue be pulled forward as the mirror is introduced into the oropharynx and positioned in such a way as to reflect the image of the vocal folds. Pulling the tongue forward has the effect of moving the epiglottis forward, thereby allowing visualization of the laryngeal structures. The patient is then asked to produce a high pitched /ee/ sound. The choice of the /ee/ vowel enhances visualization of the larynx during phonation because its production is usually characterized by superior and anterior movement of the dorsum of the tongue and the epiglottis. The reasons for the use of a high pitch are (a) the vocal folds are expected to lengthen in the phonation of a high pitch, and this lengthening maneuver tends to "open" the larynx to view, and (b) there is usually some degree of upward vertical movement of the larynx in the production of a high pitch, which brings the structures closer for viewing.

Indirect laryngoscopy is thought of as a fairly noninvasive procedure because it does not require anesthesia or surgery, nor does it cause any pain or other trauma to the patient. It does, however, have some limitations. There are patients who have very active gag reflexes and are unable to tolerate the presence of the mirror deep in the oropharynx. Anatomical variations not infrequently make it difficult to visualize the larynx adequately with the mirror exam. It is especially difficult to visualize the larynx of a young child through indirect laryngoscopy due to the anatomical relationships of the structures, which are different from and smaller than those of the mature adult. Another limitation is the inability of the patient to speak in a normal manner in the position required for this examination, thus limiting the information available relative to laryngeal physiology. Indeed, it is possible that the unnatural positioning required and the tension created in the patient may actually alter the typical laryngeal behavior of an individual, thereby rendering a less than accurate impression of phonatory behavior.

Despite these limitations, indirect laryngoscopy continues to be a very useful means of examining the larynx, especially when used in conjunction with other visualization techniques. Some otolaryngologists believe that some conditions, such as edema of the superior surface of the vocal folds, may be best visualized using the mirror exam (Brewer, personal communication).

Indirect laryngoscopy is a technique used most appropriately by otolaryngologists. Although we are aware that some speech pathologists have learned and use this examination procedure, it seems to us to be of doubtful value. The diagnosis of laryngeal pathology, a medical diagnosis, belongs rightfully to the laryngologist. As a means of monitoring progress in voice therapy, indirect laryngoscopy is not particularly productive and cannot provide information to equal that obtainable from acoustic data, perceptual data, and patients' reporting. Indirect laryngoscopy is a relatively poor way to examine laryngeal physiology, which should be the prime concern of the speech pathologist. There are few speech pathologists who see enough voice-disordered patients to gather the practice and experience to use the technique with expertise. And finally, it is our firm belief that there should be a partnership and team approach to the treatment of voice-disordered patients, which takes advantage of the special skills of each member of the team and thus makes indirect laryngoscopy performed by the speech pathologist superfluous.

Direct Laryngoscopy

Direct laryngoscopy is perhaps the most invasive of the laryngeal examination procedures. It is usually a hospital-based procedure requiring that the person be anesthetized. Direct laryngoscopy permits more detailed examination of laryngeal structures, including their actual manipulation. It is required when it becomes necessary to obtain a biopsy of a lesion and in attempts to determine the extent of a lesion. Manipulation of the arytenoid cartilages is helpful in making the distinction between a diagnosis of arytenoid ankylosis versus paralysis.

The disadvantages of direct laryngoscopy are its invasive nature, its cost, and the inability to observe laryngeal function. Prior to the relatively recent explosion of other visualization techniques, direct laryngoscopy was sometimes necessary as the only means to examine the larynx in persons for whom indirect laryngoscopy was unsuccessful.

Flexible Fiberoptic Laryngoscopy

The advent of fiberoptic technology has opened much of the human body to view in ways never before possible. Fiberscopes are used in many branches of medicine as diagnostic tools. A fiberscope, in simple terms, is a bundle of flexible fibers, some carrying light to the object to be examined and others carrying the image back to the viewer. The laryngeal fiberscope was introduced in the late 1960s (Sawashima and Hirose, 1981) and has become a standard piece of equipment for otolaryngologists.

In order to examine the larynx, the fiberscope is passed through the nasal cavity, over the soft palate, and into the oropharynx and the hypopharynx, as shown diagrammatically in Figure 7.1. Its moveable lens tip can be angled (the degree depending on the particular instrument), and the fiber bundle can be rotated to view the full larynx. The tip of the scope is usually positioned vertically, slightly above the epiglottis, but can be moved closer to the vocal folds for more detailed visualization. One of the benefits of this instrument is the flexibility possible in the positioning of the scope in the vertical dimension so as to allow visualization not only of the larynx but also of supraglottal structures and even of the velopharyngeal mechanism. Within the larynx, it is usually possible to view the anterior commissure, which is difficult to do with a mirror exam. The use of wide angle and zoom lenses also adds to visualization capabilities. The zoom lens allows for a closer look at specific laryngeal structures without discomfort to the patient, while the wide angle lens permits visualization of the entire larynx and supraglottal structures as well (depending on the vertical placement of the scope within the vocal tract). An example of a fiberoptic view of the vocal folds during respiration is seen in Figure 7.2, while Figure 7.3 shows the same larynx during phonation.

There are many advantages to this examination method. Although it may be characterized as invasive because the scope is introduced into the body, it may cause only minimal discomfort as the scope is passed through the narrowest part of the nose. As the diameter of the scope has decreased in size (and will perhaps continue to do so), discomfort to the patient has decreased. The fiberscope can be used to successfully visualize laryngeal structure and function in all but a relatively few patients. It is used with all age groups including infants, and it allows visualization of the larynx in persons with hyperactive gag reflexes and those in whom the anatomic relationships are only minimally distorted. It is possible to have the instrument coupled to a videocamera, thereby allowing for visualization of an enlarged image on a television monitor during the examination and for

FIBERSCOPE INSTRUMENTATION

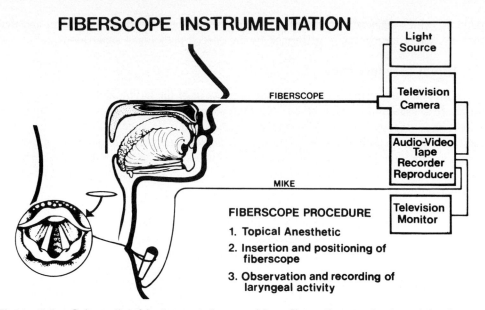

FIBERSCOPE

MIKE

Light
Source

Television
Camera

Audio-Video
Tape
Recorder
Reproducer

Television
Monitor

FIBERSCOPE PROCEDURE

1. Topical Anesthetic
2. Insertion and positioning of
   fiberscope
3. Observation and recording of
   laryngeal activity

Figure 7.1.   Schematic of instrumentation used in a fiberoptic examination of the larynx. The procedure used during the examination is listed. (From Conture, Schwartz, and Brewer, 1985.)

videotaping the examination for careful subsequent review. The image can be observed simultaneously by a number of people and has been used by some as a feedback tool during therapeutic intervention (Bastian, 1987). Videotaping provides the addition of visual documentation to the traditional verbal description and can make comparison of laryngeal conditions over time, or over a course of treatment, much more reliable. A method for computer-assisted measurement of fiberoptic images has been described by Conture, Cudahy, Caruso, Schwartz, Brewer, and Casper (1981) and was demonstrated to be useful in measuring and documenting actual intrasubject change in laryngeal physiology accom-

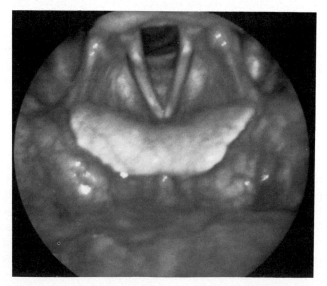

Figure 7.2.   A normal larynx during respiration. (Color photograph on page xiv by Eiji Yanagisawa, M.D.)

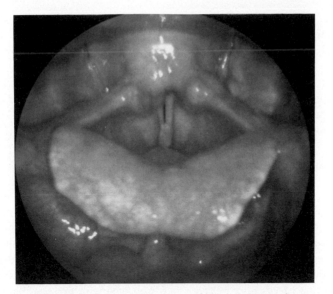

Figure 7.3. A normal larynx during phonation. (Color photograph on page xiv by Eiji Yanagisawa, M.D.)

panying the use of therapeutic techniques (Casper, Brewer, and Conture, 1981). A major advantage of fiberoptic laryngeal examination is that the patient is able to speak, sing, whistle, play a wind instrument, or simply to sit at rest, with minimal interference created by the presence of the fiberscope. This makes it possible for the patient's phonatory and nonphonatory laryngeal and supraglottal behavior to be observed.

The quality of the fiberoptic examination will be influenced by the quality of the equipment used. Casper, Brewer, and Colton, (1987b) cautioned that imaging of laryngeal structures will also be affected by factors inherent in the equipment, such as the wide angle lens distortion effect, particularly at the periphery of the image, and distortions created by the angling of the scope tip. Although these effects are not of sufficient degree to deny the overall effectiveness of the instrument, they must be taken into account when interpreting observed structural or behavioral deviations. Hibi, Bless, Hirano, and Yoshida (1988) have described the distortions as systematic and have suggested a mathematical procedure that corrects for the distortions. In addition to knowledge of the capabilities of the equipment and the skill of the examiner in handling the fiberscope, it is important to consider the sample of laryngeal and supralaryngeal behavior elicited from the patient. One of the primary advantages of this technique is that it allows such a diversity of behaviors to be explored. In examining singers who are having difficulty in a particular portion of their range or in some aspect of their singing technique relative to phonatory behavior, it is possible to watch the larynx and vocal tract as they "perform." For examination of the voice-disordered patient, a complete protocol of speech and nonspeech activities, designed to elicit habitual speech behavior, flexibility of pitch adjustments, adductory nonspeech behavior, resting state, and any other behaviors of interest, must be well thought out. In order to obtain the best visualization of the larynx during speech, stimulus sentences should be heavily loaded with the /ee/ and /oo/ vowel sounds. Whistling, a nonphonatory activity, frequently provides the opportunity to observe adductory vocal fold behavior at a slower rate than occurs in speech. A suggested protocol can be found in the Appendix. This protocol may serve only as a starting point, after which activities designed to elicit a particular behavior of interest or to attempt to change a laryngeal gesture may be added. The person who directs this aspect of the fiberoptic examination must be skilled in "reading'' the image, in understanding the physiology, and in knowing the types of vocal maneuvers that might elicit the desired changes in behavior. When the examination is videotaped and carried out as a team effort, that person is frequently the speech pathologist.

One of the limitations of the fiberoptic technique is that vibratory behavior of the vocal folds cannot be seen. The technique does not alter the speed of movement of the structures beyond what is visible with the human eye. Thus, in a certain sense, fiberoptic examination provides a relatively gross look at phonatory behavior at the vocal fold level.

Stroboscopy

Stroboscopy is a procedure that has been used to examine the larynx since 1878. It has received much greater acceptance and widespread use in some European countries and in Japan than it has in the United States. That situation seems to be changing now as recent technological advances have made the equipment more sophisticated and easier to use. Hirano (1981a) states that ''stroboscopic examination, as a routine clinical test, is the most practical technique for examination of the vibratory pattern of the vocal folds.'' Stroboscopy, indeed, permits visualization of vibratory behavior in a way otherwise not possible with the human eye, and in so doing enhances understanding of the physiological basis of voice disorders. Kitzing (1985) further points up the benefits of the stroboscopic technique for early detection of neoplasms and for differential diagnosis of laryngeal paresis and its outcome. Stroboscopy has been helpful in differentiating between functional voice problems and those caused by subtle structural abnormalities of the larynx (Bless and Brandenburg, 1983).

The stroboscopic light emits rapid pulses at a rate that can be set by the examiner or controlled by the fundamental frequency of the vocalization. If the frequency of the light pulse is the same as the vocal frequency, the resulting image will appear to be static and the vocal folds will seem to be at a standstill. At a frequency slightly less or greater than the frequency of vocal fold vibration (± 2 Hz), the image is the averaged vibratory pattern over several successive cycles and takes on the appearance of slow motion movement of the vocal folds. Each pulse of light illuminates a different point of the vibratory cycle, as schematized in Figure 7.4. These fragmented sections become fused due to the phenomenon of Talbot's law, that is, the persistence of an image on the human retina for 0.2 seconds after exposure.

Thus, stroboscopy differs from ultra-high speed photography in that it creates an optical illusion of slow motion and does not show details of each vibratory cycle, whereas high speed photography captures parts of the vibratory cycle at a very rapid rate, which appears as slow motion when the film is projected at a normal rate of 24 frames per second.

The stroboscopic image provides information about the following areas: symmetry of movement of the vocal folds, regularity or periodicity of successive vibrations, glottal closure, amplitude (horizontal excursion) of the vocal folds, presence and size of the mucosal wave, presence of any nonvibrating portions of the vocal folds, and additional observations relative to the presence of lesions and their apparent effect on the vibratory behavior. Observations of the stroboscopic image must be based on a thorough understanding of laryngeal anatomy and physiology, as well as of the changes in the mechanical characteristics of the vocal folds that result from variations in frequency and intensity. Interpretation of the observations requires understanding and knowledge of laryngeal pathologies.

The judgment of symmetry refers to the timing of the opening and closing of the folds relative to each other, as well as to the extent of lateral excursion of the folds. If the folds

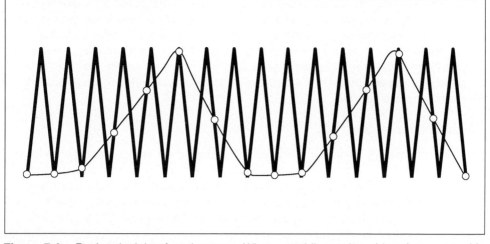

Figure 7.4. Basic principle of stroboscopy. When a rapidly moving object (represented by the high frequency waveform) is strobed by flashes at a lower frequency (curve with open circles), the rapidly moving object appears to move more slowly. (Redrawn from Kitzing, 1985.)

appear to be functioning in an equal manner during these actions, they are said to be symmetric. As noted previously, when the stroboscopic light flashes are synchronous with the fundamental frequency, the image appears to be static. Under this synchronous condition, any visible movement is evidence of irregularity of successive vocal fold vibratory cycles, or aperiodicity. Aperiodicity may be constantly present or inconsistent, in which case the image appears static part of the time. Judgments about glottal closure (the extent to which the vocal folds approximate each other) and glottal configuration during the closed phase are made during observation of phonations of normal pitch and intensity level—that is, normal or habitual for the individual. Bless, Hirano, and Feder (1987) have described seven categories of glottal closure that seem to encompass the possible variations (complete, anterior chink, irregular, bowed, posterior chink, hourglass, incomplete). Judgments of amplitude refer to the extent to which the vocal folds move horizontally. Because the extent of such movement may be different for each vocal fold, ratings are made for each individually. Again, it is important that such judgments be made during phonation of normal pitch and intensity level.

Perceptions of mucosal wave are judged on their presence or absence in whole or in part and on their extent in terms of both lateral extent and along the full length of the vocal fold. Judgments must be made for each vocal fold individually, and descriptions should be made regarding areas of absent or reduced wave.

It is possible to carry out a stroboscopic examination using a rigid endoscope or in combination with a flexible fiberoptic laryngoscope. Kitzing (1985) also describes the use of stroboscopic light in the operating microscope, combining good magnification and ''superb optic resolution'' while providing stereoscopic evaluation of the mucosal wave.

The method for obtaining stroboscopic images is not difficult. A microphone is placed or held on the patient's neck along the lateral aspect of the thyroid lamina in order to measure the fundamental frequency of the voice. The fundamental frequency of voice production controls the rate of firing of the stroboscopic light. The rigid or flexible scope is introduced, the light is activated by a foot pedal, and the patient is asked to sustain phonation of the vowel /ee/. Because vocal fold vibratory behavior will vary with frequency and loudness, it is important to obtain samples of phonation produced in various ways. The following conditions should be a part of the examination: (*a*) a minimum of 2 seconds of sustained vowel phonation at a normal pitch and loudness level; (*b*) a repeat of this, with gradually increasing loudness; (*c*) a repeat of condition 1, with a gradual elevation of pitch; (*d*) production of a chain of /ee/s with a starting and stopping of phonation between each. During the examination procedure, it is necessary for the examiner to check the settings of the equipment and alter them as necessary. Additional conditions may be necessary for some patients.

Videofluoroscopy

Videofluoroscopy, dynamic radiographic imaging of the larynx, can be a useful tool for providing information to verify or establish abnormalities in laryngeal structure or function. The projection that we have found to be most useful for evaluating phonatory behavior is the anteroposterior orientation. In this projection, it is possible to observe vocal fold adductory and abductory behaviors, the horizontal levels of the vocal folds, changes in vertical laryngeal height, the shape of the glottal arch, and other changes within the vocal tract. Advantages of this procedure, beyond the information it provides, include its relative lack of discomfort to the patient and the patient's ability to speak normally in the absence of any equipment within the vocal tract. There are some patients for whom the physical setting required for this procedure may create slight discomfort. Very heavy or broad-shouldered patients often find the space where they must sit a very close fit. Special arrangements must be made for patients who are wheelchair bound or otherwise disabled. It is particularly difficult to obtain acceptable fluoroscopic studies of patients with conditions that restrict their ability to adopt and maintain an upright head posture (tuberculosis of the spine, neuromuscular weakness, paralysis, incoordination, etc.), or those who have significant cervical spine arthritic changes that obscure visualization of the target structures. The primary disadvantage of this technique is the exposure to a certain amount of radiation that it entails. This fact alone restricts its widespread use in the assessment of phonatory behavior. However, when exploring the possible presence of a lesion and its extent, videofluoroscopic examination is widely used as a diagnostic tool.

Videofluoroscopy is the technique used in the barium swallow procedure. Patients with voice disorders whose symptoms involve dysphagia should be the subjects of a barium swallow study. The modified barium swallow described by Logemann (1983) is often the most productive of information about the nature of dysphagia, when it is present. When suspicion is raised that esophageal reflux may be creating irritation and inflammation of laryngeal structures with subsequent voice symptoms, referral for videofluoroscopic assessment of that condition may be indicated.

Ultra-High Speed Photography

This technique was developed by scientists at the Bell Telephone Laboratories in 1937, and since that time many scientists have modified and used the technique to observe vocal fold vibratory events in both normal and pathological larynges (Timcke, von Leden, and Moore, 1958, 1959; Moore and von Leden, 1958; von Leden, Moore, and Timcke, 1960; von Leden and Moore, 1961a; von Leden, LeCover, Ringel, and Isshiki, 1966; Hirano, Yoshida, Matsushita, and Nakajima, 1974; Hirano, Kakita, Kawasaki, and Matsushita, 1977; Metz, Whitehead, and Peterson, 1980). Although this technique is capable of providing excellent information about the vibratory behavior of the vocal folds, it has not found widespread acceptance clinically for a number of reasons. It requires an expensive array of equipment, the technical expertise to operate it, and the expenditure of much time both in the examination procedure and in subsequent analysis of the films; it also

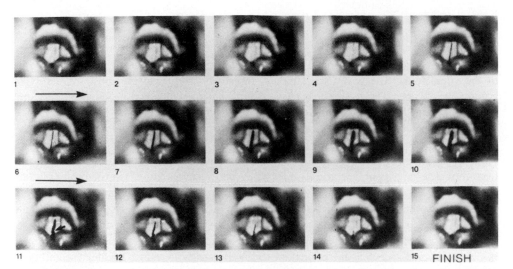

Figure 7.5. Example of a high speed motion picture sequence. This plate is a single cycle of vibration produced by a female speaker sustaining the vowel /ee/ at about 275 Hz. The film was exposed at a rate of 4000 frames per second. (From Metz, Whitehead, and Peterson, 1980.)

involves a procedure that is difficult, if not impossible, for many patients. The primary piece of equipment is a camera capable of taking pictures at a rate of 3000 frames per second or more. When films taken at these high speeds are viewed at a regular speed of 24 frames per second, the recorded events are seen in ultra-slow motion. The technique for obtaining high speed films (described by Hirano, 1981a), requires that the patient be able to position herself onto a fixed laryngeal mirror. The mirror must be positioned in such a way as to permit visualization of the vocal folds. The laryngeal mirror is used in a manner similar to indirect laryngoscopy, with the difference being that the patient must be capable of moving forward onto a fixed mirror rather than the mirror being moved into a stationary patient. An example of a high speed motion film sequence is shown in Figure 7.5.

The information obtained from high speed films is glottal area over time. That is, we can determine the amount of opening of the vocal folds during the vibratory cycle. It is also possible to determine the vibratory movement of each vocal fold, as well as the pattern of their opening.

As valuable as the information obtained from high speed films is to our understanding of the vibratory characteristics of the vocal folds, it does not seem to be a tool appropriate for routine use in the diagnosis and treatment of voice problems.

Ultrasound

Ultrasound is an imaging technique in which a high frequency current is passed through a portion of the body and partially reflected back when it strikes a change in body composition. Analysis of these reflections can be used to create an image of the part of the body of interest. It is a relatively safe procedure because the currents and frequencies used are low.

Ultrasound has been little used in the analysis of voice function. A few reports concerned with the analysis of normal voice function are available (Hamlet, 1981). Few voice clinics or laboratories possess the costly equipment and have personnel with the expertise to use it properly.

Laboratory Testing: Acoustic Studies

Fundamental Frequency

Fundamental frequency is an acoustic measure that directly reflects the vibrating rate of the vocal folds. The term "fundamental frequency" refers to the most frequently or commonly occurring frequency that characterizes a particular vocal production. The unit of measurement for fundamental frequency is the Hertz (Hz).

Fundamental frequency may be measured in a variety of ways and using any of several types of speech samples. The phonatory tasks may include sustained vowel phonation, reading, and conversational speech. The simplest of these is the sustained vowel phonation, in which the patient is instructed to produce and sustain a vowel (most commonly /ah/ or /ee/) at a comfortable, natural pitch and loudness level. The advantages of using a sustained vowel are that it can usually be sustained in a steady manner and for an adequate period of time. The uncomplicated nature of the task makes it possible to obtain accurate measures with relatively simple and inexpensive equipment. The use of a reading passage or conversational speech as the phonatory task will usually introduce greater variability of fundamental frequency, thereby making extraction of fundamental frequency a slightly more complex procedure or one that requires more expensive instrumentation. There is not full agreement as to whether the speech sample used has a significant influence on the actual measured fundamental frequency (Hirano, 1981a).

There are a variety of methods available for the measurement of fundamental frequency, ranging from the very simple to the complex and elaborate. Subjective judgments can be made through a matching procedure, but such judgments are often quite incorrect. Indeed, subjective perception of fundamental frequency, particularly in persons with disordered voice, may be misleading (Murry, 1978). Objective measurement of fundamental frequency from sustained vowel production can be carried out with the use of a frequency counter and a low pass filter (available for less than $500). A frequency counter alone would attempt to count the many frequencies that a vowel contains. A low pass filter, when appropriately set, will remove the higher components of the laryngeal tone, leaving only the fundamental frequency. The output of this equipment provides objective documentation that can be used to demonstrate and chart change.

Commercially available and easy to use pitch meters or analyzers include the Visi-Pitch (Kay Elemetrics Corp.) and the PM Pitch Analyzer (Voice Identification, Inc.). A sustained vowel or a speaking or reading sample using the patient's live voice or a recorded segment is fed into the instrument, and the fundamental frequency as a function of time is displayed on the screen. It is possible to control the total time to be displayed and thus to obtain a detailed fundamental frequency trace for short periods of time, or a less detailed trace of fundamental frequency over longer periods of time. These instruments can provide measures of other voice and speech parameters as well.

Computer programs, such as Micro Speech Lab and CSpeech, that run on IBM or IBM-compatible computers extract fundamental frequency from sustained vowels or longer speech samples. These programs can perform many more measurements than simple frequency measurements and are relatively simple to use. An example of a fundamental frequency analysis using the Micro Speech Lab program is presented in Figure 7.6.

Three summary statistics of frequency data that are useful for comparing patients to normal speakers or to themselves over a course of treatment are mean fundamental frequency, the standard deviation of fundamental frequency (pitch sigma), and frequency range. Clinically, these measures are helpful diagnostically and as documentation of pre- and posttreatment status. Mean fundamental frequency is useful to estimate the appropriateness of frequency level for the patient's age and sex. The other two statistics help to

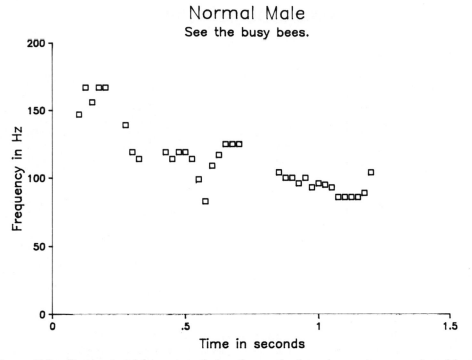

Figure 7.6. Fundamental frequency during the production of a sentence produced by a normal male speaker. Analysis was made using the Micro Speech Lab computer program.

assess and document variation of fundamental frequency during speech, or lack thereof. Speakers who are judged to be monotone would be expected to have small standard deviations and small ranges of speaking fundamental frequency.

Phonational Range

Another useful measure of the frequency characteristics of a patient's voice is phonational range, that range of frequencies from the highest to the lowest that a patient can produce. The highest and lowest frequencies are defined as the absolute limits of frequency that a patient can produce for a short period of time (approximately 1 second), without regard to intensity level or voice quality. Phonational range is said to reflect the physiological limits of the patient's voice. It is expressed in either Hertz or semitones and can be measured using any of the instrumentation discussed in the preceding section.

The absolute limits of frequency may be obtained by asking subjects to produce the highest and then the lowest sounds they can, or by using a singing scale progressing upward and downward in a stepwise fashion. Whichever technique is used, it is usually necessary to practice this task, encouraging the person to keep extending the range in both directions. The lowest and highest frequencies produced can be plotted, as shown in Figure 7.7. Kent, Kent, and Rosenbek (1987) have noted that intra- and intersubject variability on maximum performance tasks is large and may be affected by practice, motivation, or instructions. These caveats hold true for measurement of phonational range.

Vocal Intensity

Measurement of vocal intensity is useful in documenting the dynamics of the voice. Mean intensity correlates with the perception of vocal loudness, and the variability of intensity would presumably correlate with a patient's loudness variations.

Phonational Range

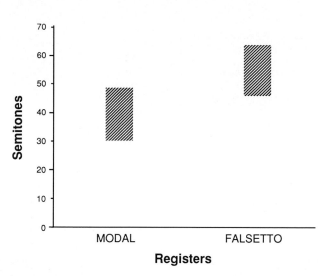

Figure 7.7. Mean phonational range of 35 male speakers. The modal register refers to that range of frequencies used most often during speech. Falsetto is a voice quality usually produced at high fundamental frequencies. (Drawn from the data of Colton, Reed, Sagerman, and Chung, 1982.)

Clinically, the mean intensity level of a patient's voice is usually a more meaningful measure than the absolute limits of intensity. However, the intensity range, frequently referred to as dynamic range, may be diagnostically important and helpful in documenting change. Patients whose mean intensity level is lower than expected for age (see Chapter 13 for some normative data on vocal intensity) and whose vocal intensity range is markedly reduced need very careful and complete examination, including, of course, audiological assessment. The case of K. B. presented in Chapter 2 is a good example of this point. Although K. B. reported that she had been constantly admonished by teachers to speak louder, this reduction in vocal intensity was not subjected to examination until she was 13 years old. The reduced vocal intensity had been assumed by teachers and others to be a behavioral manifestation, when, in fact, it was easily explained physically by the finding of congenital unilateral vocal fold paralysis.

The procedure for establishing intensity range requires that the person produce the very softest /ah/ possible and, at the other extreme, the very loudest /ah/. Patients should be asked to produce both of these sounds at a natural and comfortable frequency because frequency level will have an influence on intensity level (Colton, 1973; Coleman, Mabis, and Hinson, 1977). An example of plotting the highest and lowest sustainable intensity is shown in Figure 7.8.

Intensity can be measured from sustained vowels or connected speech. A simple intensity measurement device can be found on most tape recorders (e.g., the VU [volume unit] meter). However, this provides a very rough measure because these meters usually lack calibration in traditional intensity units (dB Sound Pressure Level). A sound level meter that is so calibrated can be purchased for less than $50 (at Radio Shack). The patient is asked to sustain a vowel at a normal loudness level with the microphone of the sound level meter held at a given distance from the mouth, and the intensity of the phonation in

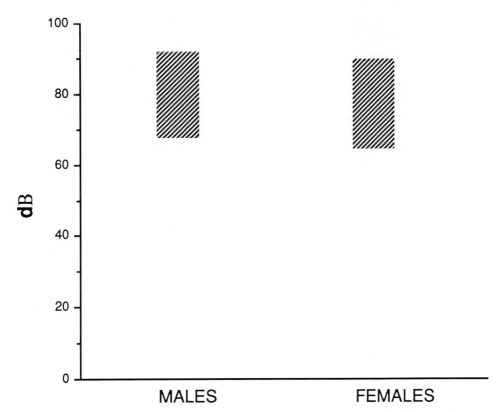

Figure 7.8. Example of intensity range measurement and portrayal. These data were collected on a sample of 35 older males (mean age = 56.17 years) and 27 females (mean age = 57.48 years) while they were phonating the vowel /a/ at 40% of their modal register frequency range. (Drawn from data from Colton, Reed, Sagerman, and Chung, 1982.)

decibels is read from the meter. This device is of little use, however, for measurement of vocal intensity during connected speech.

The Visi-Pitch and the Pitch Analyzer units described earlier can be used both to measure and to visually display vocal intensity during connected speech. Micro Speech Lab and CSpeech will display the intensity of speech production over time. It is also possible to obtain summary statistics such as average intensity level and standard deviation from these instruments and programs. It is important that the microphone used be capable of responding to all of the frequencies present in the tone whose intensity is to be measured. All sound level meters have microphones that can respond to those frequencies expected in the speech signal, as do the Visi-Pitch and Pitch Analyzer instruments. In computer programs, the sampling rate of the speech signal determines the frequencies present in the waveform and should be high enough to accurately reproduce frequencies of at least 5000 Hz (i.e., a sampling rate of 10,000 samples per second).

Another consideration when measuring vocal intensity is the distance between the speaker's lips and the microphone. The actual distance is not as important as that it be documented and consistent. Remember, sound intensity will be reduced by the square of the distance. That means a doubling of the distance will produce an intensity difference of 3 dB (or 6 dB if measuring sound pressure). The noise level of the room in which the phonation is measured must also be taken into account. It is not necessary to have a sound-isolated room, although that would be ideal. It is important to have a reasonably quiet room and to know its noise characteristics. Most rooms will have a considerable amount of ambient noise below 60 Hz. Because most speech exhibits frequencies above 100 Hz, the use of a simple high pass filter will attenuate the energy below 100 Hz and permit valid measurements to be made. Many sound level meters possess a weighting function that, in effect, carries out this filtering process. The presence of heavy drapes and floor carpeting helps to reduce noise and yield usable recordings.

Once again, it must be noted that the variability of maximum performance measures may be large. Thus, caution must be used in the interpretation of measures obtained.

Perturbation

Perturbation refers to the small, rapid, cycle-to-cycle changes of period and amplitude that occur during phonation. These changes reflect the slight differences of mass, tension, and biomechanical characteristics of the vocal folds, as well as the slight variations in their neural control (Baer, 1979). Perturbation correlates with perceived roughness or hoarseness in the voice (Wendahl, 1963, 1966) so that patients with voice problems manifesting roughness or hoarseness would be expected to show a large amount of both frequency and amplitude perturbation.

Perturbation must be measured from sustained vowel phonations in which the subject is instructed to produce a steady pitch level. Connected speech confounds the measure because linguistically produced frequency variations cannot be separated from frequency variations produced by the biomechanical characteristics of the vocal folds.

Frequency perturbation, also called jitter, is obtained by measuring the period of each cycle of vibration, subtracting it from the previous or succeeding period, averaging the differences, and dividing by the average period. If the result is multiplied by 100, jitter can be expressed as a percent change of period relative to the average period. That measure is referred to as the jitter factor. There are several other formulations for computing frequency perturbation, which make comparison of data somewhat difficult (Casper, 1983).

Frequency perturbation can be measured by the Visi-Pitch which reports it as a ratio measurement. The PM Pitch Analyzer also provides a perturbation measure that is different from and thus not directly comparable to other frequency perturbation measures. These measures are helpful for comparison of intra- or intersubject data when the same measure is being used for that comparison. The computer program CSpeech calculates frequency perturbation, and there are also many special purpose software programs that calculate perturbation. It is possible to make the measurement of frequency perturbation from oscillographic recordings, but this requires much hand measurement and is a tedious and impractical task.

Amplitude perturbation, or shimmer, refers to the small cycle-to-cycle changes of the amplitude of the vocal fold signal. As was the case for the measurement of frequency perturbation, the amplitude of each glottal cycle is measured, subtracted from the previous or following period, and averaged over all differences. Shimmer is most often expressed in average change in decibels although ratio measurements are also used.

Amplitude perturbation can be obtained directly from the CSpeech program, as well as from a number of other software programs. The measure of amplitude perturbation from the speech signal emitted at the lips is determined not only by the vocal folds but also by the resonance characteristics of the vocal tract. Thus, a measure of amplitude perturbation probably reflects the effect of the vocal tract on the speech signal, as well as the effect of the vocal folds.

Spectrograms

Spectrograms reflect the properties of the source of sound (the vibratory characteristics of the vocal folds) and the resonator (the vocal tract). In order to compare spectral

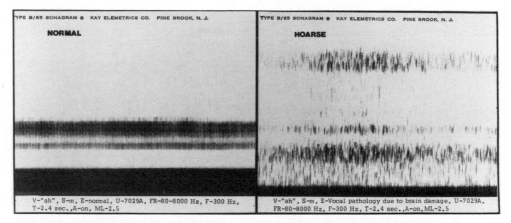

Figure 7.9. Spectrogram of a normal voice (left panel) and a hoarse voice (right panel). (Courtesy of Kay Elemetrics Co., Pine Brook, NJ.)

characteristics of a given phonation, it is important to use the same vowel. It is also necessary to have a good working knowledge of the acoustic characteristics of normal speech in order to properly interpret spectrograms obtained from voice patients.

Spectrograms are useful for analyzing and showing changes in the spectral characteristics of the vocal fold sound. Noise and weak sounds will exhibit characteristics that can easily be studied from a spectrogram. As shown in Figure 7.9, the spectrum of a hoarse voice (right panel) has considerable noise energy in the higher frequencies, whereas the normal voice on the left has little high frequency noise energy but strong low frequency periodic energy. Amplitude sections can be taken at selected points and a detailed analysis made of the spectral characteristics of the sound. Spectrograms can be stored in the patient's record for analysis and comparison with later phonatory samples.

One useful measure that can be obtained from spectrograms is harmonics-to-noise ratio. This is a measure of the energy in the harmonics of the voice signal (i.e., the frequencies produced by the vibrating vocal folds) and the noise energy in the signal. Abnormal voices will exhibit greater noise either directly (i.e., produced at the vocal folds) or indirectly as greater perturbation (Klingholz and Martin, 1985). On a spectrogram of an abnormal voice, there would be greater noise and less energy in the harmonics of the sound. The harmonics-to-noise ratio is a convenient measure to express this relationship. After treatment, the spectrogram of a voice patient would exhibit greater harmonics-to-noise ratio because greater energy in the harmonic components of the sound would be expected, along with less noise energy.

The instruments most commonly used to make spectrograms are the Kay Series of Sona-graphs (TM) and the Voice Identification instruments. Many voice clinics will not be able to afford this expensive equipment. There are, however, several computer software programs that produce acceptable spectrograms at less cost (Micro Speech Lab, Kay Elemetrics; RSL, DSPS Inc.; MacSpeech Lab, GW Instruments). The use of these programs makes it possible to obtain spectrograms routinely on voice patients and greatly speeds the process of measurement. It is also possible to compute a harmonics-to-noise ratio via computer analysis (Kojima, Gould, and Lambiase, 1979; Kojima, Gould, Lambiase, and Isshiki, 1980; Kitajima, 1981).

Acoustic Spectrum

Acoustic spectrum is a plot of the energy in each of the frequencies present in a complex tone. The amplitude section from a spectrograph is an example of acoustic spec-

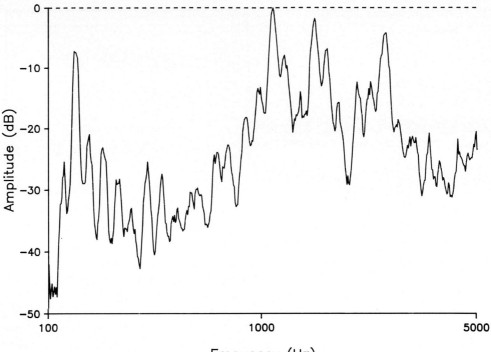

Figure 7.10. Spectral plot of a vowel produced by a normal speaker. These data were produced using Micro Speech Lab.

trum. It is possible to determine acoustic spectrum directly from the speech signal using special purpose spectrum analyzers or appropriate computer programs. Special purpose spectrum analyzers are very expensive but several computer programs are available that are not only less expensive but also more practical for clinical application. An example of a spectrum analysis produced by the Micro Speech Lab software program is shown in Figure 7.10. Such spectral profiles can be printed out for inclusion in a patient's file. Of course, it is important that the patient produce the same vowel or sound under similar conditions for each profile in order to properly interpret any spectral changes that might be obtained.

Another variant of spectrum analysis is computation of the one-third octave spectrum of the speech sample. The advantage of one-third octave spectrum is that it results in a small, manageable number of frequency bands to measure. In normal speech, there may be energy in frequencies from 100 to 5000 Hz. In a one-third octave display, the spectrum is analyzed into 10 to 20 different frequency bands, depending on the frequency range desired. Furthermore, there is a well-documented and internationally accepted body of data concerning standardization of one-third octave spectra and the characteristics of the filters. Another advantage is that one-third octave analysis is similar, although not identical to, the way in which the ear analyzes sound. In view of this, it would be expected that the results of a one-third octave analysis would correlate best with perceptual measurements of voice. Unfortunately, there are few data available on this relationship. In our judgment, the one-third octave seems to be the best choice at this time for analyzing the spectral characteristics of normal and abnormal voices.

There are several expensive one-third octave spectrum analyzers available for performing these measurements. It is also possible to extract one-third octave information from a computer-generated spectrum.

Laboratory Testing: Physiological Studies

Electroglottography

Electroglottography (EGG) is a technique for the measurement of vocal fold contact area based on the principle that tissue conducts current. A high frequency, low current signal is passed between the vocal folds via electrodes located on the external neck over the thyroid lamina. When the vocal folds touch, greater current flows than when they are open. There is a proportional variation of current when the vocal folds are less than maximally open or closed. Electroglottographic recordings can be used to determine when the vocal folds are closed and how fast they are closing. If carefully interpreted, it is possible to determine characteristics of the opening of the vocal folds from an electroglottographic recording.

Devices to record the electroglottographic signal are readily available. Currently these include the Voiscope and Laryngograph (Laryngograph, Ltd.), the SynchroVoice unit (SynchroVoice, Inc.), and the unit from FJ Electronics. For a full discussion of the measurement technique, see Baken (1987, pp. 216–227). The electrical output of the electroglottograph can easily be converted to hard copy using an oscillograph or similar graphic recording device.

The literature on EGG is primarily qualitative in nature, based on interpretation of the waveform. Several studies have related the shape of the EGG waveform to the underlying physiology of vocal fold vibration (Rothenberg, 1981; Childers, Naik, Larar, Krishnamurthy, and Moore, 1983; Painter, 1988). Information has also been reported on characteristic waveforms in patients with vocal pathology (Wechsler, 1976; Childers, Smith, and Moore, 1984; Casper, Colton, and Brewer, 1985; Colton and Brewer, 1985; Dejonckere and Lebacq, 1985). There have been only a few attempts to quantify the electroglottograph signal (Brodie, Colton, and Swisher, 1988; Rothenberg and Mahshie, 1988).

EGG reflects the state of the vocal folds in a way that can be easily demonstrated and interpreted to patients. However, a limitation of the technique is that it cannot be used with all patients. Because the technique depends on vocal fold contact, the signal is considerably diminished or even absent in patients with lack of good contact, such as those with unilateral paralysis, or aphonia. It may also be difficult to obtain a clear waveform in the presence of severe hoarseness. The thick or large necks of some patients hinder transduction of the current and result in a poor EGG tracing. Further development of EGG may greatly enhance its clinical value.

Photoglottography

Photoglottography is a technique designed to obtain estimates of variations of glottal area during phonation. Light is directed from above, usually from a fiberoptic light source passed through the nose. The light passes through the glottis and is detected by a light sensitive device usually positioned over the skin of the trachea immediately beneath the vocal folds. As the vocal folds vibrate, their area of opening will vary and so will the amount of light passing through the glottis. It is a simple, relatively noninvasive device that yields a good, but not exact, approximation of glottal area. The photoglottographic technique is complementary to the EGG signal (Baer, Lofqvist, and McGarr, 1983).

There are several measurements that can be made from photoglottographic recordings. The first, speed quotient, is the speed of the opening phase of the vocal folds divided by the speed of their closing phase. The second, open quotient, is the time of the open phase of the vocal folds divided by the total period of vibration. This term is analogous to the term "duty cycle" used in engineering. Short duty cycles, or open quotients, are usually associated with more efficient vocalizations.

There have been a few studies relating photoglottographic results to different kinds of speech and voice production (Sonnesson, 1959,1960; Vallancien, Gautheron, Pasternak, Guisez, and Paley, 1971; Harden, 1975; Hanson, Gerratt, and Ward, 1983; Hanson, Ward, Gerratt, Berci, and Berke, 1989). There is some concern that the waveform obtained from this technique is not an entirely accurate representation of the actual glottal area waveform (Wendahl and Coleman, 1967). However, it may be useful for extracting measures such as speed or open quotient, which are known to be affected by disorders of the vocal folds (Timcke et al., 1958).

Inverse Filtering

In the inverse filtering procedure, the voice signal emitted at the lips is analyzed to remove the resonant effects of the vocal tract, producing an estimate of the waveform produced at the vocal folds. According to the acoustic theory of speech production (Fant, 1960; Stevens and House, 1961), speech is the product of a sound source and a filter. That is, the sound output of the vocal folds is modified by the resonant characteristics of the vocal tract. If the resonant characteristics of the vocal tract are known, it becomes possible to retrieve the characteristics of the output of the vocal folds from the orally emitted speech signal.

Inverse filtering has been performed on the acoustic sound pressure waveform (Miller, 1959; Miller and Mathews, 1963; Sondi, 1975; Hillman and Weinberg, 1981), and on the airflow waveform (Rothenberg, 1973, 1977, 1981). We have used the airflow waveform for inverse filtering of normal and voice-disordered subjects (Colton, Brewer, and Rothenberg, 1983; Colton and Brewer, 1985; Casper et al., 1985; Brodie et al., 1988). We have also recorded the EGG signal simultaneously with the inverse filtered airflow signal in order to extract information about the vibratory characteristics of the vocal folds during the complete cycle. The techniques complement each other in that airflow will often not be present during the closed phase of the vocal folds, but the EGG provides information about vibratory characteristics of the vocal folds during that phase. Thus, with both techniques, we are able to obtain a more complete picture of vocal fold vibratory characteristics during speech.

An example of inverse filtered waveforms is shown in Figure 7.11. These traces were recorded using a small microcomputer (Commodore 128) connected to an eight-channel, eight-bit analog-to-digital (A/D) converter. Two low pass filters, one for the electroglottogram and one for the inverse filtered channels, preceded the A/D converter, along with reference voltages used for calibrating the various channels. A third channel of the A/D converter with its associated low pass filter was used to collect air pressure data recorded from the oral cavity. Using procedures described by Rothenberg (1968) and Smitheran and Hixon (1981), these pressure measurements provide estimates of the lung or subglottal air pressure used during phonation, A custom-written program was used for the collection, display, storage, and analysis of these waveforms.

Collection of electroglottographic and inverse filtered airflow waveforms is routine in our clinic. The following measures are obtained from computer-assisted analysis of the waveform: (a) each cycle's minimum and peak airflows, (b) the ratio of the time of the airflow pulse

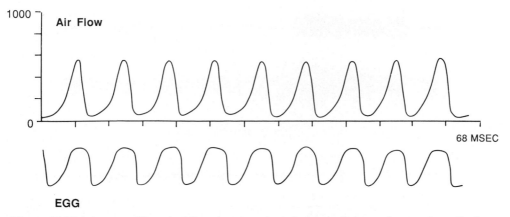

Figure 7.11. Inverse filtered airflow (top trace) and electroglottograph waveform (bottom trace) of a normal speaker. Vocal fold contact is indicated by a downward trace in the electroglottogram waveform.

relative to the total period, (c) the ratio of the closing and opening slopes of the airflow pulse, (d) the ratio of the open time to the total period of the electroglottographic waveform, (e) the closing time of the electroglottogram waveform, and (f) lung pressure. Each cycle's measurements are added to the other cycles in the data and averaged. Patient data are thus available for comparison with data collected on a small group of normal speakers.

Electromyography

Electromyography (EMG), a technique in which electrodes are inserted into specific muscles to measure their electrical activity, is used routinely by neurologists for the study of peripheral muscle function in various neuromuscular and neurological diseases. EMG is invasive and requires expertise, and precautions must be taken to safeguard the patient's well-being. For these reasons, EMG has enjoyed limited use in the diagnosis and management of voice disorders. EMG of the vocal muscles requires detailed knowledge of head and neck anatomy, along with considerable experience in manipulating needles or needle carriers within the pharynx and larynx. The muscles involved in phonation are not readily accessible. Electromyographic recording equipment is available from a variety of manufacturers and has been engineered to be medically safe. The output of the equipment, an electromyogram, is a detailed tracing of muscle activity. An example of an electromyogram is shown in Figure 7.12.

Interpretation of electromyographic recordings requires experience and practice. Onset or offset of muscle activity, the pattern of muscle activity and the overall amplitude of muscle activity are the parameters that provide the most valuable information. Electromyographic patterns of neurologically disordered patients will show greater or lesser than normal amplitudes of muscle activity, extraneous bursts of muscle activity, and slower or faster than normal muscle activation. Laryngeal electromyograms may be helpful in those patients with voice problems of suspected neurological or neuromuscular etiology.

Laboratory Testing: Respiratory Studies

Air Volumes and Capacities

Many clinicians advocate the analysis of a patient's respiratory function, including studies of lung volumes, vital capacity, residual capacity, and phonation volume. Others doubt the necessity for obtaining these data and question their value provided the patient is

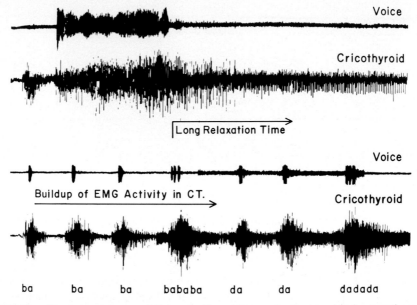

Figure 7.12. Electromyogram of the cricothyroid muscle in an elderly speaker during sustained vowel production (upper trace) and consonant-vowel syllable production (lower trace).

able to maintain adequate air volumes and airflows needed for speech. There are, of course, research issues for which such information is important.

The wet spirometer is the most common instrument used for the analysis of respiratory volumes. This device consists of an upper and a lower cannister, each with an open end. The lower cannister is filled with water. The open end of the upper cannister fits into the mouth of the lower so that an airtight seal is produced. The two cannisters are now effectively sealed, partially filled with known volumes of air and of water. A pipe, into which the patient breathes, connects to the air within the sealed cannisters. When the patient exhales, air is forced into the sealed lower cannister, the upper portion of which is allowed to move in order to accommodate the increased air volume. A pen or other marker attached to the vertically moving drum records the movement of the drum in response to the patient's breathing. Since the relationship between the air volume change and the movement of the pen is known, it is possible to obtain the volume of air used by the patient. Common measurements obtained from voice patients include tidal volume (the volume of air in an average breath), vital capacity (the volume of air that can be maximally exhaled after maximum inhalation), and total lung volume (the total volume of air in the lungs). Other volumes that may be measured are inspiratory reserve volume (the amount of air that can be inspired from the end-expiratory level of a tidal breath) and expiratory reserve volume (the amount of air that can be expired from the end-expiratory level of a tidal breath). Respiratory physiologists are also concerned with reserve volume and gas exchange, but such measurements are not performed routinely for voice patients.

A certain amount of air volume, flow, and pressure is required for speech. The respiratory system, however, can provide considerably more volume, flow, or pressure than is required for speech or even for singing. Only a small portion of the total available volume is normally used in speaking. Thus, it would seem unnecessary, and perhaps unproductive, to spend inordinate amounts of time gathering information about lung volumes for most voice patients. Information that may be more valuable is that concerning the control of the respiratory system during speech. It is necessary and vitally important that informed

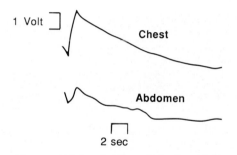

Figure 7.13.   Examples of traces obtained with an inductive plethysmograph. The top trace was obtained from the chest wall and the bottom from the abdomen. The speaker was a male who inhaled deeply and counted on a single expiratory cycle for a long as possible. Horizontal time per division is 2 seconds. Vertical amplitude scale is 1 volt per division.

decisions be made concerning the relative contributions of respiratory versus laryngeal function to the presenting voice problem. Teaching proper breathing when the problem lies elsewhere seems to us a poor use of time and money.

Respiratory Movements

It may be important to assess control of respiratory movements in some voice patients. Assessment of the movement of the thorax and abdomen during speech may provide important information about the control exerted by a voice patient. Analysis of these movements is possible using a variety of tools, including mercury-filled strain gauges (Baken, 1977), the respiratory inductive plethysmograph (Watson, 1979; Sackner, 1980; Bless, Hunker, and Weismer, 1981; Stradling, Chadwick, Quirk, and Phillips, 1985), and magnetometers (Hixon, 1987). Bless et al. (1981) provide a comparison of these techniques. Although their methods vary, all of these tools are able to monitor the movements of the chest and abdominal walls using noninvasive external devices. All are available from commercial manufacturers; there is some variation in the expertise required for their operation.

A typical recording of the movements of the chest wall and abdomen is shown in Figure 7.13. Note that the rib cage trace (upper) shows a steady decrease of circumference as exhalation progresses, with irregular but decreasing changes noted in the abdominal channel. These curves can be calibrated to produce estimates of lung volume.

Noninstrumental Testing

Critical Listening and Description

Although we have presented the voice history as a separate section, in practice there can be no separation between history taking and the voice evaluation. The initial interview, during which the history is elicited, is the point at which the evaluation begins. It affords the clinician the opportunity to listen critically not only to the content of the message but also to the vocal output. Because patients are frequently referred following laryngologic examination, it is well for the speech pathologist to always have in mind the question, are the vocal symptoms consistent with the referral diagnosis? The voice clinician's ears must always be turned on and tuned in. It is not unusual to pick up very significant clues about the presenting problem before the patient is aware that the examination is in progress.

CASE EXAMPLE A 35-year-old woman who complained of having lost her voice several weeks previously was answering all questions put to her in an aphonic whisper. During her aphonic explanation of the effect of this problem on her work, she cleared her throat. The clinician noted the entirely normal sound of the throat clearing. What information did this present?

While listening critically, the clinician should make observations about the consistency or variability in the sound of the voice and about its stability. When the voice exhibits variability or instability, it is important to be aware of the nature or pattern of that variability. For example, is the voice clear and strong initially, with gradual worsening over time? Does this happen with each sentence or two or over a more extended period of time? What is changing—quality, pitch, or loudness?

It is appropriate to make a perceptual judgment of vocal pitch, but such judgments must be made with caution and later verified with objective data. Perhaps the most important perceptual judgment to be made relative to pitch is whether or not its level is appropriate for the age and sex of the speaker. Perceptual impressions of fundamental frequency in the presence of laryngeal pathology tend to suggest lower than expected levels; however, it has been shown (Murry, 1978) that the fundamental frequency of some voice problems does not differ systematically from the norm, with the exception of reduction in phonational range in laryngeal paralysis. Another aspect of pitch to which the clinician must attend is its variability. Variations in pitch are used linguistically to mark the meaning of utterances. In the English language, pitch is expected to fall at the end of a declarative sentence and to rise to mark a question. Voices that show pitch variability are generally thought to be more ''interesting'' and less apt to lull the listener.

CASE EXAMPLE While taking the history from a 65-year-old man, the clinician was struck by an absence of inflection and a monotonic, flat, and unvarying delivery. Questions and statements were undifferentiated by the usual pitch changes. This observation, combined with noticeable slurring of speech, alerted the clinician to look for additional signs of neurological involvement. What would this absence of pitch variability suggest to you, and what other signs might you expect to find?

The loudness level of the patient's voice during assessment in presumably quiet surroundings should be another focus of the clinician's critical listening. The salient judgments to be made are whether the voice is too loud, too soft, or out of control. The consistency or variability of the loudness level are also important to note.

CASE EXAMPLE Another observation made about our 65-year-old patient mentioned above was the tendency for the loudness level of his voice to remain constant, with some decay at the end of an utterance. When asked to count and to alternate loud and soft voice for each successive number, the patient was able to comply with only the first three numbers, after which the loudness level became constant. Is this consistent with our previous observation, and why?

Descriptions of voice quality are most difficult to make. Many adjectives are used to describe voice quality, but they are difficult to quantify, and there is not widespread agreement on the meanings of voice quality terms. Some perceptions of quality can be checked against objective measures. For example, in the presence of hoarseness, there is the expectation of increased frequency perturbation (Coleman and Wendahl, 1967). Scaling of perceptions is perhaps the most valid approach to assigning a degree of objectivity to subjective judgments. Various types of scales will be discussed later in this chapter.

Those aspects of speech referred to as suprasegmentals may hold information about voice production or may add to other findings in the search for the diagnosis. The rate of speech is one such aspect. Excessively fast or laboriously slow rates may be suggestive of neurological involvement or may simply be a reflection of personality. Persons who tend to talk very rapidly often tend also to stretch vocalization to the last bit of air they can squeeze out. This style of speech is often characterized by increased tension in the respiratory and laryngeal systems. Prosody of speech may be disturbed by vocal behavior, as is the case with spastic dysphonia. If the clinician is aware of a disturbance of prosody, it is important to determine the nature of that disturbance and to describe it as accurately as possible.

Attention must be paid to any unusual vocal characteristics, such as stridor, grunts, and vocal tics. Of particular importance is the observation of stridor, inspiratory and/or expiratory noise. The presence of stridor suggests obstruction somewhere in the airway, subglottally, glottally or supraglottally. It may be a sign of a laryngeal web, an obstructing lesion, severe inflammation, or abductor vocal fold paralysis. In infants inspiratory stridor is usually symptomatic of laryngomalacia. Yet another cause of stridor may be fixation or ankylosis of the cricoarytenoid joints as a consequence of rheumatoid arthritis.

CASE EXAMPLE J. W., a 41-year-old nurse, presented for a voice evaluation with a history of 10 years of vocal difficulty and shortness of breath. She denied concern about her voice quality, which she claimed was unchanged. She believed that her vocal pitch was perhaps slightly higher than it had been but not significantly enough to be of concern. Perceptually, we were in agreement with these judgments. Her main vocal complaint was the inability to complete a whole sentence on one breath. J. W. has continued to work during this 10-year period but admitted to shortness of breath in climbing stairs or during other physical exertion. Throughout this history taking, the examiner was aware not only of her obvious shortness of breath and the disruption in the prosody of speech caused by frequent interruptions in order to renew breath supply but also of her characteristic thrusting forward of the mandible during inspiration and of audible inspiratory stridor. J. W. was immediately referred for laryngological examination, which revealed abductor vocal fold paralysis, probably as a consequence of a viral infection.

Vocal tics are characterized by sudden, unexpected, and involuntary vocalizations. They are usually thought to be a symptom of a neurological disorder. Other unusual vocal manifestations that may suggest a neurological etiology include grunts, barking sounds, and echolalia.

Critical Observations and Descriptions

It is very important that the clinician maintain eye contact with the patient and be in visual contact so as to be able to make observations of behavior that may not be audible. This requires that note taking be kept to a minimum freeing the clinician to take full advantage of all diagnostic clues. After completion of the examination, the clinician should describe all observations made.

Watch facial expression and body language. Do they match the words being spoken? How do they change in response to questions? Is the person comfortable, anxious, tense, fidgety? Is eye contact made and maintained? Are there extraneous facial or body movements? Is there tremor of the head, the hands, the jaw? Can you observe signs of neck, face, or laryngeal tension/strain? What is the emotional affect being projected? Does the person make adequate use of mouth opening and lip movement?

We suggest that observations of respiratory behavior be made during the period of eliciting the history and prior to asking the patient to engage in any specific vocal or respiratory tasks. It is important to observe respiratory behavior both during speech and at rest. Does the person have sufficient air supply to complete sentences? Does the person habitually speak until the air supply is exhausted? Does the person release exhalation prior to voice onset, or do you observe a holding of the breath in anticipation of speaking with an abrupt, sharp voice onset? Where do you observe the greatest amount of respiratory activity when the person is speaking, and when at rest? Is it clavicular, midthoracic, or abdominal/diaphragmatic?

Diagnostic Therapy

The procedures used in this part of the evaluation cannot be rigidly specified because they often depend on the symptoms presented by the patient and the observations made by the clinician up to this point. The objectives of this part of the evaluation are to explore the patient's response to different ways of producing voice, to attempt to elicit an improved voice, to test the patient's ability to manipulate parameters such as pitch, loudness, and resonance, and to test the limits of the voice. Sometimes this involves making sounds and noises that create some self-consciousness. Patients with psychogenic voice disorders often appear frightened and threatened when asked to produce ''different'' sounds, perhaps because they are uncertain of their ability to maintain control over such phonations. Each step of this process must be carried out with sensitivity and encouragement. It is also essential that the clinician demonstrate the task being required of the patient. If the patient is being asked to produce a grunt, it will ease self-consciousness if the clinician models the grunt as the patient is to do it.

The following are some diagnostic therapy tasks that might be useful.

Production of Reflexive Sounds.   These include coughing, laughing, clearing the throat, and the vocalized pause ''uh-huh.'' The clinician's ears should have been tuned in to hear these sounds if they occurred spontaneously during the interview. It is interesting then to compare the quality of the sound produced spontaneously with that elicited during this task. The rationale for using this task is to determine the quality of the phonation produced in a nonspeech task. It is most important to judge whether this elicited quality differs from the voice heard in speech in quality, pitch, or loudness. It is often necessary to work with the patient on these tasks until you are satisfied that the best sound that person is capable of, or is willing to produce, has been heard.

Altering Pitch.   Before attempting to obtain a phonational range, it is helpful to work with patients on the concept and on their ability to change pitch upward and downward. Some patients are unable to succeed on this task for reasons having to do with the nature of their problem. Others seem unable to carry it out due to difficulty in discriminating pitch changes and difficulty in matching pitches. It is important to try, during this diagnostic therapy period, to determine which of these is operative. It is helpful to engage in this activity as a practice for the actual testing of phonational range that may be carried out later. When patients exhibit difficulty in either matching a pitch or spontaneously altering pitch, we have found it useful to have them imitate animal sounds, such as the high-pitched meow of a kitten, the squeal of a mouse, or the howl of a wolf. Once again it is important to emphasize that such activities often create feelings of self-consciousness, which must be allayed by the clinician. One of the most effective methods of accomplishing this is through humor as the clinician models the desired sounds. The rationale for this activity is to test one of the limits of the voice, to explore whether the patient is capable of copying a model presented by the clinician, and to determine whether there is an overall improvement in the clarity of the sound at any point in the range. (Caution: This is not a search for an optimal pitch, which we do not believe is a viable concept, but rather an attempt to understand the physiology responsible for the vocal behavior.)

Sustaining Steady, Prolonged Phonation.   As in the previous activity, it is helpful to allow the patient some practice on this task prior to the taking of measurements. An increased level of tension is often generated in patients when they know an activity is being timed, and it is not unusual to find that they perform better in a more relaxed activity. The vowel of choice is usually /ah/. It is important for the clinician to observe carefully how the patient prepares to carry out this task and how natural or strained the phonation is, as well as noting the steadiness and length of the phonation. The rationale for this activity is to observe the patient's ability to control phonation and respiration. Vocal tremor, if present, will become more obvious on this task than during connected speech. The patient may be asked to produce such a phonation at various pitch levels as a means of continuing to explore vocal capacity.

Altering Vocal Loudness.   It is usually not difficult to elicit a very quiet sound, but people are often quite reticent to produce the loudest phonation of which they are capable while seated in a quiet office. Therefore, it may be necessary to pursue increments of loudness in steps, with the clinician providing the model. Clearly, if the patient has been referred with the diagnosis of a vocal fold lesion, inflammation, or edema, this activity should not be carried out. Some persons who have habituated very loud voice use find it difficult to lower the loudness level and ask with incredulity whether they can be heard. The rationale for this activity is to further test the limits of voice production and explore the patient's ability to manipulate isolated vocal parameters and match a model.

Phonation with Effortful Glottal Closure.   It is essential that this activity be used wisely and only with those patients for whom the activity itself will not be harmful. There are a variety of techniques that elicit effortful closure of the glottis: grunting, isometric pushing together of the palms of the hands held chest height, isometric pulling apart of linked hands held chest height, lifting a very heavy object, and attempting to raise a chair while seated on it. The person is required to phonate while tension is maintained during the activity. The rationale for the use of such a stressful phonatory act is to attempt to force vocal fold adduction and elicit a nonspeech sound that is difficult to control voluntarily. It is an activity that we have found helpful in eliciting a lowered pitch level in young boys who present with puberphonia and an improved voice in some patients with psychogenic dysphonias. Use of this procedure in therapy is discussed in Chapter 9. The intent here is to use the technique as an exploratory measure as part of the total assessment.

"Placing the Voice."   This is often referred to as placing the voice in the mask, or voice focus. As a diagnostic task, it constitutes one of the methods used in the search for the best voice a patient can produce. This technique is discussed more completely in Chapter 9.

Noninstrumental Objective Measurements

Maximum Phonation Time.   An individual's ability to sustain phonation provides some information about the control of respiratory function, glottal efficiency, and laryngeal control. When respiratory function is compromised, there will be either reduction in the amount of air available to support phonation or a problem in the control of the airflow. If the problem is at the laryngeal level, glottal resistance to airflow may be reduced due to inadequate glottal closure, or increased due to obstruction or hyperadduction. Certain problems affecting motor control of phonation may not inhibit or restrict maximum phonation time but may affect the quality of the phonation. The task is designed to test the limits of function and as such may uncover weaknesses that are not apparent at lower levels of function. Thus, for example, in the case of an individual with essential tremor, a vocal tremor may become increasingly obvious as phonation is sustained, although it may have escaped notice during speech.

The patient should be instructed to take a deep breath and sustain the vowel /ah/ for as long as possible. This should be done at a pitch and loudness level that are comfortable for the patient. A stopwatch should be used to obtain the measure, and patients should be asked to repeat the task at least three times (Hirano, 1981a), with the greatest duration being adopted as the maximum phonation time. Kent et al. (1987) caution, however, that the database for this, as well as many other maximum performance measures of speech production, may not be adequate for confident clinical use. Although Stone (1983) and others (Neiman and Edeson, 1981; Lewis, Casteel, and McMahon, 1982; Finnegan, 1984,1985) have reported instability of the maximum phonation time measure over as many as 15 trials, Bless and Hirano (1982) found that three trials were adequate if subjects were given adequate instruction and practice in the task. Corroboration of this can be found in the report that coaching and instruction led to a mean increase in maximum phonation time of 5.2 seconds for a group of 3rd-grade girls (Reich, Mason, and Polen, 1986). The available normative values for sustained phonation may be found in Chapter 13.

The ability to sustain phonation is developmental and increases from childhood to adulthood. It is logical that this should be the case in view of the physical growth of the body and increased lung capacity. Significant differences in maximum phonation time exist between the sexes, but that difference does not begin to appear until puberty, when growth spurts between the sexes differ in degree (Hirano, 1981a). There is an overall reduction of pulmonary function with aging, as well as a lessening of laryngeal efficiency (Kent et al., 1987), resulting in a decrement in maximum phonation time in the geriatric population.

S/Z Ratio. As noted previously, both respiratory and laryngeal factors play some role in determining maximum phonation time. However, the measure of maximum phonation time does not provide sufficient information to differentiate between deficits in respiratory support versus laryngeal inefficiency. In 1977 Boone introduced the s/z ratio as an expansion on the measurement of maximum phonation time. The underlying theoretical construct suggests that individuals with normal larynges should be able to sustain vocalization (i.e., /z/) for a period of time equal to that of sustained expiratory airflow without vocalization (i.e., /s/), resulting in a ratio that approximates 1. If the respiratory system is compromised and the laryngeal system is intact, there should be an equal reduction in expiratory airflow for the voiceless /s/ and the voiced /z/ components of the task, which again would yield a ratio approximating 1. However, reduced vibratory efficiency of the abnormal larynx should result in air wastage, with reduction in the ability to sustain phonation but without a reduction in duration of expiratory airflow in the absence of phonation. Thus, the s/z ratio would be greater than 1 in the presence of laryngeal abnormality. Eckel and Boone (1981), in a study of dysphonic adults with and without laryngeal pathology, obtained results that support this notion. Ninety-five percent of patients with vocal fold margin pathology studied by Eckel and Boone had s/z ratios above 1.4, while the ratios for both the normal control group and those patients with dysphonia without pathology approximated 1.

Two studies have been reported investigating the use of the s/z ratio with children, and the results have not supported the previous research. In a study of 16 children with vocal nodules, Rastatter and Hyman (1982) report s/z ratios of 1, similar to expectations in the normal population. Similar findings are reported by Hufnagle and Hufnagle (1988) in a larger study of 123 dysphonic children, of whom 69 had vocal fold nodules. Based on the results of these studies, it would appear that the s/z ratio is not sensitive to the presence of vocal fold pathology in children, nor does it separate dysphonic children (with or without pathology) from normals. Although the reason for the difference between adults and children on this measure is not entirely clear, it is theorized that the size and stiffness of the pathology in the adult subjects may have been greater than for the children, all of whom in the Hufnagle and Hufnagle study were reported to have had small to moderate size nodules that were soft in consistency. Measures of maximum duration of production of both /s/ and /z/ have been reported by Tait, Michel, and Carpenter (1980) for 53 children aged 5, 7, and 9 years with normal voices. The maximum duration times for both /s/ and /z/ reported by Rastatter and Hyman (1982) and by Hufnagle and Hufnagle for their subjects who had vocal fold nodules or were dysphonic were lower than those reported by Tait et al. for their normal subjects.

The procedure for measuring the s/z ratio is very straightforward. The patient is instructed to take a deep breath and then sustain an /s/ for as long as possible. The examiner should model the task, although it is not necessary to sustain the model maximally. The task should be repeated at least twice by the patient, with the longest duration taken as the score. The same procedure is carried out for sustaining the /z/. It is best to use a stopwatch in obtaining these measures. The ratio is obtained by dividing the maximal /s/ value by the maximal /z/ value. Available normative s/z ratio data are presented in Chapter 13.

Although this measure has been demonstrated to have some validity for adults, the cautions discussed relative to maximum phonation time measures also apply here. The s/z ratio should be used primarily as a screening measure or as one test among many others. A diagnosis of pathology should never be made based on the result of this procedure alone. However, it may alert a clinician to the need for medical examination, if that has not been done, or conversely, it may raise questions about a diagnosis of pathology if the results are not consistent. The validity of this measure for children is still open to question, and thus it should be used in that population with even greater caution.

The apparent simplicity of this measure may be somewhat deceiving. Clinically we have found that it is necessary to teach this task to patients and to allow them adequate practice before taking formal measures (Chapter 13).

Scaling. Perceptual judgments of various aspects of voice, quality in particular, are usually described as being subjective and therefore somehow invalid. However, perceptions can be quantified using well-established techniques of psychophysics and the procedure of scaling. The simplest type of quantification of qualitative or categorical variables is at the level of the nominal scale. The fundamental principle of nominal scales is equivalence; that is, all observations placed within the same category are considered to be equal. For example, voice qualities can be assigned names such as harsh, breathy, hoarse, or strident, which constitute categories. The perceptual judgment task may be to place voice samples within categories along that scale. No judgments are made or implied as to quantity or severity of the quality perceived. This is simply, as the name of the scale implies, a naming task.

However, we are usually interested in more than naming. Perhaps we want to make judgments about the degree of a quality that is present. Using our group of subjects who were nominally scaled as having hoarse voice quality, we can now engage in rank ordering them according to severity, using an ordinal scale. In this scale, numbers are used to express order of magnitude of the perception. The rank order means that higher numbers have a greater amount of a feature than lower numbers. Thus, the voice quality given a rank order of 1 has been judged to have less hoarseness than that with a rank order of 15. Ranks do not tell us how much of a feature is present or how much difference there is between ranks or even if the differences between ranks are equal. The only information we have is that at a given rank there is less or more of a feature than at the ranks above or below.

Interval scales are very common in voice quality scaling because we can use them to determine how much of a feature is present in one quality compared to another. The refinement over an ordinal scale is that the distance between adjacent points on the scale has meaning, and a given interval between measures has the same meaning anywhere along the scale. Common examples of this type of scale are degrees of temperature and calendar years. In the latter we know that as much time elapsed between 1790 and 1800 as between 1970 and 1980. The interval scale thus has a defined unit of measure. However, it does not necessarily have a defined beginning or a meaningful zero point.

The ratio scale has all the properties of the interval scale, with the added benefit of an absolute zero. Such a scale makes it possible to talk meaningfully about ratios. Examples of this type of scale are measures of length.

A visual analog scale simply presents a continuum between two anchor points, such as an undifferentiated 5-inch line-scale along which a mark is made representing the quantity of a feature judged to be present. Such a scale does not use any verbal descriptors along it and is reported by some to produce more reliable and valid judgments because it permits finer discriminations to be made (Kempster, 1984). For scoring purposes the 5-inch line in the example above could be converted into a 100-point rating scale.

The most complex scaling method is referred to as multidimensional scaling, a method for identifying the perceptual attributes of complex stimuli such as voice quality (Schiffman, Reynolds, and Young, 1981; Kempster, 1984). Algorithms of multidimensional scales represent stimuli as points on a spatial map. The difference between points is then a reflection of the judged similarity or dissimilarity of the stimuli. The closer the points, the greater the similarity of the feature being judged.

Scaling of Pitch.   Perceptual judgments of voice quality are often confounded by other perceptual attributes of the voice sample and may not always be related to a simple acoustic correlate. For example, let us examine the perception of pitch. Wolfe and Ratusnik (1988) have shown that listeners will rate the pitch of rough vowels much lower than the pitch of normally produced vowels. Consequently, vowels produced by a patient with a hoarse voice may be expected to be perceived as lower in pitch than their measured fundamental frequencies would predict. Furthermore, Wolfe and Ratusnik reported that the pitch matches they obtained were related to the acoustic measures of noise energy level and jitter ratio rather than to fundamental frequency. Thus, it appears that with respect to pitch, other abnormal perceptual (e.g., roughness, hoarseness) or acoustic (e.g., jitter, noise level, spectrum) attributes may result in inaccurate judgment. This may account for some of the discrepancies that have been noted between perceptual pitch judgments of abnormal voices and the measured acoustic correlate of fundamental frequency. Wilson, Wellen, and Kimbarow (1983) suspect that there is a skill in discriminating pitch differences in the speaking voice that is not easily developed. Their judges, described as trained and untrained, performed at chance level on a pitch discrimination task until there was at least a 20 to 29 Hz difference present between paired voice samples.

Another factor affecting the reliability and validity of perceptual judgments is the experience of the listener. Many studies in which perceptual judgments were reported used experienced listeners or listeners with extensive exposure to normal and abnormal voice qualities. How much experience is needed to produce reliable judgments is somewhat unclear. Bassich and Ludlow (1986) conducted a study using 4 judges who required 16 1/2-

hour training sessions before reaching 80% agreement with one another. These findings may help to account for the lack of difference between groups of trained and untrained listeners in distinguishing pitch differences between pairs of children's voices, as reported by Wilson et al. (1983). In this study, the trained group consisted of 10 graduate students in speech pathology, of which only 4 had had previous experience in working with patients with voice disorders.

It would seem highly unlikely that graduate students with only a brief exposure to voice disorders (usually a single academic course and perhaps an actual patient in clinic) would be able to reliably and accurately rate attributes of the voice such as pitch, loudness, and tremor. In a study reported by Colton and Estill (1981) concerned with the identification of four distinct voice qualities, the group of 6 speech pathologists performed slightly worse than the group of 15 "naive" listeners (66% versus 68%). Singers and individuals who played a musical instrument performed somewhat better than these two groups (73% for singers, 75% for instrumentalists). Although the differences between the groups were not large, these results suggest that experience in music may help a listener to make judgments concerned with voice quality attributes. At the very least, musicians may better attend to the nonlinguistic aspects of the speaker's utterance.

It is clear that perceptual judgments of vocal pitch are sufficiently unreliable to cast doubt on their use in planning treatment strategies. Determinations of the appropriateness of pitch level should be made on the measurement of its acoustic correlate, fundamental frequency, for which normative values appropriate for age and sex are available for comparison. Whenever measureable acoustic correlates of vocal attributes are available, their use is encouraged in preference to reliance on the perceptual feature.

Scaling Vocal Effort.   The effort a patient uses to vocalize may be important to assess in the examination of a voice problem. Many patients report that at the end of a day of prolonged talking, they feel vocally fatigued. They may also report that they need to expend more energy in talking than they did prior to their vocal problem. It is difficult for the clinician to know how to assess such reports and what value to give them. However, there is a way for such "feelings" to be measured, and such measures can be helpful therapeutically and in assessing the efficacy of treatment and of specific treatment techniques.

How does the clinician quantify the vocal effort a patient uses during phonation? Simply by asking the patient to produce a vocalization and afterward asking that patient to assign it a number that represents the amount of effort used. It has been shown that subjects can scale their own effort levels with this simple procedure (Lane, Catania, and Stevens, 1961; Irwin and Mills, 1965; Wright and Colton, 1972a, 1972b; Colton and Brown, 1973). Wright and Colton (1972a, 1972b) asked five normal speakers to produce the vowel /a/ at their minimum, most comfortable, and maximum effort levels. The fundamental frequency and the sound pressure level of each phonation was measured during each vocalization. The subjects were then asked to assign a number that represented the amount of effort used. They could use any number they wished, with the understanding that greater effort levels would be associated with higher numbers. This procedure is often referred to in the psychophysical literature as the method of magnitude estimation. Median results for the group are shown in Figure 7.14. The left panel shows vocal effort in assigned numbers versus SPL in decibels. In the right panel, vocal effort is compared to fundamental frequency. The solid lines connect minimum, most comfortable, and maximum effort levels. The data points between these three effort levels (squares) were generated by asking the subject to produce a phonation whose effort was halfway between minimum and most comfortable or most comfortable and maximum. Each of these intervals then was bisected again to produce the estimates of vocal effort shown in this figure.

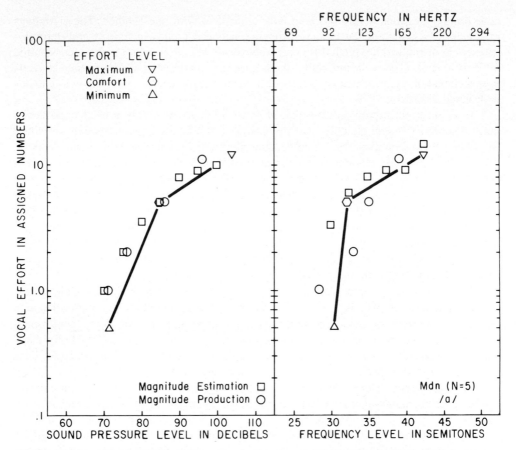

Figure 7.14. Vocal effort/sound pressure level and vocal effort/fundamental frequency relationships for five normal speakers. (Based on data reported by Wright and Colton, 1972b.)

Note how consistent the subjects were in producing and rating their effort levels, especially for effort versus SPL. The data points for magnitude production (shown by circles) were obtained by providing a number to the subject and asking him to produce a phonation with an effort level representative of the number supplied. These data are very similar to the data obtained in the magnitude estimate phase of the experiment. The vocal effort/fundamental frequency data show somewhat more variability between magnitude production and estimation than the vocal effort/SPL data. It is abundantly clear, however, that individuals can rate the effort they use to produce voice and that variations of vocal effort are manifested acoustically by variation of SPL and fundamental frequency.

   The data of Figure 7.14 clearly show that an increase of vocal effort is accompanied by an increase of both intensity and frequency. Colton and Brown (1973) have shown that speakers also exhibit systematic increases of intraoral air pressure with an increase of vocal effort. In simple consonant-vowel syllables, intraoral air pressure can be a good estimate of the pressures driving the vocal folds (Rothenberg, 1968; Smitheran and Hixon, 1981). Thus, it is not unreasonable to suspect that the magnitude of subglottal air pressure, accompanied by the consequent tension of the vocal folds, contributes to the judgments of vocal effort.

   Listeners can also rate vocal effort from recorded samples of speech (Lane et al., 1961; Warren, 1962; Brandt, Ruder, and Shipp, 1969; Moll and Peterson, 1969), but the ratings are not simply ratings of the vocal loudness (Brandt et al.). Listeners apparently use the increase of energy in the higher frequencies as cues for their judgments of vocal effort as well as the greater sound pressure levels that accompany increased effort levels. They may also internalize what they hear and relate their judgments to their own perceived efforts. It is important to understand that increased tension in the adducted vocal folds results in greater subglottal air pressure and also results in the production of increased energy in the higher frequencies. Thus, listeners and speakers appear to use similar cues, only the speaker has access to the significant physiological variable, air pressure, whereas the listener must depend solely on its acoustic manifestation, increased high frequency energy.

The concept of vocal effort, as well as its measurement, has implications for the management of voice problems, for monitoring progress, and for assessing treatment efficacy (see Chapter 9).

Voice Sample Recording

One of the easiest and simplest ways of testing a subject is to obtain a voice recording. Even if no further analysis of the recording is performed, the recording itself can be invaluable. Recording makes repeated listening possible allowing the voice clinician further opportunities to learn about the person's voice characteristics. A voice recording during the initial assessment provides a baseline record of the voice prior to intervention. This documentation can be helpful for demonstrating progress or change as a result of treatment and for judging the efficacy of treatment. A baseline recording is highly important when medical-legal issues arise. It is surprising, therefore, that so little attention is generally given to the techniques and equipment needed for producing good-quality recordings. The material presented in the following sections is based both on personal experience and on discussions by Izdebski (1981, 1983).

Tape Recorders

There are three kinds of tape recorders that can be used to make audio recordings: (*a*) reel-to-reel, (*b*) cassette, and (*c*) videotape recorders. The reel-to-reel models have an excellent frequency response and a wide dynamic range but are not often found in most voice clinics. Manufacturers of reel-to-reel units include Nigra, Ampex, and Revox. Cassette recorders are much more popular and offer the conveniences of portability and use of cassette tapes. Although inexpensive cassette recorders are available, they rarely have good frequency response or adequate dynamic range, do not produce good recordings, have high tape instability (wow and flutter), and are prone to breakdown. They are not recommended for clinical use. There are many cassette recorders costing $200 to $600 that have good to excellent characteristics and are easy to use. We include videotape recorders in this category because many of the medium-priced models, as well as the higher priced ones, have excellent frequency and dynamic ranges in the audio range, very low tape instability, and can store considerable data. Furthermore, many can record and reproduce in stereo.

In addition to good recording equipment, it is also important to use high quality tape. High quality tape has a number of advantages: (*a*) It is strong enough to withstand the starting and stopping required when many speech samples are recorded and played back, and (*b*) less of the oxide particles in the tape will rub off to affect the recording and playback heads and interfere with the motor and wheels that transport the tape. Tapes are available in 30- to 120-minute lengths. It is best to avoid the 120-minute tapes because the tape is very thin and can break easily. Cassette tapes made by TDK, Maxell, Sony,

Nakamichi, 3M, or similar manufacturers are of good quality. Tapes may also differ in type, for example, standard tape, chromium dioxide tape (a high bias tape), or metal tape (also a high bias tape). Most tape recorders are able to play back all of these types of tape. Metal tape tends to have the best response characteristics, but at considerably greater cost. Many of the good to excellent cassette recorders will have metal tape recording/reproducing capability.

Videotapes also come in various time lengths, depending on whether they are VHS or Beta format. For the VHS format, although 6-hour recordings can be made at the slowest speed setting, when using the tape for obtaining good audio recordings, it is best to use the the higher speed settings (2 or 4 hours).

Microphones

Microphones should be selected on the basis of low distortion, low sensitivity, wide frequency response (50 to 16,000 Hz), directionality, stability, and cost. Good-quality microphones can be purchased for relatively low cost, ($50 to $100). A good source for microphones is Radio Shack. Many new microphones are of the electret type, which contain a small battery and pickup element that has very good frequency and dynamic response characteristics. There are also condensor and dynamic microphones that have excellent characteristics at moderate cost. A pressure zone microphone, a relatively new type of microphone that permits recording large groups with good fidelity, is also worthy of consideration.

Environment

Recordings should be made in a quiet room, away from noisy corridors and windows that face onto busy streets. The room need not be completely sound proof, however. Carpeted floors and walls and windows hung with fabric coverings of some sort serve to reduce noise level to a significant degree. Of course, special acoustic absorbing panels can be installed, which will produce a very quiet room. The clinician should measure the noise levels within the room to make sure they are acceptable (less than 50 dB at the low frequencies) and periodically check these levels to ensure that the noise present is predominantly low frequency.

Tasks

It is important to chose a variety of tasks for the patient to carry out that will sample the full range of the patient's vocal capabilities. Sustained vowels are useful for subsequent measurement of fundamental frequency, perturbation, and spectra. Syllables and sentences should be used to sample the patient's voice under more speech-like conditions and yet yield data that can be compared at different time periods. Testing of vocal limits, that is, phonational (frequency) range and dynamic (intensity) range, can also be recorded. We usually include a standard reading passage (Rainbow Passage; Fairbanks, 1960) and a sample of conversational speech as part of our recording protocol. Of course, it is important to also record any special or unusual characteristics of a patient's vocal behavior. The speech tasks from the protocol for fiberoptic examination in the Appendix may be used for any audio recording.

Special Testing: Psychiatric, Neurological, Imaging

The linkage between personality and voice cannot be overemphasized. It is expressed in a multitude of ways by all speakers. Second only to our appearance, the voice serves as our identity, as a means of identification even in the absence of the visual presence. It serves as our emotional escape valve as we laugh, cry, scream in fear, or shout in rage. It speaks of our well-being, of our energy level, of our emotional state. We use it to cajole, to seduce, to energize, to subdue, to question, to arouse, to soothe, to scorn, to demand, to plead—in short, to create meaning for our words. And we are called upon to use our voices to impart information, to express opinions, to defend our property, our rights, ourselves, to intercede for others, to influence others, and simply to interact with others. Our voices are a road between people, the road on which the words we speak travel. Is it any wonder, then, that the road is sometimes subject to breakdown, that it gives way physically or becomes altered due to excessive tensions and stresses, that it is the scene of accidents, tie-ups, and bottlenecks? In some cases these breakdowns are minor, requiring only that someone understand the situation and arrive at a way to resolve it. However, other problems require extensive repairs and require specific types of expertise if they are to be attended to properly.

The analogies are obvious. For some people, excess tensions are felt most keenly in the laryngeal area. The effect of these tensions may take time to gradually become apparent and bothersome, or they may reach a significant level rather quickly. There is a continuum of effect, from the very mild hoarseness that tends to come on at the end of the day to the constant and all-pervasive lack of voice. The degree of the dysphonic symptoms is not necessarily correlated with the "severity" of the problem.

Clinically, patients with voice disorders of psychological origin constitute a fascinating group of people, for many of whom almost magical return of voice is not infrequent. Skill, understanding, and patience are required, but the reward for the speech pathologist is an immediate gratification that comes rarely in the practice of the profession. Specific procedures for the treatment of these kinds of problems will be discussed in Chapter 9.

For a significant number of patients, however, the basic problems are much deeper. The patient is unable to give up the symptom, or unable to do so permanently. In such cases, there is a clear need for referral for psychiatric consult or counseling. Indeed, such a referral is also often necessary and helpful for those persons who, with our help, may be able to abandon their symptoms, but for whom there continue to be problems that need attention.

CASE EXAMPLE R. W. was a young man of 16 years, referred for voice therapy with a diagnosis of dysphonia in the presence of a normal-appearing larynx. The dysphonia was in its 3rd month, and he had been out of school for that entire period of time on doctor's orders. Prior to this referral, he had already been on a regimen of voice rest and through several courses of pharmacologic treatment, with no change in symptoms. It was very difficult to engage R. W. in conversation. He responded to all questions in as few words as possible. He made only fleeting eye contact. He was a large, quite overweight, and not very attractive young man. R. W.'s voice sounded very strained and tense. Hoarseness was present. Working very slowly, with constant encouragement and praise, we were able to elicit a normal voice quality. R. W. refused to recognize this change at first, but slowly became willing to use the good voice more frequently. Within a few therapy sessions R. W. had full return of normal voice and was ready to return to school.

During the therapy sessions the need for R. W. to see a psychiatrist or psychologist was raised both with him and his mother. With return of normal voice a direct referral for such additional treatment was made. A month later R. W. returned. His voice had worsened, with a full recurrence of earlier symptoms. Our referral for psychiatric follow-up had not been carried out. R. W. was seen again for several sessions of voice therapy, during which he continued to be very closed in all respects. Once again voice was restored and once again referral for psychiatric consultation was made even more strongly. Two months later this story began to repeat itself. However, on this occasion, the mother was advised that it was not appropriate to continue this form of treatment, especially because our strong recommendation for psychiatric consultation had not been followed.

It is often necessary to move slowly when referral for psychiatric examination is being considered. A sense of trust must be built between the clinician and the patient. The clinician must be sufficiently attuned to the patient's needs to be able to approach the referral in the manner that will be most likely to be accepted. Referrals made too abruptly may be totally rejected by the patient, who may also reject the person making the referral. When that occurs, the patient may be lost to follow-up or treatment of any kind for some period of time. This is what we were hoping to avoid in the case of R. W. above. Unfortunately, even our best efforts sometimes do not bring about the desired result.

It is vitally important to consider all possible etiologies of a presenting problem before adopting the diagnosis of psychogenic voice disorder. There are a number of neurological disease processes whose early symptoms may be very similar to those presented by patients with emotionally based problems. These patients present with no visible laryngeal abnormality and with symptoms that may be mystifying and histories that may be confounding.

CASE EXAMPLE J. R., a 37-year-old woman, had been examined and treated by several otolaryngologists over a period of months with no change in her vocal status. She was then referred for a trial of voice therapy. J. R. reported a rather troubled social history involving a very difficult recent divorce preceded by a number of years in an abusive marriage during which she had suffered attempted strangulation and blows to the neck. She and her 7-year-old son were now living with a friend as she was trying to put her life in order. Her voice symptoms began during the course of the divorce process. She described a "gravelly" quality that came on gradually with any extended period of talking but that cleared when she was able to rest and be silent for a while. She denied any other physical symptoms.

The history thus far seemed to suggest a classic voice disorder of psychological etiology. During the initial evaluation, however, the clinician was impressed with this patient's attitude, forthrightness, and overall affect. Furthermore, we noted the gradual worsening of voice as the evaluation progressed, which J. R. attributed in part to having engaged in much conversation during a lengthy car trip from her home to our office. Trials of diagnostic therapy procedures were totally ineffective in eliciting improved voice quality. J. R. was subsequently referred for neurological examination and a diagnosis of myasthenia gravis was made.

Referral for neurological examination is usually well accepted by patients. It should be considered when laryngeal findings are either negative or suggestive of disordered coordination of laryngeal function, when the voice symptoms are neither consistent with nor explained by the history, when changes in vocal output cannot be altered by behavioral approaches and whenever there is a family history of neurological problems. Similarly, patients usually respond well when referred for further medical examinations, as might be indicated when gastroesophageal reflux is suspected as a key factor in the voice problem.

The past decade has seen major growth and development of increasingly sophisticated imaging technology: computerized axial tomography (CT scan), ultrasound, magnetic resonance imaging (MRI), and positive emission tomography (PET), to name a few. Although these techniques are being widely used to determine the location and extent of disease, data relevant to phonatory behavior are not yet available. At this time the primary use of these techniques for the study of laryngeal function is in the realm of research. Clinical use is limited, due not only to the limited data available but also to the limited availability of the equipment and the cost of the procedures.

Summary

The voice history is a critical part of the diagnostic process not only for the information obtained but also because of the relationship that taking it establishes between the clinician and the patient. The first section of this chapter is devoted to a discussion of the skill involved in the interview process. The content of the interview is presented in some detail and includes the following sections: the problem and its effects, the developmental history of the problem, its onset and duration, the variable or consistent nature of the problem and associated symptoms, the patient's health history, and vocational, social, and recreational histories.

The array of techniques used in the examination and testing of the voice have been described in the second and third sections of this chapter. Examination of the larynx can be carried out through both direct and indirect methods. Technological advances have substantially increased our ability to visualize not only the structure of the larynx and supraglottal vocal tract but also the dynamic physiology of both phonatory and nonphonatory behavior. The examination procedures described include indirect laryngoscopy, direct laryngoscopy, flexible fiberoptic laryngoscopy, stroboscopy, videofluoroscopy, ultra-high speed photography, and ultrasound. Advantages and disadvantages of each are discussed.

Laboratory testing procedures provide documentable and measurable evidence of vocal function. These techniques sometimes provide indirect evidence about the functional status of the larynx. They include acoustic measures of fundamental frequency and its variability, functional limits of the voice relative to frequency and intensity, periodicity and stability of the voice as evidenced by measures of perturbation, and visual evidence of the acoustic components of the voice as displayed in a spectrogram or an acoustic spectrum. Physiological studies provide further evidence and information about the larynx and the voice. These include electroglottography, photoglottography, inverse filtering of airflow, and electromyography. Testing of respiratory function is another aspect of physiological function that can add to the total data pool in selected cases.

We have chosen to include the various forms of noninstrumental evaluation of the voice, usually carried out by the speech pathologist but useful to all who examine and work with the voice-disordered patient, as part of this chapter. These noninstrumental methods include critical listening, observation, and description. Formalization of the kinds of observations that should be made, both auditory and visual, will help to focus the examiner's careful attention to the variety of clues that can be obtained about vocal function through this approach. The clinical trial involved in a diagnostic therapy approach allows the examiner to test hypotheses and extend the observations.

Objective measurements that can be made without the benefit of any equipment more sophisticated than a stopwatch are also discussed. Although fairly simple to obtain, these measurements can be extremely useful in establishing baseline measures of vocal function and subsequently to chart progress or assess the results of treatment. Within this section we have also discussed the need for suitable audio recordings and the types of equipment that are appropriate to address this need.

The final section of this chapter deals briefly with the need for additional testing, for which referral is made as indicated. Such testing may include psychiatric consultation, neurological examination, medical assessment for associated problems, and special imaging techniques.

SUGGESTED READINGS

Bernstein L, Bernstein RS,(1985), Interviewing, A Guide for Health Professionals (4th ed.), Norwalk, CT: Appleton-Century-Crofts.

Hersen M, Turner SM, (1985), Diagnostic Interviewing, New York: Plenum Press.

Levinson D, (1987), A Guide to the Clinical Interview, Philadelphia: WB Saunders.

Maple FF, (1985), Dynamic Interviewing, An Introduction to Counseling, Beverly Hills, CA: Sage Publications.

8

Surgical and Medical Management of Voice Disorders

There are three general approaches to the management of voice problems, no one of which necessarily excludes the others. These approaches are (*a*) surgical, (*b*) medical, and (*c*) behavioral. The first two will be discussed in this chapter; the behavioral approach will be discussed in Chapter 9. Although these approaches are being presented separately, it is often the case that ideal treatment requires the use of combined treatment modalities. For example, the patient who has sustained traumatic laryngeal damage in an automobile accident may first be a surgical candidate. However, after surgery and healing, this patient may well benefit from vocal rehabilitation in order to reestablish the best possible voice production.

Surgery is considered the more radical treatment approach because of the need to cut into tissues to remove body parts or abnormal growths, or to physically alter or augment the shape or position of structures. A review of surgical techniques that are currently being used in the management of laryngeal problems with a phonatory component is presented in the first section of this chapter. The medical approach to the treatment of voice disorders refers to techniques that are not invasive or do not involve surgical ablation, reconstruction, or alteration; these will be discussed in the second section.

Surgical Management

Concept of Phonosurgery

Phonosurgery refers to a collection of surgical techniques that have as their aim the improvement of voice. Some phonosurgery techniques have long been in practice. Among these are the removal of benign masses of the vocal folds, including nodules and polyps; vocal fold mediofixation and/or intrafold injection for unilateral vocal fold paralysis; and glottal reconstruction following partial laryngectomy.

Recently, however, there has been renewed interest and marked growth in phonosurgery for many other laryngeal conditions and voice disorders. There are three good reasons for this renewed interest. The first relates to a change in the focus of surgery from an emphasis on procedures designed to eradicate or ablate to those in which the goal is to conserve, reconstruct,or improve function. The second, probably concomittant reason is the recent development of surgical techniques and instruments that permit more refined surgeries, and the third is the growth of information on the anatomy, physiology, and pathology of voice, the results of which are now being seen in clinical applications.

The term ''phonosurgery'' was first used by Hans von Leden in two articles (von Leden, Yanagihara, and Werner-Kukuk, 1967; von Leden, Poyle, Goff, and Miller, 1969) discussing some surgical approaches for voice improvement. The 1970s saw marked progress in technique and growth in the use of phonosurgical procedures, primarily in Japan (Hirano, 1975; Isshiki, 1977; Saito, 1977). Since the 1980s, phonosurgery has found rapid acceptance in many countries around the world.

There are five major groups of phonosurgery: (a) removal of pathological tissue; (b) surgical correction of the position, shape, and/or tension of the vocal fold(s); (c) surgery to alter or restore laryngeal neuromuscular function; (d) surgical reconstruction for partial loss and/or deformity of the larynx; and (e) surgical reconstruction for loss of the entire larynx. Each group, except for (e), will be described in the following sections. This final group will not be included because total laryngectomy and related issues are beyond the scope of this book.

Surgical Removal of Pathological Tissue of the Phonatory Organ

The development of endolaryngeal microsurgery in the 1960s (Saito, Ogino, Ishikura, Niino, and Fukuda, 1966; Kleinsasser, 1968) opened up new avenues for phonosurgery. The operating microscope permits visualization of lesions in ways not previously possible in the living patient. It allows safe and precise removal of pathological tissue, with greater ease. Jako (1972) and Strong and Jako (1972) developed the use of the CO_2 laser in combination with the operating microscope. The use of this combined technique for removing laryngeal lesions has become widespread.

In removing vocal fold pathologies, extreme care must be taken to avoid invading normal vocal fold tissue beyond the minimum required. Normal vocal folds have a unique and delicate layered structure, as described in Chapter 3. Once this structure is destroyed, complete surgical reconstruction is usually extremely difficult, if not impossible.

Vocal Fold Nodules

The need for surgical excision of vocal fold nodules is limited because almost all nodules in children disappear spontaneously by the end of adolescence, and most nodules can be successfully treated with voice therapy. In children, surgery is indicated only in extreme cases in which the effects of the voice abnormality on the child are serious and voice therapy has not been effective. Surgical removal of nodules in adults may be indicated when voice therapy has not been effective.

When nodules are surgically removed, only the excessive tissue should be ablated. The postsurgical result should be a vocal fold with a minimal surgical wound (Fig. 8.1).

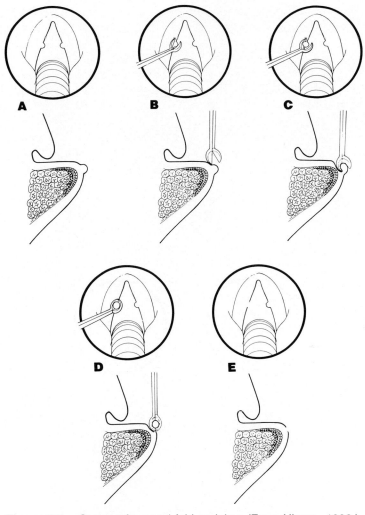

Figure 8.1. Surgery for vocal fold nodules. (From Hirano, 1988.)

Note how the small, delicate forceps are used to grasp and then cut the nodule on the left vocal fold. It is important to cut only the nodule and not extend the cut into the deeper layers of the lamina propria. Otherwise, healing will be slower, and scar tissue may develop that will interfere with normal vibration.

Vocal Fold Polyp

Fresh and small polyps are subjected to surgical treatment when they have not responded to voice therapy. For large and/or old polyps, surgery followed by voice therapy is the protocol of choice.

In surgery, only excessive mass should be removed; care should be taken not to excise healthy tissue. Again, the result should be a normal contour of the vocal fold with a minimal wound (Fig. 8.2). In this procedure, a fine knife is used to excise the upper attachments of the polyps. Then, a forcep is used to grasp and cut the remaining attachments of the polyp.

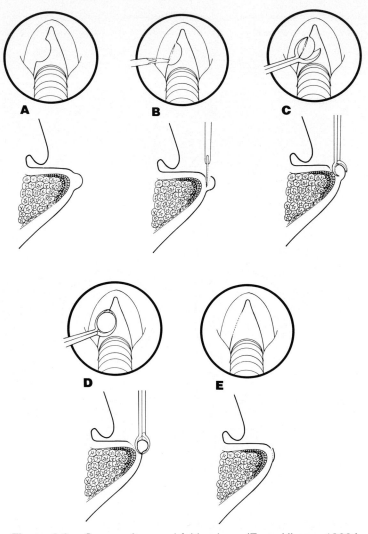

Figure 8.2. Surgery for vocal fold polyps. (From Hirano, 1988.)

Reinke's Edema

The surgical approach is indicated in almost all cases of Reinke's edema. Cigarette smoking, highly implicated as an etiological factor, should be stopped prior to surgery. Surgery should then be followed by voice therapy.

The most important principle in surgery for Reinke's edema is to preserve the mucosa at the vocal fold edge. If the mucosa is removed at the edge, stiff scar tissue may form, resulting in dysphonia. The surgical procedure involves the removal of the edematous mucosa of the upper surface of the vocal fold first (Fig. 8.3B and C). The fluid contents of the vocal fold are then sucked and pressed out of the wound (Fig. 8.3D and E). Redundant mucosa, if any, is removed (Fig. 8.3F and G).

Epidermoid Cyst

A surgical approach is indicated in all cases of epidermoid cysts. As was discussed in Chapter 4, small cysts are occasionally misdiagnosed as nodules or even completely over-

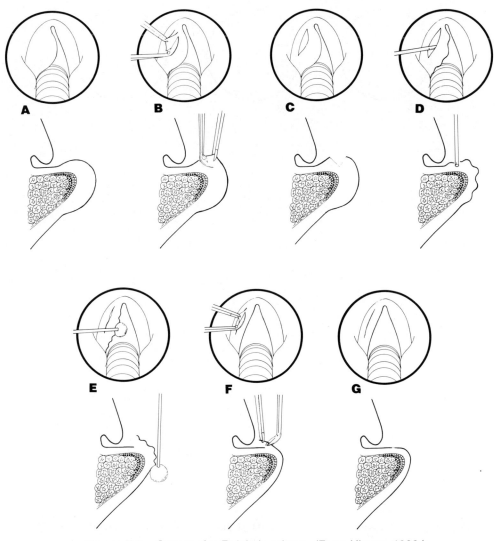

Figure 8.3.   Surgery for Reinke's edema. (From Hirano, 1988.)

looked under examination with regular light. Stroboscopy, especially when conducted with a fiberscope located close to the vocal fold, is useful in detecting such small cysts.

The ideal surgical technique is one that enucleates the cyst. A mucosal incision is made along the lateral margin or above the cyst (Fig. 8.4B). The cyst is carefully elevated from the neighboring structures and removed (Fig. 8.4C and D). A straight line incision on the upper surface of the vocal fold is the result (Fig. 8.4E).

Nonspecific Granuloma

Almost all nonspecific granulomas of the larynx are caused by either traumatic vocal behavior (contact granuloma), endotracheal intubation (intubation granuloma), or gastroesophageal reflux (see Chapter 4). They are usually located on the lateral aspect of the posterior glottis, under which the arytenoid cartilage lies. Granulomas should first be treated with nonsurgical modalities, including vocal hygiene programs, voice therapy, and

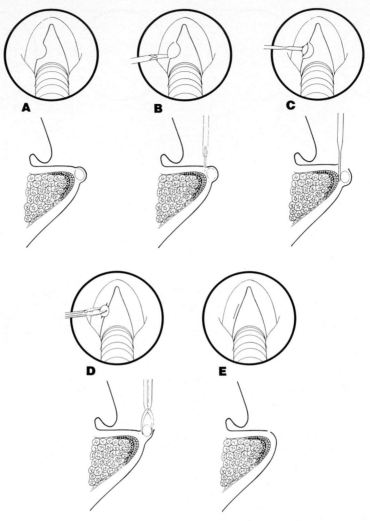

Figure 8.4. Surgery for epidermoid cyst of the vocal fold. (From Hirano, 1988.)

antireflux therapy. When nonsurgical modalities do not prove effective or the granulomas are very large, causing respiratory distress, they need to be treated surgically.

Surgery is best conducted under general anesthesia with Venturi ventilation. (Venturi ventilation refers to a technique where a fine jet of gas [oxygen, nitrogen, or appropriate combination] is directed into the trachea, replacing the usual endotracheal tube.) The major portion of the granuloma is first removed with the use of scissors and forceps, leaving the base (Fig. 8.5A and B). A laser is used to remove any material from the base (Fig. 8.5C and D). Care should be taken not to injure the arytenoid perichondrium.

Epithelial Hyperplasia and Dysplasia

Cessation of smoking occasionally results in the disappearance of hyperplastic and dysplastic epithelium. Immediate surgery can be delayed with discontinuation of smoking and periodic follow-up. If surgery is undertaken, it should be followed by cessation of smoking.

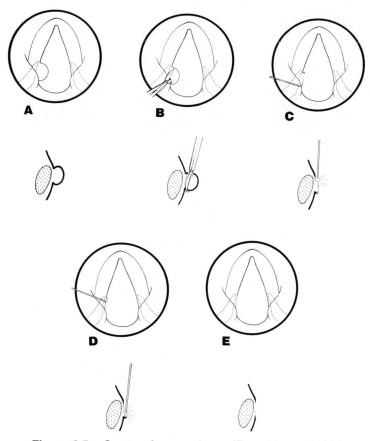

Figure 8.5. Surgery for granuloma. (From Hirano, 1988.)

The surgical procedure requires that a specimen be taken first for histological examination (Fig. 8.6B). Inclusion of the basement membrane in the specimen is essential for correct diagnosis. The remaining lesion is shaved using a CO_2 laser (Fig. 8.6C and D). This is continued until the vocal ligament is reached. The specimen is serially sectioned perpendicular to the basement membrane and studied histologically. Clinically, it is occasionally difficult to differentiate very early carcinoma from hyperplasia and dysplasia. If the histological study reveals early invasive carcinoma, further laser surgery, as described later, or radiotherapy is indicated.

Benign Neoplasms

The most frequent benign neoplasm of the larynx is papilloma. Hemangioma, fibroma, and other types of benign neoplasms are seen much less frequently. Most benign neoplasms can be removed by means of a CO_2 laser (Fig. 8.7).

Glottal Carcinoma

Glottal carcinoma confined to the membranous vocal fold (T1a classification) is a good candidate for laser excision. Treatment should be associated with discontinuation of smoking. The extent of the carcinomatous lesion is estimated by means of preoperative stroboscopy and Toluidine blue-staining under an operating microscope.

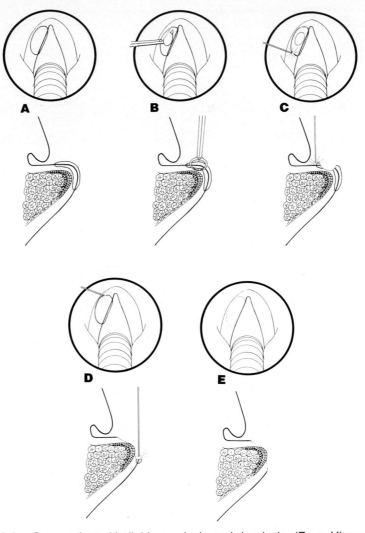

Figure 8.6. Surgery for epithelial hyperplasia and dysplasia. (From Hirano, 1988.)

An excisional biopsy is conducted by means of CO_2 laser (Fig. 8.8). A part of the thyroarytenoid muscle is usually removed. The surgical specimen is subjected to a serial section study. When histological studies reveal that cancer cells are located close to the margins of the specimens, radiotherapy, or additional surgery is indicated.

Surgical Correction of the Position, Shape, and/or Tension of the Vocal Fold

The surgical techniques in this group are used to medialize, lateralize, tense, or slacken the vocal fold, usually without direct surgical intervention to the vocal fold.

Vocal Fold Medialization

Two major groups of techniques are now in use to medialize the vocal fold edge: intrafold injection and medialization surgery.

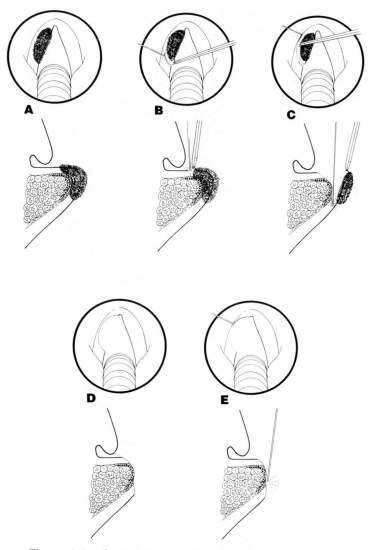

Figure 8.7. Surgery for papilloma. (From Hirano, 1988.)

Intrafold Injection. Intrafold injection is indicated most frequently to correct an incompetent glottis (i.e., the inability to close the glottis resulting from unilateral vocal fold paralysis). It is occasionally performed to correct or fill in a glottal gap accompanied by sulcus vocalis, or one caused by trauma or surgery.

Three types of injection material are currently in use: Teflon, silicone, and collagen. There are three techniques for intrafold injection: transoral injection using an indirect laryngeal mirror (Fig. 8.9), transoral injection under a direct laryngoscope (Fig. 8.10), and transcutaneous injection through the cricothyroid space (Fig. 8.11).

When injection is conducted transorally using a laryngeal mirror, the mucosa of the pharynx and larynx is anesthetized with lidocaine solution. Injection is performed while the patient sits with the mouth open and the tongue pulled forward. A curved laryngeal needle is used to administer the substance into the fold, and its effect is monitored visually and auditorily as the injection proceeds.

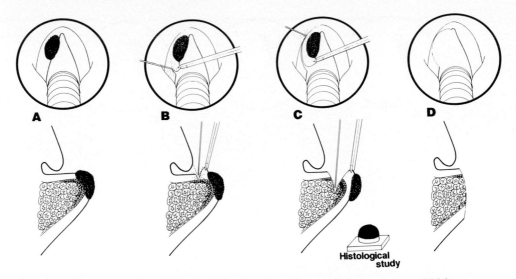

Figure 8.8.   Surgery for early glottal carcinoma. (From Hirano, 1988.)

Injection under a direct laryngoscope is performed with local mucosal anesthesia and/ or neuroleptanalgesia without endotracheal intubation. (Neuroleptanalgesia is a technique in which the patient is administered a drug that effectively abolishes memory of the procedure.) The internal branches of the bilateral superior laryngeal nerves are also anesthe-

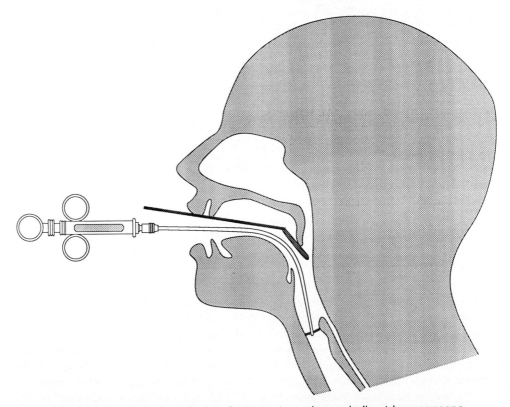

Figure 8.9.   Technique for intrafold injection using an indirect laryngoscope.

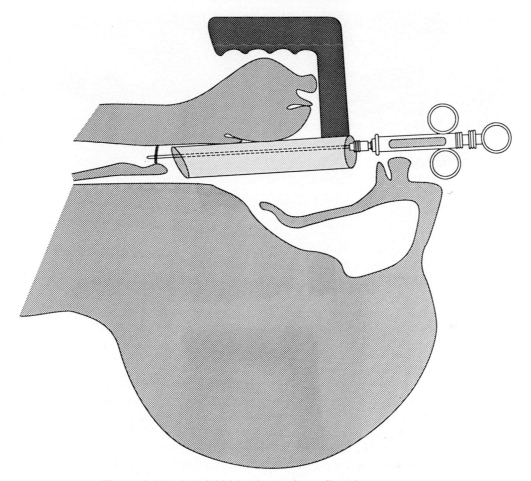

Figure 8.10.   Intrafold injection under a direct laryngoscope.

tized. The patient is placed in a supine position. The larynx is exposed with the use of a direct laryngoscope and viewed under an operating microscope. Injection is performed by means of a specially designed injection set such as the Arnold-Beuening Teflon injection set, the Nagashima silicone injection set, or the Collagen Corporation set. The effect of the injection is monitored visually and auditorily. Injection under general anesthesia with endotracheal intubation is not recommended because the effect cannot be monitored during the procedure. It is employed only for those patients who cannot undergo the procedure using local anesthesia or neuroleptanalgesia.

For transcutaneous injection, the nasal, pharyngeal, and laryngeal mucosa is anesthetized with lidocaine. The patient assumes a supine position with the anterior neck stretched. A fiberscope is inserted through the nose down to the larynx. It is coupled to a videocamera, and the fiberscopic image of the larynx is viewed on a television monitor screen. Local anesthesia is administered through the cervical skin at the cricothyroid space. The needle for intrafold injection is inserted into the larynx through the cricothyroid space. Its location is monitored by moving it back and forth medially as it proceeds. The effect of injection is monitored visually and auditorily during the procedure.

For unilateral vocal fold paralysis, Teflon or silicone is injected in the lateral portion of the thyroarytenoid muscle and/or in the space between the thyroid lamina and the

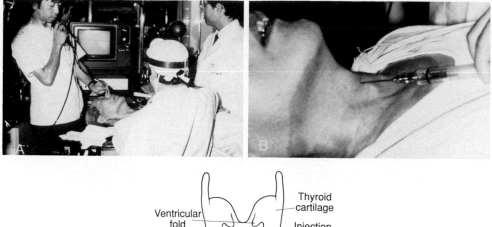

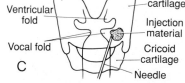

Figure 8.11.   Transcutaneous intrafold injection. **A,** An entire view during the procedure. **B,** A view of the patient's neck. **C,** Schematic presentation of the technique.

thyroarytenoid muscle (Fig. 8.12). It must not be injected in or near the mucosa of the vocal fold (Fig. 8.12A). Intramucosal Teflon or silicone stiffens the mucosa, resulting in a marked disturbance of vibration and subsequent dysphonia. Collagen, however, may be injected near the mucosa because its consistency is close to that of mucosal tissue.

In patients with sulcus vocalis, Teflon or silicone is injected in the middle of the thyroarytenoid muscle. The effect of intrafold injection for sulcus vocalis is limited because injection does not correct the sulcus itself but only reduces the glottal gap.

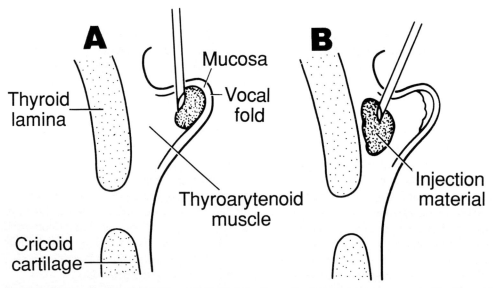

Figure 8.12.   Location of the intrafold injection. **A,** Incorrect placement. **B,** Correct placement.

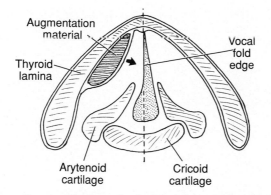

Figure 8.13. Schematic presentation of principle of surgical augmentation developed by Meurman (1952) and modified by others. (Reproduced by permission from Minoru Hirano, "Surgical Alteration of Voice Quality," in *Otolaryngology—Head and Neck Surgery, Update I*, Cummings CW, Fredrickson JM, Harker LA, Krause CJ, Schuller DE, eds. St. Louis, 1989, The C.V. Mosby Co.)

Medialization Surgery. There are many techniques to surgically medialize the vocal fold edge. They can be classified into three major types: (*a*) surgical augmentation, (*b*) medial shift of the thyroid cartilage, and (*c*) rotation of the arytenoid cartilage. Indications for the use of the first two techniques are basically the same as discussed for intrafold injection. The third type of medialization procedure is reserved almost exclusively for cases of unilateral vocal fold paralysis.

Surgical Augmentation. The basic principle of augmentation is to insert the material to be used medial to the thyroid cartilage at the level of the vocal folds, thus pushing the vocal folds medially (Meurman,1952; Sawashima, Totsuka, Kobayashi, and Hirose, 1968; Hiroto, 1976; Kleinsasser, 1987)(Fig. 8.13). A silicone block or autograph cartilage is commonly employed as the augmentation material. For a cartilage autograft, the upper part of the thyroid cartilage, nasal septum cartilage, or rib cartilage is used.

The surgery is performed under local anesthesia. A horizontal skin incision is made in the midportion of the anterior neck, and the thyroid cartilage is exposed on the paralytic side. The site of the augmentation implant can be reached with several different techniques (Fig. 8.14). In Figure 8.14A, a perichondrium incision is made along the superior edge of the thyroid cartilage whereas in Figure 8.14B a cartilage incision is made along the midline. In Figure 8.14C the site is reached via an anteroinferior approach by removing the medioinferior portion of the thyroid cartilage. In Figure 8.14D a block of cartilage is removed from the thyroid in order to reach the site for material implantation.

The augumentation material is located lateral to the vocal fold. The upper surface of the vocal fold is normally situated at the midlevel of the anterior angle of the thyroid cartilage. The posterior end of the membranous vocal fold is usually located at the anteroposterior midpoint of the thyroid lamina. Therefore, the augmentation material should be placed in the lower and anterior quadrant of the thyroid lamina. The size and location of the material is adjusted by auditorily monitoring the patient's voice during the procedure. Simultaneous visual monitoring with the use of a fiberscope is also useful. Once the material is located in the right place, it is sutured to the thyroid cartilage in order to prevent postsurgical migration.

Medial Shift of the Thyroid Cartilage. The basic principle of this technique is to medialize part of the thyroid cartilage at the level of the vocal fold, pushing the vocal fold

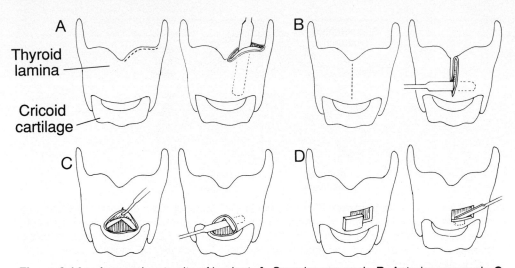

Figure 8.14. Approaches to site of implant. **A**, Superior approach. **B**, Anterior approach. **C**, Anteroinferior approach. **D**, Window technique. (Reproduced by permission from Minoru Hirano, "Surgical Alterations of Voice Quality," in *Otolaryngology—Head and Neck Surgery, Update I*, Cummings CW, Fredrickson JM, Harker LA, Krause CJ, Schuller DE, eds. St. Louis, 1989, The C.V. Mosby Co.)

edge to the midline (Isshiki, 1977; Payr, cited in Beck and Richstein, 1982; Koufman, 1986) (Fig. 8.15).

The surgery is conducted under local anesthesia. Following exposure of the thyroid lamina, a quadrangular cartilage specimen to be medialized is designed, as shown in Figure 8.16A. The upper edge is placed horizontally at the midlevel of the anterior angle of the thyroid lamina. The lower edge is located parallel to the upper edge but at a distance that is one-quarter the height of the anterior thyroid lamina. The anterior edge is positioned 5 mm from the anterior angle, and the posterior edge is located slightly posterior to the anteroposterior midpoint of the thyroid lamina.

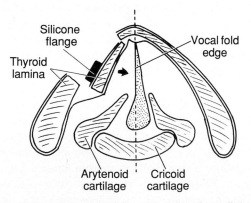

Figure 8.15. Schematic presentation of the principle of medial shift of thyroid cartilage, developed by Payr and modified by others. (Reproduced by permission from Minoru Hirano, "Surgical Alteration of Voice Quality," in *Otology—Head and Neck Surgery, Update I*, Cummings CW, Fredrickson JM, Harker LA, Krause CJ, Schuller DE, eds. St. Louis, 1989, C.V. Mosby Co.)

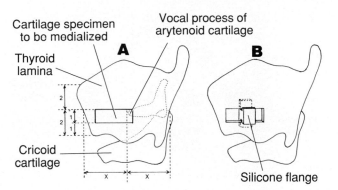

Figure 8.16. **A**, Design of cartilage specimen to be medialized. **B**, Stabilization of the shifted specimen with the use of a silicone flange developed by Isshiki and modified by others. (Reproduced by permission from Minoru Hirano, "Surgical Alteration of Voice Quality," in *Otology—Head and Neck Surgery, Update I*, Cummings CW, Fredrickson JM, Harker LA, Krause CJ, Schuller DE, eds. St. Louis, 1989, C.V. Mosby Co.)

The quadrangle is cut through the cartilage and shifted medially. The best location of the medialized specimen is determined by auditory monitoring of the voice. A combination of visual monitoring using a fiberscope and auditory monitoring is useful. The medialized segment is then fixed into place by placing a silicone flange through the window (Fig. 8.16B).

Rotation of Arytenoid Cartilage. The basic principle of this technique is to rotate the arytenoid cartilage by traction of the muscular process in the direction of the adductor muscles, medializing the tip of the vocal process to the midline (Furukawa,1967; Isshiki, 1977) (Fig. 8.17).

The surgery is conducted under local anesthesia. Following a horizontal cervical skin incision, the posterior edge of the thyroid lamina is exposed on the affected side by sectioning the thyropharyngeal muscle. The cricothyroid joint is dislocated, and the thyroid edge is retracted anteromedially. The muscular process of the arytenoid cartilage is then exposed. It is pulled anteromedioinferiorly with a nylon thread, while the patient

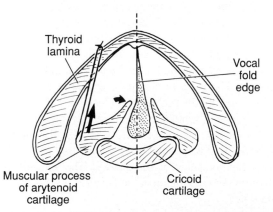

Figure 8.17. Schematic presentation of the principle of rotation of the arytenoid cartilage, as developed by Isshiki. (Reproduced by permission from Minoru Hirano, "Surgical Alteration of Voice Quality," in *Otology—Head and Neck Surgery, Update I*, Cummings CW, Fredrickson JM, Harker LA, Krause CJ, Schuller DE, eds. St. Louis, 1989, C.V. Mosby Co.)

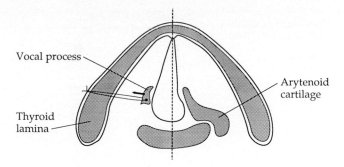

Figure 8.18.   Schematic presentation of the principle of laterofixation of the vocal folds.

phonates. When the best voice is obtained, the thread is sutured to the thyroid cartilage. Medialization of the vocal process can also be monitored visually by means of a fiberscope.

Vocal Fold Lateralization

Vocal fold lateralization is indicated in the treatment of bilateral vocal fold paralysis and in bilateral ankylosis of the cricoarytenoid joints when the vocal folds are located at or near the midline, causing dyspnea. Its purpose is to improve not the voice but the airway. It usually makes the voice worse, to a greater or lesser extent. However, when conservation of voice is part of the surgical plan, a phonosurgical approach can often help to minimize effects on the voice.

There are two major types of techniques to lateralize the vocal fold: laterofixation of the vocal fold and arytenoidectomy.

Laterofixation of the Vocal Fold.   The basic principle of laterofixation is to displace the vocal process of the arytenoid cartilage laterally, thereby widening the glottis (Fig. 8.18).

Patients requiring this surgery have usually undergone tracheostomy for relief of dyspnea. An endotracheal tube is inserted through the tracheostoma, and general anesthesia is given. Following skin incision, the arytenoid cartilage is exposed, using the same technique as that for rotation of the arytenoid cartilage. The arytenoid cartilage is dislocated from the cricoarytenoid joint, and its major portion is removed, leaving only the vocal process. The vocal process is pulled laterally with a nylon thread. The effect of lateralization is monitored with the use of a fiberscope or a direct laryngoscope. When the glottis is sufficiently opened, the thread is sutured to the thyroid cartilage.

Arytenoidectomy.   The basic principle of arytenoidectomy is to remove the arytenoid cartilage, thereby widening the posterior glottis (Fig. 8.19). Part of the mucosa covering the cartilage may also be removed. The posterior glottis, or the intercartilaginous portion of the glottis, accounts for approximately 60% of the entire glottal area (Hirano, Kurita, Kyokawa, and Sato, 1986). Therefore, a widening of the posterior glottis is very effective in improving the adequacy of the airway. The anterior glottis is widened to a much lesser extent by arytenoidectomy than the posterior glottis. This is helpful in preserving the best possible voice.

The surgery is conducted with the use of endolaryngeal microsurgery technique under general anesthesia. The CO_2 laser is very useful in this procedure because its use minimizes bleeding. The entire arytenoid cartilage is often removed, along with part of its mucosal cover.

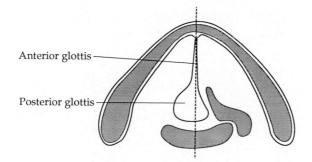
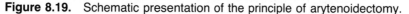

Anterior glottis

Posterior glottis

Figure 8.19.   Schematic presentation of the principle of arytenoidectomy.

Vocal Fold Tensing Surgery

The major purpose of vocal fold tensing surgery is to raise the vocal pitch. Indications for such surgery may include (*a*) excessively low pitch in females caused by a protein anabolic steroid or an androgen, or by pregnancy; (*b*) the low vocal pitch of the "sex-transferred" female; and (*c*) senile, flaccid vocal folds. Surgical techniques to tense the vocal folds have been developed during the past decade by Isshiki (1977), LeJeune, Guice, and Samuels (1983) and Tucker (1985). Data regarding the long-term functional results of vocal fold tensing are not yet available. There are two major surgical techniques to accomplish vocal fold tensing: cricothyroid approximation and anterior commissure advancement.

Cricothyroid Approximation.   The basic principle of cricothyroid approximation is to create a permanent approximation of the cricoid arch to the thryoid cartilage anteriorly, simulating the function of the cricothyroid muscle (Isshiki, 1977) (Fig. 8.20). Recall that contraction of the cricothyroid muscle results in the approximation of the cartilages and that in so doing the vocal folds are lengthened and tensed. Both the decreased mass of the folds and the increased tension under which they are held result in a faster vibratory rate, and thus a higher pitch is produced.

The surgery is best conducted under local anesthesia so that the pitch of the voice can be monitored during the procedure. However, if the patient is unable to tolerate the procedure, general anesthesia is given. Following horizontal cervical skin incision, the thyroid and cricoid cartilages are exposed. They are approximated anteriorly by means of nylon sutures (Fig. 8.20). Stretching of the vocal fold can be visually monitored with the use of a fiberscope.

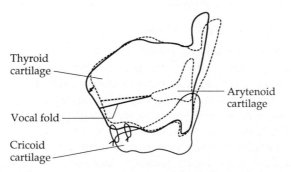

Thyroid cartilage

Arytenoid cartilage

Vocal fold

Cricoid cartilage

Figure 8.20.   Schematic presentation of the principle of cricothyroid approximation, as developed by Isshiki.

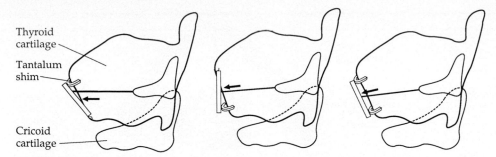

Figure 8.21. Schematic presentation of the principle of anterior commissure advancement, as developed by LeJeune and Tucker.

Anterior Commissure Advancement. The basic principle of anterior commissure advancement is to stretch the vocal folds by advancing the anterior commissure anteriorly relative to the arytenoid cartilages (LeJune et al., 1983; Tucker, 1985).

The surgery may best be performed under local anesthesia, but general anesthesia is employed when the patient cannot tolerate the procedure. Following a horizontal cervical skin incision, the thyroid cartilage is exposed. A vertical cartilage flap is made in the midportion of the thyroid cartilage. The flap may be inferiorly based, superiorly based, or sectioned both superiorly and inferiorly. The flap is advanced anteriorly and stabilized in place by inserting a shim of tantalum posterior to the flap (Fig. 8.21). When local anesthesia is employed, changes in vocal pitch are auditorily monitored during surgery. Vocal fold stretching can be visually monitored by means of a fiberscope.

Vocal Fold Slackening Surgery

The major purpose of vocal fold slackening surgery is to reduce the tension of the vocal folds (Isshiki, 1977). This is the reverse of the vocal fold tensing procedure described above. The indications for this procedure are not yet well established, and its use is in the experimental stage.

In order to slacken the vocal folds, it is necessary to move the anterior commissure closer to the arytenoid cartilage. The surgery may best be performed under local anesthesia because auditory monitoring of voice change is available during surgery. When the patient cannot tolerate the procedure, general anesthesia may be used. The thyroid cartilage is exposed in the same way as for anterior commissure advancement. A vertical cartilage flap is made in the midportion of the thyroid cartilage and pushed back (Fig. 8.22).

Surgery to Alter Laryngeal Neuromuscular Function

Neuromuscular Surgery for Vocal Fold Paralysis

The ideal treatment for vocal fold paralysis would be to restore normal innervation of all laryngeal muscles. This is, however, not possible in cases of axonotmesis and neurotmesis. One of the major problems in the neurosurgical treatment of vocal fold paralysis results from the fact that the recurrent laryngeal nerve contains both adductor and abductor fibers. Simple nerve anastomosis or nerve graft of the recurrent laryngeal nerve causes misdirected reinnervation, as shown in Figure 8.23. Some neurons that originally innervated one of the adductor muscles now may innervate the abductor muscles, while some neurons that were originally for abductor innervation now act to innervate the adductor muscles, causing a disturbance in vocal fold mobility (Siribodhi, Sundmaker, Atkins, and Bonner,1963; Hiroto, Hirano, and Tomita, 1968).

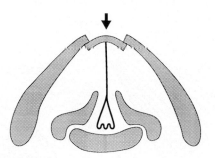

Figure 8.22. Schematic presentation of the principle of anterior commissure pushback, as developed by Isshiki.

Many experimental and clinical attempts have been made to avoid the problems resulting from misdirection of regenerated nerve fibers. Some of them will be described in the following paragraphs.

The procedures that are most frequently in use employ a nerve-muscle pedicle (Fig. 8.24) obtained from the ansa hypoglossi nerve that innervates the omohyoid, sternothyroid, and sternohyoid muscles (Tucker, 1978; Tucker and Rusnov, 1981). One of the muscles (along with its nerve) is chosen as the donor. In cases of bilateral abductor paralysis in which the vocal folds are fixed near the midline, causing dyspnea, the nerve-muscle pedicle is implanted into the porterior cricoarytenoid (PCA) muscle, whose primary function is to abduct the vocal folds. For unilateral paralysis, the nerve-muscle pedicle is implanted into the lateral cricoarytenoid (LCA) muscle.

Other surgical approaches for bilateral paralysis have been reported and include anastomosis of the split phrenic nerve to the PCA or to the nerve branch innervating the PCA (Crumley, 1983) and anastomsis of the split vagus nerve to the nerve branch of the PCA (Miehlke and Arold, 1982).

Recurrent Laryngeal Nerve Section for Spasmodic Dysphonia

Since 1976 when Dedo first reported unilateral section of the recurrent laryngeal nerve (RLN) for spasmodic dysphonia (Dedo, 1976), the procedure and various modifications of it have been carried out by many laryngologists. The immediate postsurgical results have been reported to be highly successful and appreciated by many patients (Dedo, 1976; Dedo, Izdebski, and Townsend, 1977; Barton, 1979; Wilson, Oldring, and Mueller, 1980; Dedo and Izdebski, 1981) but the long-term results appear to be conflicting (Wilson et al., 1980; Aronson and DeSanto, 1981; Fritzell, Feuer, Haglund, Knutsson, and Schiratzki, 1982; Aronson and DeSanto, 1983; Chevrie-Muller, Arabia-Guidet, and Pfauwadel, 1987). While some surgeons continue to perform the procedure, others have abandoned it due to the finding of return of symptoms in time despite continued paralysis

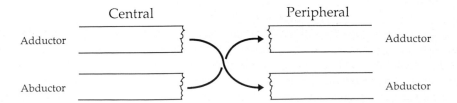

Figure 8.23. Schematic presentation of misdirected reinnervation in the recurrent laryngeal nerve.

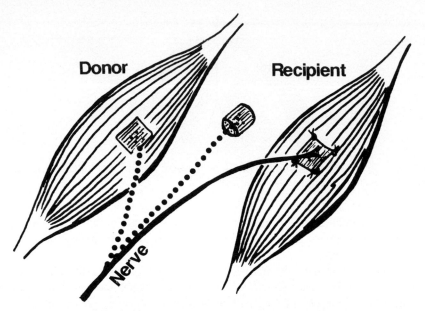

Figure 8.24. Nerve-muscle pedicle procedure.

of the vocal fold caused by the sectioning procedure. Other techniques for reducing the spasmodic episodes have been tried (Henschen and Burton, 1978; Hartman and Vishwanat, 1984; Blitzer, Brin, Fahn, and Lovelace, 1988), but the results have been disappointing or there has been insufficient time to evaluate the results.

For example, Blitzer et al. (1988) reported on their results using botulinum toxin for the relief of the dystonic spasms in spasmodic dysphonia. Injections were made into the vocalis-thyroartenoid muscle of five patients. All patients experienced immediate relief of the spasms, with breathy dysphonia and aspiration present within the first 5 days after injection. The voice remained relatively normal for a period of 3 to 6 months, at which time the dysphonic symptoms reappeared. Because of the limited duration of the relief of symptoms, continued injections of the toxin must be considered in order to provide long-term relief. The long-term effects of botulinum toxin are unknown, either in terms of the muscle into which it is injected or the body as a whole. Thus, further experience is needed with this mode of symptom relief for spasmodic dysphonia before its efficacy in the treatment of this debilitating voice problem can be evaluated.

Surgical Reconstruction for Partial Loss and/or Deformity of the Larynx

Overview

The surgical procedures that fall into this category vary vastly. They can be classified into four major groups: (*a*) surgical reconstruction following partial laryngectomy, (*b*) surgical repair for trauma of the larynx, (*c*) surgery for cicatricious stenosis of the larynx, and (*d*) surgery for congenital deformities of the larynx. Many of the patients who require surgical reconstuction exhibit problems in breathing and/or swallowing, as well as voice disorders. All of these problems must be taken into consideration when surgical treatment is undertaken. It is therefore imperative that phonosurgeons have a thorough understanding of the physiology and pathophysiology of breathing and swallowing, as well as of phonation.

Because the focus of this book is on phonation, the only specific condition to be addressed in this section will be phonosurgery for anterior glottal web, where voice is the major concern.

Anterior Glottal Web

Anterior glottal web forms as a congenital malformation or is caused by trauma, including surgical trauma. There are two major surgical techniques for its removal: endolaryngeal surgery and surgery under thyrotomy.

Endolaryngeal Surgery. Thin and/or small webs are successfully treated with the endolaryngeal approach. The surgery is conducted under general anesthesia. The vocal folds are exposed under a direct laryngoscope and viewed with an operating microscope. The web is sectioned at the midline or partly removed. A CO_2 laser is useful for this purpose (Fig. 8.25A). After removal of the web, a silicone plate is placed in the glottis in order to prevent postsurgical reunion of the vocal folds. To do this, a tiny horizontal skin incision is first made in front of the thyroid cartilage. A hypodermic needle threaded with a piece of nylon thread is inserted through the incision into the laryngeal cavity, above the thyroid cartilage (Fig. 8.25B). The nylon thread is pulled out of the patient's mouth through the laryngoscope. A second piece of nylon thread is inserted in the same way but below the thyroid cartilage and is pulled out through the laryngoscope. The two pieces of nylon thread are sutured to a silicone plate at the outside of the mouth (Fig. 8.25C). The silcone plate is placed in the glottis through the laryngoscope as the two pieces of nylon thread are pulled through the skin incision. The nylon thread is sutured in front of the thyroid cartilage (Fig. 8.25D). The skin incision is closed. A superior view of the glottis immediately after surgery is shown in Figure 8.25E. The silicone plate is removed endolaryngeally 2 to 4 weeks after surgery.

Thyrotomy. Surgery under thyrotomy is indicated for thick and extensive webs. The surgery is usually conducted under general anesthesia. Following a vertical or horizontal cervical skin incision, the thyroid cartilage is exposed and sectioned vertically at the midline. When marked scar tissue exists in the web, it is carefully removed; the covering epithelium is preserved. The wound at the sectioned web is sutured and closed (Fig. 8.26). The larynx and the wound are closed in layers.

Medical Management

Edema, Inflammation, Irritation of the Vocal Folds

Through differential diagnostic examination, acute laryngeal problems in which the vocal folds and laryngeal structures demonstrate redness, swelling, or the appearance of irritation may be determined to be the result of infection, allergy, drainage from the nose, reaction to noxious agents, gastroesophageal reflux, or directly related to recent episodes of abuse. Clearly, the diagnosis will determine the treatment. In the presence of infection, the use of antibiotic drugs is common and should be accompanied by a reduction in voice usage for the period of time that the acute symptoms are present. When an allergic reaction appears to be the cause of the tissue changes that are being mirrored in the voice, it is important to determine the source of that reaction. Elimination or avoidance of the allergenic agents or desensitization of the body's reaction should restore the tissues to a healthy condition and eliminate the voice problem. Both the identification of and treatment for

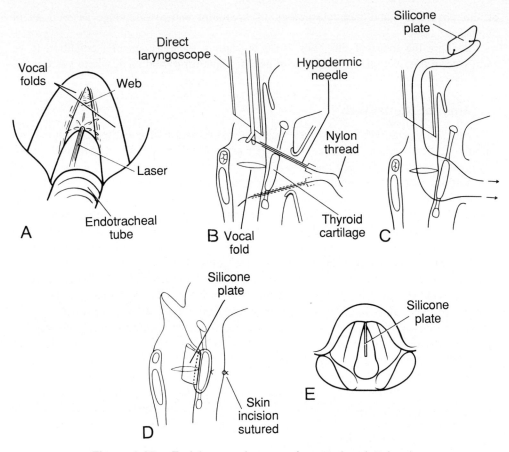

Figure 8.25.   Endolaryngeal surgery for anterior glottal web.

allergies can, of course, be a rather long process. As long as the vocal folds appear to be edematous or inflamed, the voice must be used sparingly in both amount and loudness dimensions. Some detective work might be involved in determining whether exposure to noxious agents is responsible for the observed irritation of the mucosa.

It is well recognized that the smoke of tobacco or illegal substances is irritating to laryngeal mucosa. The obvious treatment is cessation of the behavior. Because physical addiction may be involved, the person's ability to abandon the habit may be very limited. Many patients need much support, encouragement, and special assistance through a variety of treatment programs in order to stop smoking. The doctor's recommendation, although carrying much weight, is often insufficient and should be followed with concrete offers of help or specific referral to sources of such help.

It is now recognized that a nonsmoker's exposure to tobacco smoke may be sufficient to cause eye, nose, throat, and respiratory tract irritation (U.S. Dept. of Health, Education and Human Services, 1986). Professional voice users, singers and actors in particular, may often find it necessary to perform in environments heavy with tobacco smoke. There are no known antidotes to the irritant effects of tobacco smoke, but other methods of relieving irritation may be attempted. However, it must be made clear to the patient that continued use of the voice in the presence of edematous or inflamed vocal folds creates increased risk for further and perhaps more lasting damage to the tissues and the voice. Passive smoking—involuntary exposure to cigarette smoke—may also take place in the

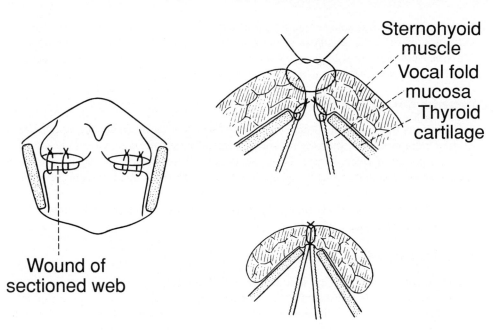

Figure 8.26.   Surgery for anterior glottal web under thyrotomy.

home and the workplace. Recognition of this effect may lead to appropriate environmental adjustments.

It is also possible that a person may have experienced exposure to other noxious agents. Relief from such exposure should result in resolution of the irritation, although there is not a great deal of information about such effects. Inhalation of certain gases can result in burns of and trauma to the mucosa of the respiratory tract (see Chapter 6).

Another environmental factor that may have an irritating effect on laryngeal mucosa is very dry air. Both heating and cooling systems in houses, public buildings, and airplanes often provide insufficient humidification. Breathing this air may result in dehydration of the vocal folds, increasing their stiffness and disrupting normal vibratory behavior (Brewer, Brodnitz, Gould, Lawrence, Monaghan, Pratt, Titze, and Vaughan, 1979). The obvious treatment for this situation consists of environmental manipulation, increasing the humidification of the air, rather than direct treatment of the condition itself. In the case of airplane travel, it is especially important for the professional voice user to be counseled against use of the voice in performance too soon after extensive flights.

The suspicion of gastroesophageal reflux as the etiology of mucosal irritation is raised when that irritation most obviously affects the posterior portions of the larynx, when the history reveals that the voice symptoms are at their worst first thing in the morning, and when the symptoms include an acidic taste in the mouth, heartburn, frequent burping, and the like. Patients with this condition should receive a thorough work-up. Treatment will include a combination of environmental adjustments, such as elevation of the head of the bed (not the use of additional pillows), pharmacologic management, and dietary constraints.

When vocal abuse appears to be the cause of the laryngeal problem, pharmacologic treatment should be limited. In the case of a professional voice user who must perform, corticosteroids are occasionally used to reduce edema and inflammation. This treatment must be viewed as an emergency measure, and it must be recognized to be primarily palliative in effect. (See Chapter 4 for a discussion of the effects of drugs on the voice.) In instances of acute vocal abuse, elimination of the abusive behaviors and some degree of modification of voice use should serve to resolve the problem. However, referral for training in voice use and vocal hygiene would be important to avoid recurrence of such episodes or the development of a more chronic condition.

Chronic Changes

Conditions that result in chronic changes in laryngeal tissue frequently require combined treatment protocols. In many instances, surgical intervention may be necessary, followed by a period of voice therapy. Other situations call for medical management through drugs and environmental changes, perhaps combined with voice therapy. And for some, a trial course of voice therapy may be the first treatment option, to be followed by other courses of treatment only if necessary. Patients with chronic changes of laryngeal tissue must be monitored closely, often for many years.

Neurological Conditions

Pharmacologic management is sometimes available for the relief or control of symptoms in certain neurological disturbances. For example, pyridostigmine is used to control the symptoms of muscle weakness in myasthenia gravis (Ravits, 1988), and levodopa (Larodopa) or carbidopa-levodopa (Sinemet) are used in the management of Parkinson's disease (Merritt, 1979). Because these drugs have beneficial effects in reducing some of the abnormal characteristics of the disease, they may also be found to improve the voice and speech. There are numerous other drugs used in similar ways in the treatment of the many progressively debilitating neurological diseases.

Summary

In the first section of this chapter, a review of phonosurgical techniques currently in use for the treatment of voice problems is presented. Phonosurgical techniques are divided into four categories: (*a*) removal of pathological tissue; (*b*) correction of the position, shape, and/or tension of the vocal folds; (*c*) surgery to restore laryngeal neuromuscular function; and (*d*) reconstruction for a partial loss or deformity of the larynx. A brief description of the techniques currently used by otolaryngologists is given in order to aid the reader in understanding of the advantages and disadvantages of the techniques.

In the second section of this chapter, some of the techniques used in the medical management of voice problems are reviewed. Many of these techniques involve the use of drugs for the relief of symptoms, as well as for treating the original cause(s) of the voice problem. Allergies are often implicated as a cause of voice problems. Other medical techniques include counseling and simple behavioral modification techniques to encourage the patient to change habits (smoking, drinking), lifestyle, or the environment.

9

Vocal Rehabilitation

Goal of Voice Therapy

The specific goal of voice therapy will vary from patient to patient. Nevertheless, in general, the goal of voice therapy is to restore the best voice possible, a voice that will be functional for purposes of employment and general communication. The patient must be the final arbiter of what constitutes acceptable voice. However, it is important for both the patient and the clinician to recognize that restoring voice to the way it previously sounded or to some idealized goal may not be possible. When irreversible alterations have occurred in laryngeal structure or physiology, the voice may never return to what it once had been. This realization is particularly traumatic for persons who have relied heavily on their vocal skills for their livelihood or as their primary source of pleasure.

Concept of Normal Voice

An accepted definition of normal voice does not exist. There are no established standards, and no boundaries of accepted norms have been set. Attempting to set such standards might be likened to defining what constitutes normal appearance. Voice, like appearance, comes in so many varieties. Cultural, environmental, and individual factors contribute to the determination of what is designated normal. And voice, again like appearance, does not stay constant. It changes throughout the life-span; it changes in reaction to emotion; it changes in response to environment; it reflects the state of health of the body and of the mind. It would be extremely difficult, if not impossible, to have a single definition that would encompass all of the ways that a normal voice can sound. Normal is not a single state but rather exists on a continuum.

Some normative data have been gathered about specific acoustic vocal parameters (see Chapter 13). Usually these data provide ranges within which voices that have been judged as normal have been found to fall. Often even these data are suspect, since investigators remind us that both intra- and intersubject variability may be very large (Kent, Kent, and Rosenbek, 1987).

It is perhaps easier to attempt to define the abnormal. The voice that is so reduced in volume that normal-hearing listeners have difficulty hearing it is abnormal. The voice that is so different in pitch level as to be incongruent with the age or sex of the speaker may be judged to be abnormal. The voice that lacks the flexibility to alter pitch or loudness or that has a quality that calls attention to itself in an unpleasant manner or that is so loud that we are aware of it whether we choose to be or not suggests something outside of our internalized norms.

The lack of a definition of normal voice creates problems in setting therapeutic goals and in describing abnormality and its degree of severity. There is no complete and objective template against which to measure and compare it. This is one of the major obstacles in clinical research confounding collection of objective, quantifiable data. If a voice improves, how can we measure that improvement—what can we compare it to? Which of the vocal attributes have contributed to its improvement? How much better is it? Is it normal? Is it normal for that patient?

This last question raises another aspect of the concept of normalcy of voice, that is, how did a particular voice-disordered patient's voice sound before it became disordered? It is usually the case that the only voice known to the clinician and available for any measurement is the disordered voice. This can create problems if at a given point during therapy the clinician judges a patient's vocal productions to be quite acceptable but the patient continues to be unhappy, claiming they are different from the remembered normal voice. Or the opposite may occur if the clinician continues to seek a better voice when the patient reports that the voice being produced sounds right and normal.

The Underlying Bases of Vocal Rehabilitation

Voice therapy must be rooted in and derived from an understanding of laryngeal anatomy and phonatory physiology. It is necessary to understand what is wrong in order to know how to fix it. When there is a hole in a bucket, it is important to understand the effect of that hole, not only to know that the hole is there. That understanding may lead to more than a single approach to fixing the problem. And it may be very important to understand how the hole developed in order to prevent it from recurring despite it's having been fixed once.

Accurate diagnosis is critical to treatment planning. The diagnosis should provide the voice therapist with the information necessary to plan a course of treatment. However, patients are often referred for voice therapy with minimal diagnostic information. When that is the case, requests should be directed to the otolaryngologist for as detailed information as is available. Voice symptoms and signs in combination with information derived from a complete history and voice assessment must be compatible with the referral diagnosis. Communication between the speech pathologist and the referring laryngologist will be helpful in clarifying terminology and observations, as well as in developing a treatment plan.

The relationship between the person and the voice must be understood and incorporated into the therapy program. This is true whether or not the voice problem is psychogenic. Emotionality, stress, and anxiety may be components of many voice problems, both in terms of their etiologies and the reactions they engender. Individual reactions to voice problems may very well determine the response to treatment and the patient's ability to follow a therapy plan.

Freed from constraints imposed by organic lesions, stress factors, or abusive habits, the larynx will usually function well. Thus, it is often possible to eliminate the constraint through voice therapy and thereby to correct the voice problem. It is not always necessary to teach patients every aspect of voice production, as if they had never done it correctly before.

Guidelines for Voice Therapy

A simplified explanation of normal vocal physiology and of the patient's specific deviance from it can be critical. For most patients, the idea of voice therapy is an unfamiliar one. They do not understand how, after many years of speaking without difficulty, they can now be speaking improperly. They have little appreciation for the connection between various vocal behaviors and their own particular problem. What they really would like is for the doctor to prescribe some type of medication that, taken three times a day, would cure the problem. Instead, they learn that they must assume some responsibility for dealing with the problem. In order to do so, they must begin by gaining some knowledge. Without an understanding of the nature of the problem, the patient's approach to therapy will often be highly skeptical.

Throughout therapy it is important to encourage the patient to verbalize perceptions of how the voice sounds and feels. This provides information for the clinician, but more important, it sensitizes the patient to the voice and increases self-awareness. It encourages a process of self-discovery that is exciting and motivating for the patient as changes are perceived. For the clinician, the patient's verbalizations provide information about how the patient views the problem, how tuned in to the problem the patient is, and perhaps help to shape the therapy plan.

The use of both auditory and visual feedback during therapy can be extremely helpful. Auditory feedback can be provided by the judicious use of tape recording (using good-quality equipment). Visual feedback may take a variety of forms, including the use of instruments such as the Visi-Pitch (Kay Elemetrics Corp.) or the PM Pitch Analyzers (Voice Identification, Inc.). This type of instrumentation, as well as other computer software, permits visualization of a model and of the patient's attempt to match that model. Visual feedback may also involve the use of the fiberoptic laryngoscope connected to a videotape recorder and monitor during the therapy process (Bastian, 1985,1987). The patient is taught to identify certain desirable or undesirable laryngeal behaviors and has the benefit of the visual image to assist in shaping laryngeal activity. Spectrograms, electroglottograms, and other printouts of acoustic or physiologic data can be used for demonstration and explanation but do not lend themselves as easily to direct therapeutic use. Biofeedback using surface electrodes over laryngeal muscles has been reported with inconclusive results (Prosek, Montgomery, Walden, and Schwartz, 1978; Stemple, Weiler, Whitehead, and Komray, 1980). Because this method, as currently used, is incapable of differentiating between the activity of those muscles that need to be active and those that should be relaxed, and because we have no data to specify how much activity is normal and how much is hyperfunctional for any given muscle during phonation, the meaning of electromyographic biofeedback is uncertain.

Another form of feedback is the use of instruments that monitor a behavior and supply a signal when a preset level of that behavior has been surpassed. For example, the

Voice Intensity Controller (VIC), described by Holbrook, Rolnick, and Bailey (1974), is a small unit capable of being worn by a patient to monitor vocal intensity. A small throat microphone is affixed to the neck, an earphone is worn in the ear, and the unit fits into a pocket. The permissible intensity is preset. When that level is exceeded, a tone is emitted in the earphone. The use of this feedback device has been found to be very effective in modifying vocal loudness in a short period of time (Holbrook et al., 1974).

Therapy should move gradually from one step or activity to the next. It is important to give the patient adequate time to practice a technique and to master it. Familiarity with a technique and a sense of having learned it provides a sense of accomplishment for the patient. Furthermore, if the behavior is but one phase of a progression, the patient needs to have a solid foundation on which to build. There is a fine line here between overdoing a good thing and moving on too quickly, which must be recognized. To help make this transition, it is wise to begin to introduce a new technique while continuing to incorporate practice on those already learned. It is also important to give a technique a chance to work. The clinician must not allow the patient's anxiety and desire for instant results to affect clinical judgment. In the initial stages of therapy, it is often necessary to experiment with techniques and approaches. The patient should be made aware of this process in order to avoid feelings of uncertainty and confusion.

The clinician should always model therapy tasks for the patient. We often ask patients to produce sounds or engage in activities that might seem strange to them. Moreover, we ask them to do so in the presence of another person, the clinician. This raises the patient's level of self-consciousness significantly. In order to minimize such feelings, as well as to demonstrate clearly what the patient is being asked to do, the clinician must demonstrate therapeutic tasks. When a task is demonstrated, it must be done just as you wish the patient to do it. If the request is for the patient to produce the loudest "hey" possible, it will not do to have the clinician model it quietly. Because it is often difficult to verbally explain or describe a vocal behavior, modeling it takes on greater importance. A demonstration, like the proverbial picture, is worth a thousand words.

It is helpful to tape record therapy sessions in whole or in part. Doing so provides a record of the patient's voice and the therapy session. Memory for voice is very fleeting, and both the clinician and the patient may readily forget what the voice sounded like at a given point. When therapy seems to be taking longer than the patient expected, or when it appears that little progress has been made, the playing of an earlier tape recording may be very helpful in providing some perspective. Another valuable use for tape recorded sessions is as home practice material. Patients often report that without the clinician's model or their own from a previous time, they are not sure that they are practicing correctly. The tape recorded session provides the structure they need.

Patients must be carefully instructed in what to practice, for how long and how often. It is helpful to have the patient demonstrate the exercise or activity to be practiced before leaving the therapy session. Because talking is an activity that is so pervasive yet so rarely attended to by most speakers, we have found it effective to recommend frequent practice sessions of limited duration. This approach seems to help the patient focus on the voice frequently. Furthermore, there is usually some follow-up or generalization of practice for a period of time immediately after it has been done. Frequent practice periods capitalize on this "overflow effect" because it occurs more frequently.

The prognostic statement made at the initiation of a program of vocal rehabilitation must be viewed as an educated guess about the outcome of therapy. It must be realistic but must not be sealed in concrete. It should be modified appropriately as therapy progresses.

The variety of factors that will enter into the development of a prognostic statement will be discussed later in this chapter.

Not all patients are appropriate candidates for a voice therapy approach, for reasons other than the nature of the pathology present. A patient must recognize that a problem is present, and must be willing to undertake a therapy program and to follow the regimen. Some find it extremely difficult to abandon abusive habits because of lifestyle, employment, or personality factors. Even when explicitly directed to do so, smokers may be unable to stop or even to significantly reduce this habit. The irritation created by continued smoking may be sufficient to maintain a condition and sabotage any positive effects that can be brought about through changed phonatory behavior. The therapeutic process is a complex one, and patient behavior may unwittingly pose a major hindrance to progress. Despite apparent cooperation, the patient may be exhibiting a variety of behaviors described by McFarlane, Fujiki, and Brinton (1984) as exemplifying the "reluctant client."

Prognostic Considerations

Many factors enter into the consideration of a prognosis. Because voice therapy requires full patient participation, it is often difficult to predict its anticipated outcome. In determining whether a patient is an appropriate candidate for a voice therapy approach and arriving at a prognosis, the clinician should consider the following factors. First, the patient must recognize that there is a problem. People possess internal references about how they should feel, what is normal for them, and what they should sound like. A voice that sounds abnormal to us may not sound particularly deviant to the person with the voice. Second, the patient must be willing to follow a therapy plan including regular practice periods as required. This is difficult for those seeking the quick cure for which they do not have to assume responsibility. Third, there must be a willingness to give up abusive habits and to alter or eliminate some voice use, at least temporarily. This is easier said than done for most people. Changing manner and amount of talking involves changes in lifestyle, in everyday habits, and even, it may seem, personality. Fourth, psychiatric problems, if present, may interfere with the ability to modify vocal behavior. A voice problem may be a manifestation of a psychiatric problem. Amelioration of the voice problem may be possible temporarily, but it will not deal with the problem (recall the case of R. W., Chapter 7). Fifth, the patient's voice disorder must be amenable to change through a voice therapy approach. For some voice problems, surgical or medical management may be the first or sole step. For other patients, the nature of the disorder may preclude any real possibility of success through voice therapy. The patient and the speech-language pathologist must be able to recognize the limitations of voice therapy. Sixth, appropriateness of the patient's expectations must be considered. If a person has an essentially normal voice but wishes to sound like another person, voice therapy is not indicated. Seventh, it is necessary to give full consideration to the patient's laryngeal condition and general health status. Some patients are insistent upon attaining full return of premorbid voice. The nature of the disorder and the resultant laryngeal changes may be such that this expectation may be unrealistic. The vocal folds may be damaged to the extent that normal phonation is not possible. Patients may have other health problems that may limit their ability to participate in voice therapy or may place constraints on their ability to control phonatory behavior. Finally, the speech-language pathologist must have an adequate understanding of the problem, feel competent in handling it, and be able to establish a good relationship with the patient.

Voice Therapy in the Management of Changes in Laryngeal Tissue or Structure

Vocal rehabilitation may play a primary role, as either the sole treatment modality of choice or simultaneously with other treatment, or a secondary role, as a follow-up treatment after a primary approach has been carried out.

When Is Voice Therapy Alone Appropriate ?

It is unfortunate that there is a paucity of hard data to support a position on this question. Theoretical constructs and clinical experience are the primary bases on which therapeutic judgments are made.

Perhaps the most agreement exists about the treatment of vocal fold nodules. Prominent authorities in the treatment of voice, in the fields of both otolaryngology and speech-language pathology, generally agree that the initial treatment of choice for symptomatic vocal nodules in adults is voice therapy (Vaughan, 1982; Boone, 1983; Aronson, 1985; Bastian, 1986; Gould, 1987; Sataloff, 1987a, 1987b, 1987c; Hirano, Chapter 8, this book). The option for surgical intervention is not compromised or eliminated by the more conservative approach of at least a 6- to 8-week period of voice therapy. Some authorities make a distinction between early nodules, which appear to be soft and reddish, and nodules that have been present for months or years and are large, hard, and white. Voice therapy as the initial treatment is recommended for the former, and surgical removal followed by a period of voice therapy is most commonly recommended for the latter (Arnold, 1973; Boone, 1983; Case, 1984). Sataloff (1987b) states that even nodules that appear to be large and fibrotic may disappear, regress, or become asymptomatic through a course of voice therapy. Other authors suggest that decisions regarding choice of treatment have to be made on an individual basis but that vocal reeducation must be part of any treatment (Moore, Hicks, and Abbott, 1985). Once again, it should be remembered that a trial period of voice therapy does not in any way compromise the option for surgical removal. Prater and Swift (1984) point out that voice therapy is more cost-effective than surgery, results in less time lost from work, and is nontraumatic. Furthermore, the learning that takes place during the therapy program will serve to eliminate vocal abuse and will be readily transferrable to postoperative voice use should surgery become necessary. It is agreed that vocal nodules may well recur if vocal abuse is not eliminated through a vocal rehabilitation program.

Less agreement exists about the need for and value of any treatment for vocal nodules in children. Vaughan (1982) and Hirano (Chapter 8) report that vocal nodules in children resolve spontaneously in early adolescence and therefore usually require no treatment. Hirano, however, recognizes that the vocal symptoms resulting from vocal nodules can potentially create significant emotional problems for a child, in which case voice therapy is advocated. Surgical removal of vocal nodules in children is contraindicated (Arnold, 1973; DeWeese and Saunders, 1982; Ballenger, 1985). Most speech-language pathologists believe that youngsters with aberrant voices due to vocal nodules can be effectively helped to eliminate vocally abusive behaviors and thereby the nodules themselves (Teter, 1976; Boone, 1983; Johnson, 1983; Wilson, 1987) and that such treatment should not be withheld. The psychosocial effects of aberrant voice on a young child can be quite significant.

The controversy about the role of the speech pathologist in the treatment of voice disorders in children has recently been taken up by Sander (1989—against) and Kahane and Mayo (1989—for). While Sander claims that young children experience resolution of voice problems at puberty without the benefit of any treatment, Kahane and Mayo cite reports that adult vocal deviations are frequently traceable to patterns set in childhood (Pahn, 1966; Cooper, 1973) and, further, that the incidence of voice disorders in school children in the middle school grades (6th through 9th grades) may be higher than has previously been reported (Warr-Leeper, McShea, and Leeper, 1979). Kahane and Mayo present a compelling argument for the development of prevention programs and cite the positive result of such a program reported by Nilson and Schneiderman (1983).

Vocal fold polyps are usually thought to be the result of vocal abuse, sometimes caused by a single or intense period of trauma during which small blood vessels rupture. They are also thought to be amenable to a voice therapy approach, particularly the sessile, or broad-based, polyp. Just as with vocal nodules, opinions about the preferred mode of treatment are mixed, but also, as is the case with nodules, little is lost when a period of voice therapy is the initial treatment provided.

When Should Voice Therapy Be Combined with Other Treatment?

Contact ulcers and granulomas have frequently been thought to result from a specific type of vocally abusive phonation. Recent studies and reports provide additional insight into the underlying pathophysiology of contact ulcers (Cherry and Margulies, 1968; Delahunty and Cherry, 1968; Delahunty, 1972; Chodosh, 1977; Ward, Zwitman, Hanson, and Berci, 1980). Ward and Berci (1982) cite the chronic irritation caused by hiatal hernia and gastroesophageal reflux as the basic problem, which in turn causes chronic coughing and harsh and frequent throat clearing. It is these abusive behaviors, coughing and throat clearing, that then initiate contact ulcer and granuloma formation. Response to medical treatment as reported by Hallewell and Cole (1970) was very successful in 21 of 22 cases. Chronic nonspecific laryngitis, pharyngitis, and pachydermia laryngis are included in the family of problems with this underlying pathophysiology. Voice therapy is appropriate as one part of the treatment regimen in order to eliminate laryngeally abusive behaviors. However, appropriate medical evaluation of and treatment for a possible gastroesophageal reflux condition also needs to be part of the total treatment protocol. Surgical treatment without the other components of care is frequently unsuccessful in the long-term, as the condition recurs.

Polypoid changes of the vocal folds (Reinke's edema) are highly related to long-term, excessive smoking and to age (Hirano, Kurita, Matsuo, and Nagata, 1980). Although a component of vocal abuse may also be present and may aggravate the condition, these lesions are generally not caused by abuse and not responsive to voice therapy. However, many patients will benefit from a course of voice therapy following surgical excision of the lesion.

There are numerous other laryngeal lesions that are not caused by vocal abuse and that require medical and surgical intervention. However, vocally abusive habits may result as the patient attempts to compensate for a poorly functioning mechanism. Those habits may persist beyond resolution of the pathology, and a period of voice therapy may be required. A specific group of patients that would be included in this category are those with papillomatosis, requiring frequent surgical removal over a period of years. The condition of the mucosal cover of the vocal folds following numerous surgeries will be a most important factor in determining the quality of voice that will be possible.

Goals of Voice Therapy

When voice therapy is undertaken as the treatment modality of choice in the presence of mucosal and voice changes, the primary goals are, of course, to restore the mucosa to a healthy condition and to regain clear and full vocal function. Subgoals include identification and elimination of all abusive behaviors through the reduction of laryngeal tensions, institution of a vocal hygiene program, environmental manipulation, easy voice production, and establishment of improved vocal habits. Other goals may include identification of patient needs that require other forms of attention and appropriate referral.

When voice therapy is an adjunct or secondary treatment modality, the goals will depend heavily on the laryngeal status of the patient. The primary goal may be to restore healthy function and return of good voice, or it may be to help the patient find the best voice of which she is capable. The limits on that voice may be imposed by permanent changes in the shape or structure of the mucosa. Subgoals, in addition to those noted above, may include helping the patient to accept a changed voice, exploration of the adequacy of the voice for all necessary speaking situations, and suggesting environmental adjustments as necessary.

Nature of Therapeutic Intervention

Vocal rehabilitation must address a variety of factors. Patients are often called upon to make changes in the manner in which they produce voice, the various ways in which they use voice (e.g., singing, lecturing, etc.), and the environments in which they may use voice. These changes are all very closely linked to how individuals see themselves and how they interact with others. Recognition of the highly sensitive nature of the therapeutic process and the impact that it may have on the patient cannot be overemphasized.

Voice Therapy in the Management of Misuse and Abuse Problems

When Is Voice Therapy Alone Appropriate?

Voice therapy is almost always the treatment modality of choice for voice problems stemming from behaviors that have been identified as misuse or abuse of the laryngeal mechanism. However, it has been our experience that these patients, who may have negative laryngological examinations or minimal signs of laryngeal irritation, frequently receive up to 3 months or more of medical treatment prior to referral for voice evaluation. It is not uncommon for patients in these categories to be treated with antibiotics, antihistamines, decongestants, tranquilizers, and even corticosteroids, or to be sent home with some fairly nonspecific advice about relaxing or reducing voice use. Due to the effects on laryngeal mucosa of some medications, the actual voice symptoms may worsen over the course of the treatment, rather than improve (see Chapter 4). Recognition of the problem is critical to obtaining effective treatment.

Some patients may not be appropriate candidates for a voice therapy approach due to social/emotional problems beyond the scope of practice of the speech-language pathologist. However, it is within the speech-language pathologist's expertise to recognize such conditions and to make recommendations for or to arrange appropriate referral. Patients who do not recognize that a problem exists or who are incapable or unwilling to change habits or lifestyle will also be poor candidates for therapy.

Goals of Voice Therapy

The primary therapeutic goals are to identify and eliminate behaviors that constitute misuse or abuse and to replace them with acceptable patterns of voice production. Full return of normal voice is anticipated, especially when there is no evidence of mucosal tissue change. Subgoals in the treatment of vocal abuse and misuse might include reduction of laryngeal tensions, decrease of vocal loudness, decrease in amount of talking, adjusting environmental factors, and others. For those voice problems that appear to be psychogenic, a goal of therapy may be to help the patient understand the dynamics that initiated and sustained the voice problem.

Nature of Therapeutic Intervention

As stated in the previous section, therapy directed toward the elimination of vocally abusive behavior requires that the patient change habits of voice production. Those habits, even if not of very long standing, nevertheless may be quite tenacious. In addition to altering the way in which voice is produced, it may be necessary for the patient to make some sacrifices in the ways the voice is used. The changes that need to be made may be imposed by the therapy process, rather than as limitations caused by the problem itself. For example, the patient who enjoys singing in a church choir may need to forego that activity at least temporarily. The college professor who has never used amplification despite having to lecture to very large classes in large rooms with poor acoustics may need to do so. These are difficult changes for people to make. The therapeutic process may involve discussion of personal and interpersonal concerns that require understanding, the ability to listen well, and a nonjudgmental attitude. It is also essential for the clinician to be able to provide support and encouragement in helping a patient to accept a changed or restored voice.

Voice Therapy in the Management of Neurological Problems

Voice problems are but one of the dysarthric components of disability that may accompany certain neuromuscular disorders. With the possible exceptions of unilateral vocal fold paralysis (usually peripheral nerve damage) and spastic dysphonia (etiology still questioned), it is unusual for the voice disorder to be the primary disability. It is possible that the earliest symptoms of a neurological condition may be exhibited in changes or aberrations of phonation. However, the degree of impairment of various motor systems may undergo changes, both relative and absolute, in progressively debilitating neurological disorders, such that other symptoms may become increasingly debilitating. For example, dysphonia may be an early and isolated symptom in Parkinson's disease. However, as the disease progresses, other symptoms may become apparent, and the degree of severity of the various areas of disability caused by the disease may shift. Thus, although voice symptoms will not go away (indeed, they may worsen), symptoms affecting locomotion and gross motor acts may become more severely handicapping to the individual. Voice therapy will usually play an adjunct role in the management of voice disorders in progressive neurological disease, along with whatever medical treatment may be available. The speech-language pathologist may well be involved with these patients in working on the related disabilities of dysarthria (articulation and resonation), apraxia, aphasia, and dysphagia, as they exist.

There is some controversy concerning the role of voice therapy in the management of unilateral vocal fold paralysis. Data to support the efficacy of vocal rehabilitation is unavailable. The literature suggests that a great deal of spontaneous recovery and/or compensation occurs (Tucker, 1980). The major portion of such recovery occurs within 6 months of onset, although there are reports of recovery up to a year beyond onset (Ward and Berci,

1982). The phonosurgical approach of Teflon injection (Hirano, Chapter 8) has been used with significant success in individuals who have failed to show spontaneous recovery of vocal fold function and/or voice (Lewy, 1976; Reich and Lerman, 1978; Tucker, 1980; Hammarberg, Fritzell, and Schiratzki, 1984). The issue of voice therapy procedures recommended for treatment of unilateral vocal fold paralysis will be discussed further in the section on unresolved issues and myths.

Another area of continued controversy is that of spastic dysphonia. Controversy rages about the etiology of this puzzling condition, as well as about its treatment. Historically, the strain/struggle voice of the patient with spastic dysphonia was first thought to be entirely psychologically based (Arnold, 1959). This view has been modified at least to the extent that most authors now believe that more than a single etiology may exist but that a neurological basis for the disorder exists in most cases. The need for very thorough differential diagnosis is also well accepted in order to differentiate between types of spastic dysphonia (adductor versus abductor) and possible etiologies. Voice therapy continues to be a viable option, if only on a trial basis, to determine whether relief can be obtained through that process. Freeman (1988) recently suggested that a therapy procedure based on speech on inhalation has been successful in the treatment of a number of patients with spasmodic dysphonia. Complete data on that approach are not yet available.

Goals of Voice Therapy

Voice therapy can offer no cures when neuromotor disability is involved. However, through voice therapy, patients may sometimes be able to learn to produce the best voice possible and in some instances to exert a degree of voluntary control over the production of voice that may allow them to remain communicatively functional in occupational and social settings for a period of time (Rosenfield,1987). The speech-language pathologist can also be helpful in assessing the effects of medications on the patient's voice and speech production. If functional verbal communication is not a viable option, voice therapy becomes inappropriate, and the goal then must be to provide the patient with a means of nonverbal communication.

Nature of Therapeutic Intervention

The manner in which voice is produced may receive very direct attention, particularly in cases of vocal fold paralysis and sometimes of spastic dysphonia. More attention may be directed to suprasegmental factors such as utilizing breath groups, prosody, rate, and marking for stress and inflection, in work with other neurologically based disorders. Patients may have adopted particular patterns of voice use in an attempt to compensate for alterations in control of the voice. Some of these compensatory behaviors may be helpful, while others may not. Changes in how the voice is used are imposed on the individual by the nature of the disability. For example, the inability to increase loudness will restrict the environments in which the person can communicate effectively. Manipulation of environmental factors may be of some assistance. Hanson and Metter (1980) describe the use of a small, wearable, delayed auditory feedback (DAF) device in the treatment of a patient with progressive supranuclear palsy and severe hypokinetic dysarthria. They report that the patient, who was noted to have weak vocal intensity, demonstrated an increase of vocal intensity with the introduction of 100 milliseconds of DAF in both reading and counting aloud conditions, and that this increase was maintained in follow-up testing after a 3-month period of daily use of the device. Desired changes were also noted in a reduction of speech rate and increased speech intelligibilty. The therapeutic process may often be more difficult and less rewarding for neurologically impaired patients and for voice clinicians than it is for the types of patients discussed in earlier sections. It is incumbent on the clinician to recognize the limitations of the therapeutic approach and not to promise what cannot be delivered but to make every effort to help the patient arrive at the best means of communication possible.

Voice Therapy of Special Voice Problems

A number of voice problems that do not readily fit the above categories but that may appropriately require a period of vocal rehabilitation will be covered in this section.

The Transsexual Voice

The voice problem most immediately associated with a sex change is that of inappropriate pitch. In the case of change from a woman to a man, this problem is usually eliminated when male hormones are administered; these tend to increase laryngeal mass and thus lower fundamental frequency. However, no drugs are available to reduce the mass of the vocal folds, so that a man changing to a woman will not experience elevation of pitch secondary to hormone therapy. The incongruity of a masculine voice in a woman can present a significant psychological barrier. Therapeutic attempts to elevate speaking fundamental frequency should be undertaken, with care being taken to recognize the physiologic limits of the larynx. The use of breathy phonation can be helpful in giving the illusion of a higher pitch without the risk of inviting laryngeal trauma.

However, in addition to differences in pitch between men and women, there are differences in other speech patterns, habits, and mannerisms. This has been demonstrated experimentally by Coleman (1971, 1973, 1976) who found that female voices are still recognized as female even when the pitch difference between male and female voice is removed. Some of the difference between male and female voice is vowel quality, in that the relative sizes of the oral and pharyngeal cavities are different in the two sexes. Other differences include those of stress, inflection, timing, and even choice and use of words. Changes in these areas will go far in feminizing a voice even in the presence of a low speaking fundamental frequency. The actress Lauren Bacall presents a good model of someone whose voice is low in pitch and yet whose style is entirely feminine. A program of voice therapy designed to make the man-to-woman change should include careful study of this and other models of feminine low pitched speech. The goal of therapy should be to make those changes that will be effective in changing the overall image, rather than to work on artificial changes, such as pitch change, that may never become natural and that in fact may court laryngeal problems.

Voice Problems Due to Endocrine Disorders or Hormone Imbalance

Hypothyroidism

Hypothyroidism is a condition that can come on at any age. The symptoms may develop gradually over a lengthy period of time. As a result, their effect may not be recognized until a critical level of symptomatology has been reached. Change in the voice may be one such symptom. Typically, the voice of the patient with hypothyroidism is hoarse and has gradually lowered in pitch due to increased mass (edema) of the vocal folds. The diagnostician, thus, must be alert to this as a possible diagnosis when vocal fold edema is noted and does not appear to be related to factors of vocal abuse. Referral for testing should be pursued, and voice therapy is not indicated.

Virilization

This term is used to refer to the increase in size and mass of the vocal folds that occurs in women as the result of excessive secretion of the androgenic hormones or due to ingestion of androgen-containing hormones in treatment for menopausal symptoms or other problems. Damste (1967) described these changes and also showed them to be frequently irreversible. Voice therapy is contraindicated.

Menstruation, Pregnancy, and Birth Control Pill Use

Most of the voice-related negative effects of hormonal changes associated with the menstrual cycle occur in the pre- or early menstrual days. Excess loading of the vocal folds with fluid changes their mass and thus may affect vibratory behavior. This is usually not problematic for the average speaker but may present a problem for the professional singer. Submucosal hemorrhages in the larynx are common. Diuretics should be avoided because they do not free the protein-bound submucosal fluid (Sataloff, 1987b). Voice therapy is never indicated, but the clinician should be aware of the possibility of some subtle voice changes in female patients during these time periods.

Pregnancy may also result in change in the voice. During pregnancy the woman's endocrinological state undergoes great change. If a change in voice occurs, it is usually irreversible (Sataloff, 1987b). There are no drugs available to counteract the normal physiologic effects of either the menstrual period or pregnancy, and voice therapy is of no value in these cases. Voice clinicians must be aware, however, that such changes may be reported by patients.

A very small number of women appear to experience changes in the voice as a result of the use of birth control pills (Simkin, 1964). The quality and range of the voice may show these effects. Once again, they are usually not noted by the average speaker but may create problems for the singer. These voice changes are reversible when use of the pills is terminated.

Paradoxical Vocal Fold Motion/Laryngeal Spasms

This is a relatively rare disability, which can easily be mistaken for asthma and treated accordingly, even to the point of tracheostomy. A 1983 study reported in the *New England Journal of Medicine* (Christopher, Wood, Eckert, Blager, Raney, and Souhrada) described five patients 14 to 68 years of age, of whom four were male and one female, who presented with paroxysms of wheezing and dyspnea and had initially been diagnosed as severe, uncontrollable asthmatics. However, the patients failed to respond to standard therapy for asthma and, indeed, did not test positively for the expected symptoms of asthma. All patients had a chronic history of repeated ''attacks,'' ranging from 1 to 13 years. One patient had undergone eight tracheotomy procedures. All patients on laryngological examination during the spasm were found to have adduction of both true and ventricular folds during the full respiratory cycle and exhibited both inspiratory and expiratory stridor. Laryngeal function was normal during asymptomatic periods. Inhalation of a mixture of helium (80%) and oxygen (20%) was found to be effective in relieving at least the acute symptoms and frequently resulted in symptom reduction even after cessation of the treatment. All patients were found to have psychological problems, and all were referred for both speech therapy and psychological counseling. Follow-up ranged from 3 to 21 months, and no patient had had recurrence of the symptoms.

Other varieties of paradoxical vocal fold motion have been reported, in which the vocal folds seem to behave in a manner opposite to the normal, that is, adduction is observed during deep inspiration, and there is at least slight abduction on expiration (Rogers and Stell, 1978; Kellman and Leopold, 1982). One such patient had undergone tracheotomy twice for relief of symptoms that had been diagnosed as laryngospasm. Patients were reported to show significant reduction, if not elimination, of symptoms in response to various interventions, including speech therapy, intravenous injection of diazepam or of a placebo, hypnosis, and verbal support. Although voice symptoms ranging from aphonia to weak or hoarse voice may be present, restoring the airway is of primary importance. Voice therapy may be helpful in teaching these patients methods of relaxation and specific breathing techniques. However, psychological treatment must also be part of the treatment protocol.

Voice Therapy Techniques: Associated Physiology and Indications for Use

Introductory Comments

It is important to recognize that the manner in which a therapeutic technique is used will vary from clinician to clinician. Furthermore, with experience each clinician will develop and perfect those techniques found to be most useful and effective. Clinicians bring their own personalities and approaches to the clinical process, and the techniques that fit that style and produce a level of comfort and confidence are the ones that are most likely to be adopted and well used.

It is the philosophy of this book that an understanding of laryngeal anatomy and phonatory physiology is basic to being a skilled voice clinician. Therapeutic techniques are only valid when they are used knowledgeably. The clinician must develop the knowledge base and the skill to determine what therapeutic approaches make sense for the individual patient. Indeed, a skilled clinician may make up a technique never tried before but something that makes sense for a given person.

> **CASE EXAMPLE**   J. M. was a patient whose use of ventricular phonation was felt to be of psychological origin. A variety of techniques had been tried to elicit clear voice, but to no avail. She was then instructed to simply blow through her fingers while holding them in front of her mouth and to feel the airstream. She was to sustain that airstream steadily for at least 5 seconds. After a few trials of blowing, she was told to add a very slight bit of sound to the blowing while she continued to feel the airstream on her fingers. She successfully produced acceptable voice quality in doing this. Very gradually the good voice was shaped into speech, with no return of the ventricular phonation. This was a technique the clinician had never used previously.

There is nothing magical in the technique. For this patient, a way had been found to allow her to release laryngeal tension and produce easy voice. In this example, as in many others that might be cited, the clinician had a working hypothesis, perhaps unspoken, relating the technique to be used to the physiological effect that is desired. A patient may respond favorably to a number of approaches, all of which have the same goal. There is not a single technique that is always effective with all people. The clinician must understand what the patient is doing that is undesirable and then ask the question: "How can I get this patient to alter that specific behavior?"

Returning to the case example above, the clinician knew from previous fiberoptic laryngoscopic studies of this patient that the ventricular phonation was produced with tight squeezing of the whole larynx, including supraglottal structures. Perceptually, the voice sounded tight and strained, in addition to being very hoarse. It also seemed that this particular patient "froze" and became very tense when asked to try any new activity that required phonation. Therefore, she was asked to carry out an activity, blowing, that does not require phonation and was therefore not threatening. The addition of feeling the airstream captured J. M.'s attention and provided tangible, nonphonatory feedback. If J. M. continued to concentrate on this smooth, constant airstream, phonation would begin softly and easily in perhaps a breathy manner. The introduction of tension and strain would surely interrupt or markedly change the airflow. For these various reasons it was hypothesized that if the patient was able to carry out the instructions, there was a good chance that she would do so with good voice.

There are few techniques that are specific to a single voice disorder because there is so much similarity in laryngeal physiology across many disorders. For example, patients who misuse their voices and those who have abused them to the point of creating mucosal changes may be engaging in the same form of vocal behavior, from the physiological point of view. Thus, many of the same therapeutic techniques may be used in each instance. The specific type of misuse or abuse (i.e., talking too much versus talking too loud) will differ from patient to patient, and that issue must be addressed individually. However, the suggested means of changing those patterns may be similar across patients.

A major lack in voice research is documentation of the efficacy of therapeutic techniques. This lack, although decried by many (Moore,1977; Reed, 1980; Ludlow and Hart, 1981; Johnson, 1985; Perkins, 1985), is not easily corrected. Problems of terminology, of definition, of qualitative and quantitative assessment procedures, and of well-established normal standards (as discussed previously) plague the researcher who wishes to address the issue. Brewer and McCall (1974) used the fiberoptic laryngoscope to demonstrate visible changes in laryngeal physiology as patients were instructed in a therapeutic technique. Johnson (1985) reports on the efficacy of his particular program of reducing vocal abuse (VARP), which utilizes a highly structured behavior modification approach. Casper, Brewer, and Conture (1981) reported on computer-assisted measurement of specific intrasubject changes in laryngeal physiology, visible on fiberoptic images, that were felt to be the result of therapeutic intervention. The procedure, although workable, was fairly time consuming, and the results could be interpreted only relative to that individual's performance. Such research is helpful, but the approach does not lend itself to all voice problems. In the case example cited earlier, a new technique was used, and although in this case it proved to be effective, it would not necessarily be an appropriate or effective procedure with other cases of psychogenic dysphonia. If the research question to be answered is concerned not with specific techniques but rather with the question of whether the voice improved as a result of therapy, there must be some agreement on quantitative or qualitative parameters of assessment that would substantiate improved status. Such standards do not yet exist.

Thus, we are left with a variety of therapy techniques whose efficacy is acclaimed by many authors. The most often used of these will be discussed in the following section, which not only will describe how they are done but also will give at least a theoretical rationale of why clinically they seem to be of value. The authors want to caution again that the techniques are only as good as the clinician who is making use of them. Clinicians should use them wisely but should continue to question their efficacy and search for ways to demonstrate it.

There is no particular meaning to be assigned to the order in which these techniques are presented. There is also no intent to make this an all-inclusive list. Indeed, most clinicians adapt procedures to fit their personal styles and develop unique ones, as do most voice coaches. The challenge is to be able to think through a problem in such a way that it is possible to devise techniques to use based on an understanding of the type of vocal behavior that you wish to elicit. No single technique will be equally effective with all people.

Therapy Techniques

Breathy Phonation: The Confidential Voice

This technique is being described first because we have found it to be widely appropriate and easy for patients to learn and to use, and it has resulted in clinical successes. The voice is described to patients as being the softest (intensity) they can produce, much like the voice you would use to exchange a confidence with a friend when you do not wish others nearby to hear. It is not a whisper, because there is some voice present. It is important to make sure that the patient does not reduce mouth movement or lower pitch in using this confidential voice. Very few instructions need be given about how to produce the desired voice beyond what has been described plus the clinician's presentation of a model. The patient is instructed to use this voice for all speaking and is forewarned that it will be inaudible in any noisy environment. All loud talking is thus eliminated temporarily. It is also important to instruct the patient that fewer words per breath will be possible because of the increased expenditure of air. Furthermore, because one effect of the increased airflow may be a drying of the mucosa, we suggest that the patient increase fluid intake. This technique is appropriate for patients who need to eliminate vocal abuse or misuse. It is helpful as part of a vocal hygiene program whenever a period of modified voice rest or reduction of voice use is indicated.

Rationale: We have observed laryngeal physiology fiberoptically as we have asked patients and normal speakers to use this voice and have noted the desired effect (Casper, Colton, Brewer, and Woo, 1989). The glottis remains very slightly open, thus reducing the force of contact and of medial compression of the vocal folds. The larynx seems to remain vertically at about the resting level. There is an absence of any appearance of laryngeal tightness or squeezing, and the closed phase of the glottal cycle is reduced. In some patients there may be a tendency to produce breathiness with a posterior glottal chink and Y appearance. Thus, with one maneuver the patient is provided with a type of voice production that eliminates abuse yet allows continued voice use, albeit different and reduced. It is a holistic approach that does not require that the act of speaking be broken down into its component parts, with each addressed separately and then put back together. We have also found it rather simple for patients to move gradually from the breathy, confidential voice to increased voicing without returning to abusive patterns.

Sigh, Aspirate Initiation, Easy Initiation of Phonation

These three techniques are combined under one heading because they are variations on a theme sharing a common rationale. For the sigh the patient is instructed to produce the most relaxed, effortless, natural sigh possible. Whether or not voicing is present does not matter initially, but as this is practiced it is hoped that some voicing emerges naturally and easily. In a natural, spontaneous sigh it is not uncommon to release some air audibly before the actual voicing begins, then to produce just minimal voicing in terms of loudness and duration, and to finish the sigh with audible expiration of the rest of the breath supply. It is important that the patient not hold the breath after the inspiration. There must be a continuous flow from inhalation to exhalation, otherwise there is a tendency to close the glottis tightly as the breath is held.

From the sigh it is easy to have the patient practice aspirate initiation of voicing, using words that begin with an /h/. This should be done in a slightly exaggerated manner so that the /h/ is held and the voicing is initiated much as in the sigh and with a breathy quality. As the patient becomes adept at this maneuver, it is possible to omit the actual production of the /h/ yet continue the effortless gliding into easy initiation of phonation.

Rationale: These techniques reduce laryngeal and vocal tract tensions, reduce the force of vocal fold contact and of medial compression, teach easy coordination of airflow and phonation, counteract abusive habits of tension and glottal attack, and foster resting level laryngeal posture. They may be very helpful for patients who have difficulty in learning to use a breathy voice for general conversation and appear to need more direct step-by-step work to learn to reduce tensions. In a fiberoptic and stroboscopic study of aspirate initiation of phonation, Casper et al. (1989) observed the expected physiological characteristics described above.

Yawn/Sigh

The patient is instructed to simulate a real yawn, or if possible, to actually trigger a real yawn. The yawn is completed with a sigh, making sure to allow air to be released in a relaxed way. This is not always easy for patients to do. We tend to be socialized into hiding and stifling public yawns. It is sometimes helpful to instruct the patient to open the mouth very wide, pull the tongue back and inhale long and deeply. Initiation of voicing should be carried out with this same oral posture, with a gradual closing of the mouth as the yawn and sigh progress. It is well to suggest that patients become aware of natural yawns and try to concentrate on how they feel when they occur spontaneously. As the patient learns the technique and can identify the tension reduction, a gradual shaping of the yawn/sigh into production of words, then phrases, and finally sentences should proceed slowly. The yawn should be gradually eliminated.

Rationale: In a true vegetative yawn, the larynx lowers dramatically (Casper et al., 1989). This change can be observed fiberoptically. The physiology of a yawn is incompatible with the excessive laryngeal tensions that many patients exhibit. Easy, natural airflow and phonation are fostered. The intent is to eliminate abusive initiation and maintenance of phonation and to reduce laryngeal tensions.

Chewing

The act of chewing as a therapy technique was described by Froeschels in 1952. The technique requires that the patient practice the motions of chewing in an exaggerated manner and then sequentially, over time, add voicing, random sounds, words, phrases, sentences, and conversation while gradually reducing the degree of exaggeration of the mouth movements. As the technique is described, it is very important to help the patient imitate the chewing act quite exactly. This must involve constant movement of the tongue. Exaggeration of the act requires that the mouth be open while chewing. The resulting sounds produced when the activity is carried out correctly should be very variable. If the sound produced tends to be a repetitive, unchanging "yam yam," the chewing is being done with inadequate tongue movement. It has been our experience that it is difficult for patients to learn to do this chewing. As with yawning, we have been socialized into chewing as unobtrusively as possible, and certainly with the mouth closed. If this technique is to be used, the clinician must be adept at and comfortable with modeling it for the patient. It is often helpful for the clinician to do the activity along with the patient, thereby reducing self-consciousness. The use of chewable substances can help the patient identify the components of the chewing act. It then becomes somewhat easier to carry out that activity based on recall and imagery and without the actual substance in the mouth. (Caution: It is not a good idea for the clinician to provide chewable material. If you wish to use this idea, suggest that the patient bring crackers, gum, or other chewable foods to the therapy session.) Each step of chewing as a therapy approach must be mastered before the next level is introduced. Thus, the patient must learn to chew in the most exaggerated manner while producing voicing and random sounds before being asked to practice words. It is important to realize that articulatory clarity will be reduced in the early stages of using this technique as the focus remains on the chewing motion. Use of words and phrases that begin with vowels may be the easiest to begin practice. As the patient progresses and longer utterances are introduced, the chewing motions are almost eliminated, but excess tensions associated with phonation should not be evident.

Rationale: In adopting this technique, Froeschels sought a natural vegetative movement onto which phonation could be added without changing the totality of the act and without adding tensions or other negative behaviors the patient had habituated into the speaking act. The chewing motion has a tendency to release excess tensions in the vocal tract and laryngeal area, and when done correctly encourages mouth opening and reduction of mandibular tensions. These behaviors in turn foster easy onset of phonation without making that a specific focus of attention.

Chant-Talk

The name of this technique describes a manner of speaking that is a cross between speaking and singing or, from the singer's point of view, a form of singing that is a cross between singing and speaking. We tend to think of it as having limited frequency variability yet the flow of song. It can be used as a therapeutic technique in a number of different ways. Most simply, the patient can be asked to chant an utterance rather than speak it. If this is effective in eliciting effortless phonation of a good quality, the technique can be extended in practice with gradual reduction of the sing-song quality of the chant. If a particular "voice placement" or "focus" is sought, this chanting can be one of a variety of ways of finding that focus. For example, using Cooper's "um-hum" technique (1973; see also the "um-hum" therapy technique below), the patient may be asked to sustain that sound and chant the counting of numbers, or series of words or a sentence. It may be helpful for some patients to locate and identify the desired vocal sound through this chanting approach.

Rationale: The chanting of an utterance encourages an easy flow of phonation, reducing the tendency toward hard glottal attack and increased force of vocal fold contact. There may be some increased proprioceptive feedback as vibrations are felt through the nose and cheek areas, thus helping the patient to reduce focus on the larynx. It is also felt that if the voice is produced in this manner, there is usually a reduction in laryngeal and vocal tract tensions. Because chanting differs from talking and is usually a new way for patients to produce voice, it may be easier for them to alter voice production through this activity than to attempt to do so in speaking, wherein the habits are entrenched.

Hum and Nasal Consonants

This is another technique designed to teach easy voice production through a "natural" approach. The patient is asked to produce a hum and to be able to feel the resonance of that hum in the nose and cheeks. The pitch of the voice is generally not of direct concern, although it may seem to change as the patient searches for an easily produced, fully resonant sound. The hum is sustained, and the patient practices this until the target sound is produced without difficulty. It is often instructive to then ask the patient to lower the jaw, keeping the lips closed, while sustaining the hum. This results in an almost palpable forward movement of the focus of the voice, with a tickling sensation often being reported around the lips and along the palate. One of the authors was instructed by a voice coach to "hook" the sound in the back of the throat in order to master this kind of voice quality. The sound used for practice was the /ng/. Bear in mind that the sound being sought is not a nasal sound but rather a sound that might best be described as the "twang" that is typical of country Western singing (Colton and Estill, 1981). Gradually the production of these sounds is shaped into speech by first using nonsense syllables and words heavily loaded with the nasal consonants. Although the early practice of this technique may result in greater nasal resonance than is desirable, that is temporary and normalizes as speech is introduced. This technique can easily be combined with the chant-talk technique.

Rationale: As described in the rationale for chant-talk, the act of humming is different from speaking and thus may not be encumbered with undesirable habituated behaviors. A hum encourages easy initiation of phonation and provides proprioceptive feedback of nasal and facial vibration, thus refocusing the patient's preoccupation with the laryngeal area. The continuant nasal consonant promotes ease of sustained phonation, and it can easily be coordinated with the idea of smooth airflow from inhalation through exhalation. The "twang" sound also produces a mode of vocal fold vibration that produces a greater number of harmonics and thus a richer sound (Colton and Estill, 1981).

Digital Manipulation, Pressure, and Massage

Aronson (1985) has described a technique that involves direct physical manipulation and massage of the laryngeal area. The clinician must identify the tips of the hyoid bone and exert light pressure in a circular motion in that area. The clinician then moves the fingers into the thyrohyoid space and carries out the circular motion massage, moving posteriorly from the thyroid notch area. The massage is then done on the posterior borders of the thyroid cartilage. With the fingers along the superior border of the thyroid cartilage, the clinician begins to gently exert pressure in a downward manner in order to move the larynx down. There should be an increase in the thyrohyoid space. During these maneuvers the patient is asked to phonate vowels. When a positive change in the voice is noted (clearer quality and lowered pitch), the focus shifts to the production of that voice with, and then without, the manipulation. This entire activity needs to be carried out with care and with recognition that some pain might result. Patients must be reassured that the pain is temporary and is like any muscular pain associated with excessive tension and its reduction through direct manipulation and massage. According to Aronson, this technique may be effective in eliciting normal voice in a single therapy session in cases of dysphonia due to increased musculoskeletal tensions. However, when the condition has been of long standing, a longer course of treatment using this technique may be necessary.

Rationale: This technique is based on the need to reduce cramping in the extrinsic and intrinsic laryngeal muscles, which is believed to be the cause of dysphonia in many patients. The massaging of muscles induces relaxation, and the technique promotes a lowered laryngeal position, permitting ease of phonation. In using this technique, it is particularly important that the clinician understand and be able to identify the specific disturbance of phonatory physiology exhibited by a patient. Many but not all voice patients who are classified as having a hyperfunctional voice disorder speak with the larynx in an elevated posture. Care must be taken not to exert undue effort in pushing the larynx lower than is comfortable for the patient.

Boone (1983) has described a method of digital pressure that is very different in both intent and technique from that described above. Boone suggests that digital pressure be applied as a gentle inward push on the anterior aspect of the thyroid cartilage while a patient sustains a vowel. This pressure should result in lowered fundamental frequency and can be used to elicit and then habituate this lowered pitch, when that is a therapeutic goal.

Rationale: Applying pressure as described tilts the thyroid cartilage posteriorly and in so doing shortens vocal fold length and increases mass. This then results in a lowered fundamental frequency of vibration, perceived as lowered pitch. Once elicited in this manner, the lowered pitch becomes the target to be practiced and produced voluntarily.

Easy Production of Falsetto or High Pitched Sounds

This technique is yet another one that tends to shift the patient away from habituated patterns of voice use. It is especially helpful for patients who demonstrate anteroposterior laryngeal squeezing and for some who are said to be using ventricular phonation. It may require trial and error and much suggestion on the part of the clinician in order to facilitate the patient's ability to produce a high pitched sound. The use of imagery can be very helpful (see "Imagery," below). It is important to observe that there is a continuous flow from inhalation through exhalation, as the patient may have the tendency to increase tension and hold the breath prior to initiation of voicing. When the patient learns to easily produce the high pitched vowels at will, that sound can be sustained and the pitch gradually lowered in a glissando to the comfortable speaking level, without a change in voice quality. The patient is then asked to produce a sustained vowel at that targeted speaking pitch, maintaining the improved quality. As this is established, it can be shaped into speech. There is no attempt to specify a pitch level beyond that which is identified by the patient as comfortable and normal sounding.

Rationale: Easy production of the upper frequency range is most commonly produced by a lengthening of the vocal folds, decreasing their mass. It cannot be done using ventricular phonation, for example. Therefore, if a high pitched sound is elicited from a patient who has been using ventricular phonation, the technique has successfully shifted the patient out of that phonatory mode. The same rationale may be applied to patients who tend to constrict the larynx in the anteroposterior dimension or to those whose aberrant voice production behaviors are psychologically based. For the latter, the change in laryngeal physiology from what they are doing to that required for the production of the upper frequency range, if successful, may be sufficient to restore normal phonatory function, which can then be maintained as pitch is normalized.

Imagery

The use of imagery can be very helpful in describing how a particular type of sound should be produced. For example, statements of imagery such as "Make it feel as if your voice is floating effortlessly out of your throat and up into your head" can describe to the patient a way that effortless voicing might feel. Patients should be encouraged to provide their own imagery as they release tensions and change their manner of initiating phonation. The use of imagery can be combined with many of the other techniques, as it can help patients keep in mind what they are attempting to do. Imagery is often used in those techniques designated by some as "placing the voice" or finding a "focus" for the voice. It has been reported that professional singers and actors use imagery concerning their breathing, which although often in contradiction to known physiological fact, works well for them (Hixon, 1987; Watson, Hixon, and Maher, 1987).

Rationale: The physiology of imagery is receiving increasing attention as its use in the training of athletes and in fighting disease is increasing (Keaton, 1983; Ungerleider, 1986). It has been used in singing pedagogy for many years, and its effectiveness is per-

haps attested to by legions of superb performers. We use it in voice therapy to help a patient understand something about how to produce voice or what quality to attempt to produce, when other types of explanations are either not possible or have not been effective. Imagery, although perhaps not physiologically correct, can describe what seems to happen in a very subjective, sensory way. It is important that both the clinician and the patient recognize that the imagery being used is a means to an end, not necessarily as an accurate explanation of the desired physiology.

Pushing, Pulling, Isometrics

These techniques are placed together because they are used interchangeably to produce the same end result. Pushing refers to any of the many ways that patients may be encouraged to push against the wall, push down on the chair, and so on, while pulling refers to the opposite maneuvers of pulling up on a very heavy desk, pulling up on the chair one is sitting in, and the like. Isometric forms of these activities include placing the palms of the hands together at chest height and pressing them together or locking the fingers of the hands together at chest height and pulling them apart. Whichever method is used, the patient is instructed to phonate at the point of maximum pull or push. The sound produced will be a forceful grunt and should be demonstrated by the clinician. All of the varieties of these techniques are designed to force hyperfunction of the mechanism. They can often be used with surprising success in eliciting a low pitched phonation in cases of puberphonia and in eliciting voicing in patients who present with psychogenic aphonia. Once the patient has learned to carry out the push or pull, the same effect can be obtained by holding the breath, bearing down, and grunting. As the desired voicing is produced, the patient is instructed to sustain that sound as the force of the maneuver is gradually released. In a gradual stepwise fashion, the targeted sound is practiced with less and less need for the forceful push or pull activity.

Rationale: These maneuvers are designed to create effort closure of the glottis with the larynx in a lowered position. As such they are the opposite of hypofunction. Furthermore, the posture of the laryngeal mechanism is determined by the activity and dictates a particular type of vocalization. This shifts the individual from the usual manner of vocal production and introduces a behavior difficult to counteract. If tension is released prior to phonation, then the technique will be ineffective. Traditionally these types of procedures have been recommended for use in cases of unilateral vocal fold paralysis. The rationale has been that the effort closure forces a crossing of the midline of the unaffected vocal fold to approximate the paralyzed fold. This has not been our experience. Further discussion of this topic will be found later in this chapter under "Unresolved Issues and Myths." This technique should be used cautiously and sparingly in recognition of its potentially abusive nature.

Laughing, Coughing, Throat Clearing, Gargling, and Other Reflexive Acts

In the attempt to elicit voice from the aphonic patient or to find a normal voice for the dysphonic patient in the absence of positive laryngologic findings, the use of any of the above can be extremely effective. Indeed, it is important for the clinician to listen for spontaneous laughing, coughing, vocalized pauses, or throat clearing during general conversation with the patient. Patients are not aware that the mechanism used for producing the above sounds is the same as is used for producing the speaking voice. Thus, when asked to produce these sounds, they may do so and give evidence of normal voicing. The skilled clinician can make use of that sound by shaping it into speech in a gradual manner.

Some patients will, of course, produce these sounds in a dysphonic manner when doing so in response to a request, but normal voicing may occur if they happen spontaneously. Again, it takes the skill of the clinician to utilize all instances of good voicing to reestablishing normal voice.

Rationale: These behaviors are so automatic that the patient may perform them unconsciously. Thus, they may be accompanied by much better voicing than is heard in speech. Because they are not speech behaviors, their production may be free of habituated but undesirable phonatory speech behaviors. The inability to elicit an improved voice using these behaviors is also a meaningful finding. Although throat clearing and coughing can be abusive to the laryngeal mechanism, they can be used judiciously in the search for normal voicing.

"Um-hum"

In this technique the patient is instructed to say "um-hum," the vocalized utterance used by a listener to indicate agreement with the speaker, in a naturally spontaneous and sincere manner. This production is then shaped by adding single words, as in "um-hum one." Gradually this is extended through the use of increasingly longer utterances until the patient is able to produce the targeted voice without needing the starting "um-hum."

Rationale: According to Cooper (1984) this simple utterance, if said as naturally as possible, results in producing a voice at the appropriate pitch level and with the correct focus for the individual. Vibration should be perceptible along the bridge and sides of the nose and down to the lips. This technique, similar to the one previously described, capitalizes on a phonatory act that is almost reflexive in nature. The fact that a nasal component is present in the consonant /m/ adds to the appropriate focusing of the voice.

Whispering

Whispering is the act of moving the articulators to form words in the presence of rapid airflow but the absence of phonation. Very little instruction is usually required to elicit whispering. A quiet whisper can be used when vocal rest or minimal voice use is part of the treatment plan. It is sometimes instructive to ask patients who habitually use excessive loudness to limit themselves to a quiet whisper for part (or parts) of each day. The pronounced contrast between the whisper and the habitual loudness level may help to focus the patient's awareness and make loudness reduction to an acceptable level easier to accomplish.

Rationale: Despite many caveats in the literature to the effect that whispering is harmful, there is no experimental evidence to support that notion. Indeed, there is evidence that suggests otherwise. This issue is addressed more completely in the section "Unresolved Issues and Myths."

Breathing

It is sometimes helpful for direct attention to be paid to respiration. By focusing on the breathing, tensions that may be generalized throughout the chest as well as the larynx and vocal tract can be reduced. Patients should be instructed as simply as possible to sit at rest and allow their breathing to function normally. Remember that the diaphragm is a muscle of inhalation and functions during the inspiratory cycle (Fig. 9.1). But at high lung volumes it may be necessary to contract the diaphragm in order to prevent the rapid, unwanted descent of the ribcage, producing greater than needed subglottal pressures that will produce louder and uncontrolled voice production. As shown in Figure 9.1, a number of muscles are activated during a speaking event. At high lung volumes, the muscles acti-

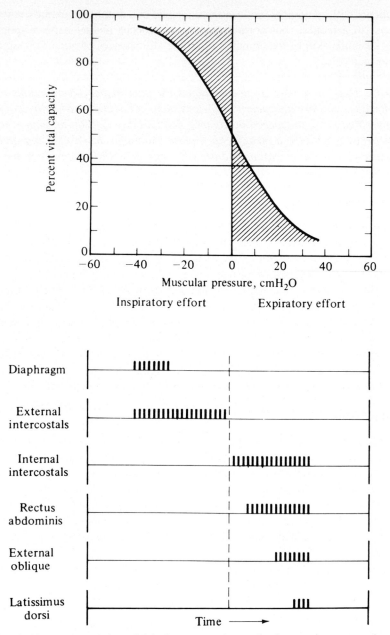

Figure 9.1.   In the upper portion of this figure are shown the lung volume-muscle pressure relationships during the production of a sustained vowel. At high lung volumes, a large amount of inspiratory muscle pressure is needed to counteract the large lung pressures that are created. As lung volume decreases, less inspiratory effort is needed, until resting lung volume is reached (point where the curve crosses the vertical line in the middle of the graph). At still lower lung volumes, expiratory muscle effort is needed to produce the necessary subglottal pressures for speech. In the panel below, a schematic of muscle activity in the diaphragm, external intercostals, internal intercostals, rectus abdominis, external oblique, and latissimus dorsi is shown in relationship to the pressure relationships shown above. (From Hixon TJ, (1973), Respiratory function in speech. In: Normal Aspects of Speech, Hearing, and Language, Minifie F, Hixon T, Williams F (eds.), Englewood Cliffs, NJ, Prentice Hall, Inc., © 1973, p 107.)

vated will be inspiratory, but as lung volume falls, expiratory musculature will be needed to provide the proper air pressure to drive the vocal folds. Excess muscle activity in the respiratory musculature will prevent the smooth coordination of the respiratory system and the steady maintainance of subglottal air pressure and phonation. The clinician should observe the patient's breathing pattern at rest and, assuming that it is normal, instruct the patient to gently place one hand on the area of the diaphragm/abdomen and the other on the upper chest, while continuing to breathe quietly. The patient should be able to identify slight outward movement of the diaphragm/abdomen area on inhalation and imperceptible movement of the upper chest. The patient's attention also needs to be directed to the continuous movement in the respiratory cycle from inspiration through expiration. As soon as this effortless breathing has been established, the patient should be instructed to breathe in a little more deeply and to release the exhalatory cycle as a sigh, without changing the rate or manner of breathing. Thus, the focus on breathing leads easily into incorporation of the sigh, the yawn-sigh, aspirate initiation of phonation, and so on. Throughout this type of practice the patient should continue to monitor the ease with which voice is introduced without tension. As the patient learns to do these activities easily, the task can continue to be altered so that the inhalatory stage of breathing occurs more quickly, as it does during speech, while the exhalatory stage is lengthened. When adding the latter refinement, it is important that the patient not introduce tensions and attempts to extend exhalation beyond the available air supply. The clinician must determine whether the work on breathing has helped the patient to also reduce or eliminate laryngeal tensions. It is important that the patient be instructed in the generalization of the improved respiratory control to conversational speech. The clinician must remember that average conversational utterances on one continuous respiration tend to be very short, about 5 seconds (Boone, 1988), and that, therefore, nonprofessional voice users do not need to inhale as deeply as do professional voice users in singing, acting, or public speaking. The amount of therapeutic time devoted to work on breathing and, indeed, the need for any such attention, must be decided on a case-by-case basis.

Extended training in breath support and breath control will be helpful to the professional voice user. Many activities or exercises can be designed to accomplish this, but they must be done with an understanding of the process and recognition of the need to build control in a gradual way, as in any activity of muscle building and training.

Rationale: The respiratory system is the power source for the voice. The systems involved in phonation are closely intertwined, and tensions in one system cannot easily be isolated from the rest. Thus, reducing respiratory tensions and assuring a continuous flow from inspiration through expiration assists in reducing laryngeal tensions and avoiding closure of the glottis prior to the initiation of phonation. Most patients, with the exception of those who have chronic obstructive lung disease or neuromotor impairment of the control of respiration, tend to have normal respiration and adequate air supply for speech. This topic will be discussed further in the section on unresolved issues and myths. Singers, actors, and other professional voice users may have demands placed on voice use that require greater control of increased volumes of air. This group of voice users will need more extended training in the management of breath support and breath control than the average speaker.

Relaxation

A variety of techniques are used to teach generalized relaxation. These include progressive relaxation in which the patient is instructed to concentrate on specific parts of the body one at a time and then through imagery and suggestion to release the tensions present

(Jacobsen, 1938). Another part of the technique involves purposefully tensing a specific body area, followed by a release of that tension. The neck is very vulnerable to muscle tightening in tense individuals (Nagler,1987). A popular activity for relaxation of neck tension has been the head roll in which the patient is instructed to very, very slowly allow the head to be rotated 360 degrees. However, it has been suggested that circular rotation of any part of the spine may not be helpful to the intervertebral disks, and the following exercises are recommended instead (Nagler):

1. While holding the left elbow in the right hand, pull it over to the right side, hold, then relax. Do the same with the other arm, and repeat the sequence three times for each arm.
2. Place the hands, palms in, on the upper chest, with elbows out to the sides. Circle the elbows in one direction and then reverse. Repeat three times.

Rationale: The rationale for engaging in relaxation therapy as one segment of a vocal rehabilitation program is primarily to release excess tensions in systems that have to do with phonation. However, it must be recognized that most of our talking is done in states other than complete relaxation. Thus, it is important to use these techniques in specific ways and then to incorporate them into healthy patterns of phonation.

Phonating on Inhalation

The technique for creating voice in this way is just as described by the title. The patient is instructed and shown how to make sound in the reverse of the normal pattern, that is, as air is being drawn into the lungs. This is usually a fairly simple sound for most people to make. The most common use of this technique involves practice in going directly from the voice produced on inhalation into voice produced on exhalation. If this technique is successful in eliciting an improved voice quality in the exhalatory phase, then it can be continued with gradual reduction in the need to start the phonation on inhalation. A different use of phonation on inhalation has recently been described by Freeman (1988), in which patients with severe voice disorders (e.g., spastic dysphonia and phonatory apraxia) were taught to speak on inhalation without switching back to the exhalatory mode and were reported to have made significant improvement in their ability to communicate vocally. That form of treatment is still in its preliminary stages, and a full description of how to train the inhalatory sound into conversational speech has not yet been offered.

Rationale: Voice produced on inhalation is said to be produced by the true vocal folds (Lehmann, 1965; Williams, Farquharson, and Anthony, 1975). Thus, in patients who are using ventricular fold phonation or those who are improperly using the vocal folds, it is theorized that this technique will stimulate more appropriate physiology. It is difficult for patients to control the behavior of inhalatory phonation because it is such a new and different behavior for them. As a result, the vocal folds will very normally be brought into play, and if that posture can be maintained by the patient when the direction of the flow of air is reversed, normal voice should result. The rationale for improved voice on inhalation in cases of spastic dysphonia remains unclear at this time.

Vocal Hygiene

This category will include techniques that should be incorporated into most voice therapy programs. Vocal hygiene may constitute the entire rehabilitation program, or it may be but one part of the program. In most instances of misuse and abuse of the voice, it should be a routine part of the program, and training in vocal hygiene as a preventive measure should be the final stage of voice therapy after a successful outcome has been attained (Fig. 9.2).

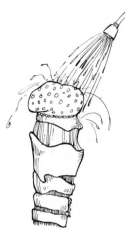

Figure 9.2. Vocal hygiene.

Reducing the Amount of Talking.   Patients should be counseled about the need to significantly curtail the amount of talking they do, for perhaps only a specified period of time. This is sometimes referred to as modified vocal rest. Instructions should be as detailed as needed and should include all restrictions on voice use. If patients are able to eliminate all but essential talking, that is usually sufficient. Other restrictions having to do with loudness of voice will tend to reduce voice usage as well. It may be helpful to use therapy time to work out a plan for where and when the voice will have to be used. Other behavior modification approaches, such as charting when, where, and for how long voice was used, may help accomplish this reduction in the amount of talking. The topic of complete voice rest will be discussed in greater detail in the section on unresolved issues and myths.

Reducing Loudness.   This may involve eliminating all use of the voice when an intensity level above that permitted by a soft breathy voice is required. Such a restriction will not allow yelling for the dog or for children playing outside or upstairs, or talking in a car, above a television or radio, above machinery or other noise in an employment setting, at a cocktail party or in a bar with loud music playing, and so on. Such reduction of loudness is necessary when there have been mucosal changes, whether evidenced by inflammation, edema, or vocal nodules.

There are some patients whose primary vocal abuse is the routine use of excessive loudness. This often requires different techniques and is not an easy pattern to alter. We all have a vocal image in our minds, which includes a loudness level. Patients who are excessively loud often do not believe that people will be able to hear them if they speak more softly. They must be willing to test out whether this is the case by engaging in intensity reduction activities. A useful device known as the Voice Intensity Controller (VIC, Behavioral Controls , Inc.) is small enough to be worn by the patient and preset to beep when a specific loudness level has been exceeded. Visual feedback of loudness can also be provided with the use of the Visi-Pitch (Kay Elemetrics Corp), The PM Pitch Analyzer (Voice Identification, Inc.), and the Vocal Loudness Indicator (LinguiSystems).

Identifying and Reducing or Eliminating Vocal Abuse.   All potentially abusive behaviors and abusive vocal use should be identified and eliminated if possible, or at least reduced to a minimum. Exploration of abuses needs to be very thorough. Abuses may include smoking of legal or illegal substances, use of certain drugs, spending large amounts of time in dry, dusty, or smoke-filled environments, exposure to airborne irritants, frequent habitual throat clearing, constant cough, and excessive drinking of alcoholic beverages, as well as the abusive behaviors of excessive talking, excessive loudness, and excessive strain discussed elsewhere. All identified abuses need to be discussed, and specific plans need to be made as to how they will be reduced or eliminated. Patients should be required to monitor their performance on the agreed upon plan.

Environmental Manipulation. Whenever it seems appropriate, changes can be made in the environment to help patients function with reduced voice use or to make the environment itself more hospitable. For example, humidification can be increased by the use of room humidifiers, amplification can be used when there are demands on vocal loudness, whistles or bells can be adopted by teachers to obtain attention in place of typically loud voice use, the television volume can be muted when it is necessary to talk, and so on. Creativity is sometimes required in order to plan environmental changes. People may be resistant to changing their habitual modes of functioning. It is often necessary to work through this resistance and for the clinician to find ways to encourage patients to adopt the plans and give them a fair trial.

Rationale: *The rationale for all of these activities is that they reduce either the force or the amount of vocal fold contact, or both. In so doing, they potentially eliminate irritation of the mucosa and reduce habitually abusive behaviors.*

Energizing the Voice

This technique is a difficult one to describe because of the abstractness of the concept. It is perhaps analogous to the car engine that is chugging along on only three spark plugs rather than all six. It is akin to the desire to "set a match" under someone who is too low keyed, too subdued and laid back. It is appropriate for use with patients who are known to have normal metabolic states and a normal ear, nose, and throat examination and who are not psychiatrically depressed. It includes (*a*) the use of adequate mouth opening and movement of the articulators, (*b*) the use of more inflection or variability of pitch, (*c*) the use of adequate loudness level and increased variability of loudness as appropriate to mark meaning, and (*d*) the use of a "well-placed" and well-supported (respiration) voice. Use of the many methods of accomplishing this will vary depending on the age, personality, and speaking needs of the patient. The use of scripted material from plays or other sources can be helpful, as can exercises such as practicing the role of a drill sergeant, calling out cadences, practicing in a large room, moving and using the whole body while counting, and so forth. Care must be taken so that the patient does not simply begin to shout. Whatever exercise or material is used, the patient must have specific goals that have been explained and practiced at lower levels of difficulty first. Many of these activities are often better carried out with the patient and the clinician standing some distance away from each other. Increasing mouth opening requires much work and practice. It is often helpful for the patient to practice very exaggerated movements first while receiving feedback from a mirror. The exaggeration is reduced gradually to the point where oral use is adequate. At that point, the increased mouth opening should no longer feel unusual or bizarre to the patient. Variability in pitch and loudness can be aided by the use of instruments that provide visual feedback (Visi-Pitch, PM Pitch Analyzer, etc.) until such time as the patient has improved auditory sensitivity to and discrimination of these parameters.

Rationale: *Some patients complain about having "weak" voices that do not carry, that do not convey the desired image, and that seem to fatigue as the day goes by. In the absence of hormonal imbalance, serious psychiatric problems laryngeal abnormality, or other organic problems, it is necessary to examine how the patient is speaking. All of the behaviors described above can be detrimental to the production of voice, and all can be changed behaviorally. It is clear that personality factors may be heavily involved, and the clinician must always keep this in mind.*

Vocal Effort

The concept and technique of measuring vocal effort was described in Chapter 7. It is a simple concept that can be adapted for use as a therapy technique. It requires that the patient assign a number to represent the amount of effort being expended to talk. (The only stipulation is that the numbers used increase with an increase of effort.) In order to obtain a comparative scale for that patient, have him produce phonations at a minimum effort level, a comfortable effort level, and at a maximum effort level. For example, if a patient has complained of feeling that it is a strain to talk, suggest that he talk with a degree of effort corresponding to a number just slightly above the number he assigned to his minimum effort level. Patients can learn to internally monitor their effort levels and modify their behavior accordingly, thereby achieving an increased measure of control over phonation. They are able to experiment with how they produce sound in order to achieve a more efficient and vocally less tiring, and probably less abusive, mode of phonation. Yet another benefit of this technique is the ease with which progress can be tracked. After a period of use of either reduced or increased effort (whichever was the goal), patients can again be asked to assign a number to their habitual phonations. This can be compared to the previous judgment.

Rationale: Because it has been determined that patients are able to estimate vocal effort and that their estimates are manifested acoustically by variation in sound pressure level and fundamental frequency (Wright and Colton, 1972a, 1972b; Colton and Brown, 1973), in therapy this approach accomplishes desired goals in a holistic manner without fragmenting the various components of producing voice. It is also a technique that is easy for patients to understand and to retain in memory, thereby increasing the likelihood that they will be able to put it to use. It does not require extensive practice and provides almost immediate reinforcement both through a sense of accomplishment and control and awareness of the reduction in strain.

Criteria for Termination of Therapy

Elimination or Reduction of Vocally Asymptomatic Tissue Changes

For some patients, a significant reduction in the size, extent, or severity of mucosal pathology may lead to essentially normal voice. We have known of patients who although totally asymptomatic for voice problems were found (during routine ear, nose, and throat examination) to have vocal fold nodules. These patients were not only vocally asymptomatic at the time of the examination but denied experiencing any change in voice in the past. It appears that certain small lesions may be so situated as to have minimal effect on glottal closure or on mucosal vibratory behavior, leaving the voice perceptually unchanged. This then may also be the case with a patient who has normal-sounding voice and full vocal range despite the continued presence of some mucosal pathology. Training in vocal hygiene prior to termination of treatment is essential for this type of patient in order to prevent a recurrence or worsening of the laryngeal condition. The patient who experiences full resolution and elimination of signs of pathology and return of good voice is obviously also a candidate for termination of voice therapy.

Improved Voice of a Quality Acceptable to Patient

In clinical practice, a patient may experience a degree of improvement that is looked upon by the clinician as only a point along the road to the "best" voice but that is accepted by the patient as being totally adequate. This may be a form of resistance to therapy, or it may be related to the expense incurred in continuation of the therapy, or it may reflect the patient's view and expectation quite precisely. At some point it is important for the clinician to raise the self-directed question, "Whose needs am I interested in fulfilling, mine or this patient's?"

There are also many situations in which restoration of normal voice is not a realistic goal. For those patients, the attainment of an acceptable voice should signal the consideration of termination of therapy.

Elimination of Physical Symptoms of Pain, Discomfort, and Fatigue

Patients sometimes complain of these sensory symptoms more vigorously than they do of their voice symptoms. Indeed, the voice symptoms may be fairly minimal perceptually. Thus, for such patients, the relief of pain, discomfort, and fatigue associated with phonation is the goal, and attainment of that goal may be the proper time to terminate therapy. Incidentally, when these symptoms are relieved, patients have usually changed phonatory behavior in ways that are also reflected in improved voice production.

Habituation of Changed Vocal Behaviors with No Return of Symptoms

When a patient has fully adopted the desired vocal behaviors and no longer complains of any of the initial phonatory problems that brought him to treatment, therapy should be terminated.

Lack of Improvement after an Appropriate Therapy Trial

Voice therapy is generally not a long-term process. Some improvement should be perceptually discernible with most voice patients within a month or two of therapy, assuming at least one session per week. If that is not the case, the clinician should review the case thoroughly. Every attempt should be made to resist adopting the facile excuse that the patient is resistant to therapy and is not practicing. Indeed, that may sometimes be the case, but it is incumbent upon the clinician to fully explore all other possibilities as well. These may include an erroneous initial diagnosis, an inappropriate therapeutic approach, the presence of psychological factors that do not allow the patient to abandon a symptom, environmental or medical factors helping to maintain a problem that have not been identified or dealt with, or the presence of a condition that is not responsive to a voice therapy approach. Possible actions to be taken would include consultation with the referring physician, referral to a voice laboratory for additional testing, reassessment and alteration of the therapy approach, and referral for additional consultations (neurological, psychiatric, etc.). It may well be that after all of the appropriate steps have been taken, a decision to terminate therapy may be the correct one.

Documentation of the therapy process, beginning with the evaluation and all test data, is essential in helping to determine and to support the decision to terminate therapy. If the data reveal positive changes that might be expected with a successful course of therapy, being able to reveal and explain the data to the patient will inspire an added measure of confidence—confidence the patient has in the clinician and self-confidence the patient gains based on the progress made. If the data are negative, revealing essentially no change, the door is opened for discussion of possible reason, and support is lent to the need for additional testing or examination.

Unresolved Issues and Myths

Clavicular Breathing: The Cause of Voice Problems?

After many years of experience in examining and working with voice-disordered patients, we are struck by the absence of clavicular breathing as a symptom or a sign. This is especially so in view of the frequent mention of this breathing pattern in many texts. Moreover, despite the claims, there is an absence of data to support this notion.

Clavicular breathing may be present in patients whose respiratory function is compromised as a result of chronic obstructive airway disease or neurological impairment. It may also be apparent in persons who are anxious and extremely tense. It is difficult to understand what the nature of the pathophysiology would be for an otherwise healthy individual to develop true clavicular breathing.

It is often the case, indeed it happens almost universally, that when people are asked to take a deep breath during examination, they will lift the shoulders and give a good example of clavicular breathing. However, if the patient's breathing pattern is carefully observed (without comment) during general conversation and at rest, we would submit that clavicular breathing will rarely be seen. That is not to say that a patient's manner of voice production may not include some effect on respiratory function. It is difficult to isolate excess tension only to the larynx and supraglottal vocal tract. Increased generalized thoracic tensions, thus, might be a part of the total voice production behavior, disrupting effective respiratory support for phonation. This should not be interpreted, however, as a basic respiratory problem or abnormality.

Talking from the Diaphragm

Talking from the diaphragm seems to have become a phrase known to all whether or not any understanding of its meaning is attached to its utterance. It no doubt stems from singing pedagogy and early elocution training. If taken literally, it is physiologically impossible. However, it seems to be understood to mean that exhalation may be controlled in some way by the diaphragm. Physiologically, we know that the diaphragm is the primary muscle of inspiration, acting to enlarge the thoracic cavity in the vertical dimension. It is not an active muscle of expiration. When it is important to fully enlarge the thoracic cavity in order to be able to fill the lungs, then it would seem to be of value to spend time working on "diaphragmatic breathing." In addition, it has been shown that the diaphragm is active during the initial expiratory phase of respiration when phonation is begun on high lung volumes (Hixon, 1987). There is no doubt that professional voice users should be well trained in respiratory control. However, the average speaker is rarely called upon to have that degree of control. The normal speaker adjusts inspiration (speed and amount) and expiration (rate) to the demands of the utterance (Bless and Miller, 1972). Daniloff, Schuckers, and Feth (1980) state that speakers tend to breathe deeper when the utterance ahead is a long one, and less deeply when the anticipated utterance is short. In soft speech, the average duration of expiratory airflow is reported to be 2.4 to 3.5 seconds, as compared with the well-trained singer's ability to phonate loudly for more than 15 to 20 seconds (Daniloff et al.). It is at high (or low) lung volumes that greater muscular control of respiration needs to be exercised. However, for normal speech activity, great diaphragmatic breaths are not required.

It is our impression that a great deal more emphasis has been placed on "teaching" or "correcting" breathing than is usually necessary in working with the voice-disordered patient who is not a professional voice user. Occasionally, attention to easy and relaxed breathing can be helpful in reducing tensions and diverting focus from the larynx. We would suggest that more attention should be paid to the ways in which the speaker uses the air supply. For example, does the person release a lot of the available air supply before initiating phonation? Or does he keep talking after the easily available air supply has been exhausted, and in so doing increase tension? Or does she tend to stop in midsentence without releasing the air supply or replenishing it before starting up again? Is there a tendency to hold the breath before starting to talk? Direct work on such behaviors will help to indirectly change respiratory behavior.

Ventricular Phonation: Diagnosis or Description?

The term "dysphonia plica ventricularis," or dysphonia resulting from ventricular fold phonation, has typically been used as a diagnosis. We suggest that it is really a description based on visual observation, through indirect, fiberoptic, or stroboscopic laryngoscopy, of greater than expected approximation of the ventricular folds during phonation. The descriptive term does not reveal the underlying etiology of the behavior. The name given to this problem, "ventricular phonation," implies that the ventricular folds are the actual source of sound, which would suggest that the true vocal folds are not fully adducting. However, we have observed full true vocal fold adduction in the presence of compression of the ventricular folds, suggesting perhaps that the ventricular folds, rather than being the source of sound, may produce a damping effect on the sound emitted at the true vocal fold level or a restraining effect on the vibratory behavior of the true vocal folds.

Caution should be exercised in diagnosing ventricular phonation based on indirect mirror examination alone. The positioning of the oropharyngeal structures required for indirect laryngoscopy, with the tongue held firmly in a fully protruded posture, may result in laryngeal adjustments that may not be typical for that person during conversational speech. Fiberoptic examination allows for habitual phonatory physiology to be observed.

Much is yet to be learned about the physiology, acoustics, and etiology of ventricular phonation. When the observation of excessive ventricular fold activity is made, it is necessary to continue the process of differential diagnosis in an attempt to uncover its etiology.

Unilateral Vocal Fold Paralysis: Does It Cross the Midline?

It has been stated for many years that the compensatory behavior involved in the restoration of good voice in the presence of unilateral vocal fold paralysis is a crossing beyond the midline of the uninvolved fold to make contact with the paralyzed fold. As a result, the goal of therapeutic procedures that have been espoused for use with this population has been a strengthening of the normal vocal fold through activities of forceful effort closure of the glottis. There have been scant data to support either the crossover effect or the efficacy of this or any other forms of vocal rehabilitation in the presence of unilateral vocal fold paralysis. The question must also be raised as to whether return of voice has been in some instances inappropriately credited to the therapy program when the patient has, in fact, experienced spontaneous return of function (as is often the case with an idiopathic paralysis). Or perhaps the therapy hastened or assisted the return of function. Answers to these speculations are unavailable. And, indeed, there are those cases who, despite continued paralysis, have experienced return of good voice. How? What makes the difference between those who experience return of voice in the presence of paralysis and those whose voices continue to be aberrant?

Although the notion of the crossover effect is an appealing one, we have been impressed by the lack its occurrence in patients we have examined fiberoptically (Casper, Colton, and Brewer, 1985), whether or not they exhibited return of voice. We explored whether the crossover could be elicited through various voice therapy maneuvers and failed to observe its occurrence in the few patients we studied. Schematic representations based on information obtained from high speed films of the behavior of the vocal folds in the presence of unilateral paralysis have shown that the glottis remains open, with the normal vocal fold approaching the midline but not crossing it, while the affected fold has a motion described as being like a "flag flapping in the wind" (Hirano, Kakita, Kawasaki, and Matsushita, 1977).

Paralysis of the vocal fold not only results in its inability to be moved by contraction of the affected muscle(s) but also changes its level and shape. These parameters—the level, tension, thickness, and eventual position relative to midline—of a paralyzed vocal fold will be determined by a variety of factors, including muscle fibrosis and contractures (Ballenger, 1985). These effects must be better understood in order to be factored into an understanding of the variability of vocal performance in the presence of paralysis.

In our own experience, we have not been impressed by the results obtained in voice therapy using effort closure techniques. Indeed, many patients have reported such exercises to be fatiguing to the voice and seeming to result in poorer vocal performance for a period of time during and after their execution. In view of these many concerns, we feel constrained not to recommend the routine use of such exercises in these cases. Other techniques have been incidentally reported to be effective in producing clearer and less breathy voice. Among these is the use of a high pitch or falsetto. When the superior branch of the recurrent laryngeal nerve is intact and functional, stretching and thinning of the affected vocal fold will still occur due to the action of the cricothyroid muscle. This action has a component of adduction and results in greater approximation of the folds and increased tension in the lax paralyzed fold. The problem with this technique is that the effect and the improved voice quality that it allows is not transferrable to a modal register phonation at an acceptable frequency level for general communication. Methods of treating unilateral vocal fold paralysis through the use of phonosurgical techniques were described in Chapter 8.

The Myth of Optimum Pitch

The concept of an optimum pitch dates back to at least 1940, when it was described by Fairbanks. It has been defined variously as (a) that pitch at which the voice has good quality and maximum intensity with the least effort, (b) that pitch at which there is a "vocal swell," and (c) a biologically determined ideal pitch for an individual, determined by the anatomic and physiological characteristics of individual larynges. The methods for its determination have also varied somewhat, and include

1. Listening for that pitch at which the quality of the voice is best and intensity is the greatest
2. Counting the number of musical notes in a person's full range (optimum pitch will be that which is 25% of the way up from the bottom of the range)
3. Using the same technique as in no. 2 above and going up one-third of the way from the bottom of the range
4. Having the patient say "um-hum" naturally, with the lips closed and a rising inflection, while feeling the oronasopharyngeal surfaces for the most resonant frequency

5. Finding the pitch at which the sustained phonation of the vowel /ah/ is the longest and loudest
6. Finding the lowest pitch a person can produce and counting at least four notes up the scale
7. Listening for the pitch of the sigh of a yawn/sigh maneuver, which is said to represent a person's optimal pitch

Experimental attempts have been made to explore the claims made about optimum pitch. In 1958 Thurman measured intensity at the various frequencies as subjects hummed a scale. Only 11% of the highest intensity levels occurred within the range of frequencies that might be considered to be appropriate for an adult's optimum pitch. A number of other investigators have examined frequency-intensity relationships (Damste, 1970; Komiyama, 1972; Coleman, Mabis, and Hinson, 1977), and have reported maximum intensity occurring about 70% up from the subject's lowest sustainable frequency (not the 25% to 30% claimed for optimum pitch). Vocal efficiency, another tenet of optimum pitch, can be measured as the ratio of the total output (acoustic) power over the total input (aerodynamic) power at the glottis. Van den Berg (1956), using a catheter between the vocal folds to obtain a direct measure of subglottal pressure and an esophageal catheter for an indirect measure, found a positive relationship between subglottal pressure and sound pressure level (SPL). He converted the SPL into speech power in watts to measure laryngeal efficiency at various frequencies and intensities. If optimum pitch exists, the expectation would be that an increased output power would be obtained for the same level of input power at a given frequency. This did not occur. Using slightly different methodology, Isshiki (1964) reported results similar to van den Berg's. House (1959) demonstrated an important contribution of the vocal tract when he reported that a perceptible change in overall intensity occurred when a vocal harmonic coincided with the center of a vocal tract resonance. The so-called "vocal swell" thus does not appear to be related to the concept of laryngeal efficiency. Another line of questioning was pursued by Stone (1983) when he questioned the perceptibility of the intensity change that was claimed to mark the optimum pitch. He found that the intensity changes between 100 and 200 Hz, the range between which optimum pitch would be expected for adult males, were very minimal and thus imperceptible. Similar to previous reports, Stone also found greatest intensity for half of his subjects to occur at frequencies well above the level at which optimum pitch would be anticipated. And still further, using the Fairbanks method for measuring optimum pitch, Stone reported that in 23 of 30 trials (N = 10 × 3 trials each), the "optimal pitch" fell above the speaker's modal pitch. Minifie (1984) reported that the efficiency of the power conversion increased with intensity rather than with frequency. This author could find no evidence to support the concept of an optimal pitch as being most efficient. All of the studies cited thus far used normal-speaking subjects. However, Ludlow, Connor, and Coulter (1984) explored the viability of the optimum pitch concept in patients with laryngeal pathology. Their results suggest that vocal function is best at the frequencies in the upper 50% of the speaking range for normal speakers, but not for those with laryngeal pathology. They interpret their findings to mean that a set of lawful relationships exists between several measures of phonatory function, and frequency in normal speakers, which are disturbed in the presence of pathology. Pathology compromises phonatory function, limiting it to a particular range in frequencies. Thus, in pathological states it is the disturbance of the lawful relationships that is meaningful rather than the existence of a particular fundamental frequency range at which phonation can be expected with least effort.

These data all seem to substantially reject the notion of an optimum pitch, at least as currently defined. Finally, it is important to be wary of subjective perceptions of pitch level. Murry (1978) demonstrated that judgments of pitch in dysphonic voices may be confounded by other voice signal parameters, such as loudness, effort, and voice quality.

He found a reduction in phonational range in patients with laryngeal paralysis but did not find speaking fundamental frequency in dysphonic patients to be significantly lower than in the normal-speaking population. In Chapter 5 it was reported that a prominent perceptual characteristic of voice in Huntington's disease was low pitch. However, actual measurements of fundamental frequency in this population showed it to be within the normal range. Wilson, Wellen, and Kimbarow (1983) demonstrated that trained listeners were not better than untrained listeners in judgments of perceived fundamental frequency (pitch) of children's voices and that neither group could identify differences of less than 20 Hz at better than chance level. It is also important to recognize that raising pitch level may appear to reduce breathiness or hoarseness, but that this happens at the expense of, not for the benefit of, the larynx. The extra effort put forth by the patient may serve to override some of the vocal symptoms. Reduction of loudness is physiologically a much sounder approach. It seems quite logical that even an optimum pitch, if there were one, could be used in improper, abusive ways.

It is the philosophical approach of this book that if phonatory physiology is normalized, the voice that emerges will be at an appropriate pitch level for that individual. Therefore, approaching the rehabilitation of disordered voice by attempting to impose an arbitrary pitch level seems inappropriate, perhaps incorrect, and often unproductive.

Whispering: Is It Harmful?

Some authors believe that whispering should be avoided during periods of voice rest or as a therapeutic technique because they claim that it results in vocal fold adduction that is undesirable, or that extreme glottal friction characterizes the whisper, and that is undesirable. Are there available experimental data to support these contentions? There have been a number of investigations of laryngeal configurations during whisper (Pressman, 1942; Pressman and Kelemen, 1955; Hamlet, 1972; Monoson and Zemlin,1984; Zemlin, 1988; Solomon, McCall, Trosset, and Gray, 1989), describing a variety of configurations including (*a*) lack of complete adduction along the full length of the glottis, (*b*) an inverted V shape, (*c*) a bowed appearance, (*d*) a Y shape with a posterior chink, (*e*) a bimodal (anterior and posterior) chink, (*f*) a parallel configuration with some adduction, and (*g*) toeing in of the vocal processes. Various reasons have been suggested for these differences in glottal configuration. Some have suggested that the glottal shape is a function of the effort involved in the whisper, others suggest it has to do with the type of whisper (quiet versus forceful whisper), while yet others claim a relationship to the phonetic context.

Monoson and Zemlin (1984) compared laryngeal appearance (high-speed films), electromyograms, acoustic, and airflow data for four conditions: quiet whisper, forced whisper, breathy phonation, and conversational phonation. Glottal configurations varied to some extent among the conditions and were believed to be at least partially determined by the effort level involved. Vibratory behavior was absent in both whisper conditions and present in both breathy and conversational phonation. Airflow was greatest in forced whispering, which was felt to be due in part to an increase in activity of the expiratory muscles in that condition. The data do not support the thesis that whispering is an abusive behavior. However, the increases in expiratory muscle activity and in airflow attributed to the forced whisper suggest an increase in effort and perhaps in tension.

Solomon et al. (1989) report on a study of laryngeal configurations for two types of whispering (high effort and low effort) in 10 speakers using consonant-vowel units and running speech. The laryngeal configurations were visualized via a fiberoptic bronchoscope and videotaped for analysis. Significant individual variability was reported. Intrasubject inconsistency was also noted, although most subjects exhibited a preferred configuration. A medium-sized glottal opening was described for most subjects, with a large glottal size occurring more frequently in the high effort whisper than in the low effort whisper. Although some constriction of supraglottal structures was reported, it apparently occurred less than half of the time, even in high effort whispering. The glottal configurations described by these authors were primarily of two types: a straight edge, parallel configuration or a toeing in of the vocal processes. It is still not clear how such approximation of the vocal folds occurs during whisper, although these authors report observation of more contact during running speech than in the production of consonant vowel units. Four of the 10 subjects displayed the straight margin configuration of the glottis, and these same subjects did not approximate the vocal folds. These authors suggest that the determination regarding the use of whisper as a therapeutic technique or during periods of vocal rest should be made on an individual basis, depending on the type of glottal configuration assumed for whisper by that patient. The efficacy of whispering as a therapeutic approach was not addressed in this study. Hufnagle and Hufnagle (1982) reported that patients demonstrated improved voice quality following a period of whispering, suggesting therefore that the behavior is not harmful and, indeed, may be helpful.

There is not yet sufficient evidence available to state unequivocally that whispering is not harmful. However, our clinical intuition suggests that it may be helpful for some patients, with a few caveats. Because the high effort forced whisper tends to suggest increased tension and effort somewhere in the system, and because tension and force are precisely the behaviors that most patients need to reduce or eliminate, it seems to us that the use of the forced whisper could be counterproductive. It is also important that the patient recognize that whispering may have a drying effect on the mucosa of the vocal folds, which should be counteracted by an increase of fluid intake.

The available evidence about the whisper is not nearly as frightening as some of the strongly stated admonitions against its use. However, much remains to be learned about the mechanism of whispering. The amount of force in medial compression of the folds when they appear to make contact during whispering has not been addressed and remains an open question, as does the degree of expiratory muscle effort involved.

Prevention of Voice Problems

We can discuss the prevention of voice problems by addressing both primary prevention—preventing the occurrence of the problem in the first place—or secondary prevention—preventing the recurrence of a problem. An understanding of the deleterious effects of cigarette smoking has been effective in convincing many people to change their habits and eliminate smoking. Throughout American society, steps have been taken to minimize the spread of the effects of inhaling environmental cigarette smoke by establishing prohibitions against smoking in theaters, planes, certain sections of restaurants, and other places of public gathering. Much more needs to be done, however, as it appears that in absolute numbers, the population of smokers has not decreased significantly. The evidence linking smoking with laryngeal cancer is impressive.

Greater strides need to be made in recognizing the aversive effects of certain noxious gases. However, in the absence of widespread information, it behooves professionals to suggest safeguards that individuals may take when knowingly exposed to a variety of potentially harmful agents.

Education is the primary need in decreasing vocal abuse and misuse. We know that cheerleading constitutes a very stressful, abusive use of the voice that often results in mucosal damage. However, this knowledge seems not to have penetrated the cheerleading world so that training in voice use and voice conservation might be provided. There are other abusive activities that could be similarly identified. Some, such as rock singing in the presence of highly amplified sound, are probably not amenable to change. Despite, or perhaps due to, laryngeal pathology such as nodes or polyps, some rock singers have a "sound" uniquely theirs that would not be possible without abuse.

Another group of people who would benefit from increased education about the voice are choir singers. Many have untrained voices and abuse them with regularity but without awareness. Choir directors frequently have limited backgrounds in vocal pedagogy and are thus ill-equipped to train their choirs in healthy habits of singing and voice use. This becomes increasingly critical when the choir is composed of or includes prepubertal children.

Primary prevention through education needs to be increased in the public schools so that children learn to recognize beginning signs of vocal abuse and are trained in voice conservation. In addition to education of the children, all school personnel should have a greater understanding of vocal abuse, its harmful effects, and ways to avoid or eliminate it. Such education not only would be helpful to them in managing their own voice production but also would make them more capable of identifying the problem in children. Such a program, which had impressive results, is described by Nilson and Schneiderman (1983). Their program was directed at 2nd and 3rd grade students and their teachers and included discussion of the vocal mechanism and voice production, voice qualities both normal and abnormal, and learning to identify vocal abuse. Both the children and the teachers were found to have gained and retained significant knowledge about the voice, and when the children who had been part of the program were retested for voice, no new cases of dysphonia were identified. A primary prevention plan has been proposed by Flynn (1983), and Marge (1984) has addressed prevention of voice disorders as one area under the broader topic of prevention of communication disorders.

Secondary prevention, for those who have experienced even a single episode of vocal disturbance that required treatment, is essential. It is incumbent upon laryngologists who successfully treat a patient with a preventable problem that they either take the time to clearly instruct the patient in a program of vocal hygiene or refer that patient to a speech-language pathologist for such education and counseling. Indeed, failure to do so might leave the door open for medical-legal problems.

Malpractice

In the current litigious climate, it is important that all those who treat patients with voice problems, including speech-language pathologists, recognize how they may be vulnerable to malpractice actions and take appropriate steps to safeguard themselves. Instances of persons with voice problems bringing suit against otolaryngologists or speech-language pathologists and of speech-language pathologists being called upon to testify as "expert witnesses" in suits brought against others have already occurred. During the years 1980 to 1985, there was a 10% increase in claims against speech-language pathologists (Kooper and Sullivan, 1986).

Prime candidates to bring such suits are persons who claim that the treatment provided, surgical or otherwise, created or resulted in a permanent condition no better or worse than the original problem, and that they had not been advised of the possibility of that outcome. Others might claim damages for a missed diagnosis that resulted in unnecessary treatment and/or delayed initiation of appropriate treatment. The extent of liability for a disabling condition appears to be directly related to the severity of the injury as measured by its duration (Kooper and Sullivan, 1986). Thus, if a voice disorder is present and is not expected to abate or change over the person's life-span, its severity will be judged to be greater if the patient is 25 years old than if she is 85. The extent of liability will be related to the perception of the degree of severity of the problem.

It is of utmost importance that very complete, dated records be maintained on each patient. Such records should contain the results of all testing and examination, case history material, statements of diagnosis or a listing of the differential diagnosis if full exploration has not been completed, a treatment plan, statements of prognosis specific to planned treatment modalities, and a record of all contacts with the patient or about the patient. Furthermore, whenever surgical intervention is planned, a recorded sample of the patient's voice should be a part of the record. A second recording should be made postoperatively, with additional recordings made periodically as changes in voice occur. The speech-language pathologist should make audio recordings of the patient's voice at the time of the initial visit and periodically after that.

Those who work with voice-disordered patients, when called upon to testify in court as an expert witness, must establish their expertise. They must be knowledgeable and articulate about phonatory physiology, as well as about testing and treatment procedures, the nature of voice disorders, and the emotional ramifications of disturbed communication skills or loss of the source of a livelihood. The primary question to which they will be expected to respond deals with the acceptability of the treatment that was provided in the case. This does not require that the witness agree with the course of treatment, as long as it is an accepted form of treatment for the problem.

Summary

Vocal rehabilitation in its broadest sense is discussed in this chapter. Concepts, principles, and guidelines basic to vocal rehabilitation receive attention, then specific therapeutic techniques are presented. The role of voice therapy in the treatment of voice disorders, the appropriate goals of such treatment, and the nature of the therapeutic process is proposed for the various categories of voice disorders, such as those associated with mucosal changes, those involving misuse and abuse, and those with neurological involvement. A section is devoted to discussion of some special voice problems that do not fit into the above categories. The discussion of specific therapeutic techniques includes a description of how they are done, with suggestions and cautions gained from clinical practice. A rationale is presented for each technique that relates its physiological implications to the disturbed physiology typical of the voice disorders to which it is applicable. The considerations that must be taken into account in developing a prognostic statement are discussed, and some criteria for termination of therapy are suggested. The authors raise some issues in vocal rehabilitation that are based on unresolved questions and for which no substantiating data are available and question the continued use of optimum pitch as a viable concept. Discussions of the prevention of voice disorders and of malpractice concerns complete the chapter.

10

Anatomy of the Vocal Mechanism

Introduction

In the human body, structure determines function. That is, the shape and form of a structure determine the manner in which the structure will operate. Thus, it is important to understand the anatomy of a structure in order to understand how it works. Such is the case for understanding the larynx and voice production.

A brief review of the anatomy of the larynx will be presented in this chapter. The focus will be on functional anatomy, that is, the determination of how a structure functions based on its anatomy. It is not the intent of this chapter to present full anatomic details of structures, their articulation with other structures, and their blood and nerve supply. Such details may be found in many complete anatomy texts (Dickson and Maue-Dickson, 1982; Zemlin, 1988). Rather, it is our purpose to present those details needed to understand the structure and how it functions in voice production. This information is presented so that clinicians can rapidly review a segment of anatomy and use that information to better understand a given voice problem. It is hoped that this section will be actively used during the process of differential diagnosis and in the management plan. Anatomy need not be memorized if it is understood and if reference materials are consulted in a meaningful manner.

We will begin our discussion of laryngeal anatomy from the outside and proceed to the inside. That is, we will first consider the extrinsic muscles of the larynx, then move inward to the cartilages of the larynx and the intrinsic muscles. Then a brief overview of the internal structures and cavities of the larynx will be presented. Finally, we will consider the body cover model of the vocal fold structure and look at laryngeal anatomy as viewed through a flexible fiberoptic laryngoscope.

Extrinsic Muscles of the Larynx

The extrinsic muscles of the larynx are those muscles that have one attachment to a structure within the larynx and one attachment to a structure outside the larynx. It is necessary to understand that the hyoid bone, which is a rather distinct structure, is considered to be part of the larynx. Some of its features are shown in the upper panel of Figure 10.1. All extrinsic muscles have their laryngeal attachments on the hyoid bone. The attachments outside of the larynx include many different structures, such as the mandible, the mastoid, and structures in the thorax. Recall that in anatomy the origin of a muscle refers to its least moveable attachment, whereas the insertion refers to its more moveable attachment.

There are eight extrinsic muscles, four that lie below the hyoid bone and four that lie above it. For those reasons, they are divided into the suprahyoid and infrahyoid groups. The muscles that comprise these two groups are listed in Table 10.1 and shown in Figure 10.1.

Suprahyoid Group

Note how the suprahyoid group forms a sling supporting the hyoid bone and, secondarily, the larynx. The anterior part of the sling is formed by a portion of the digastric (anterior belly), the geniohyoid, and the mylohyoid. When contracted, this group of muscles pulls the hyoid bone (and thus the larynx) forward. These muscles are active during the production of a front vowel or a consonant that requires a high front tongue position. The posterior belly of the digastric and the stylohyoid form the rear part of the sling. Their contraction pulls the hyoid posteriorly. Note that the angle of pull is steep for this muscle group, whereas the angle of pull of the anterior muscle group is shallow. Thus, the action of the posterior group is to pull up on the larynx, while the anterior muscle group exerts a pull on the hyoid bone that is more forward than upward.

Infrahyoid Group

This group is made up of four muscles: the thyrohyoid, sternohyoid, omohyoid, and sternothyroid. With the exception of the thyrohyoid, the other muscles in this group have attachments from the hyoid to structures below the larynx. As a result, their contraction has the effect of pulling the larynx downward. The lowered laryngeal position results in a lengthening of the vocal tract, which has a primary effect on vocal resonance characteristics affecting the formant frequencies. A more direct effect on the voice may result from the restriction of thyroid cartilage movement that is caused by contraction of this muscle group. This restriction of movement has directly to do with vocal fold length, mass, and tension, and thereby affects vocal pitch regulation. Other muscles are also involved in pitch regulation, and they will be discussed later.

The thyrohyoid muscle connects to the larynx, and its action contributes to determining the angle of the thyroid with respect to the cricoid cartilage. If the thyroid cartilage is fixed (by other muscles) so that it cannot move, then contraction of the thyrohyoid would contribute to pulling the hyoid bone down. If, however, the hyoid bone is fixed (by contraction of muscles above it), then contraction of the thyrohyoid would pull upward on the thyroid, increasing the distance between it and the cricoid cartilage (especially anteriorly). Thus, most of the effect of the thyrohyoid muscle is to rock the thyroid cartilage upward and in so doing to potentially alter length, mass, and tension of the vocal folds, thereby affecting the pitch of the voice.

Positioning of the larynx in the vertical dimension during speaking is primarily related to vowel or consonant production. There is some variation of position in singing, and good singers may vary the vertical position of the larynx considerably, depending on their

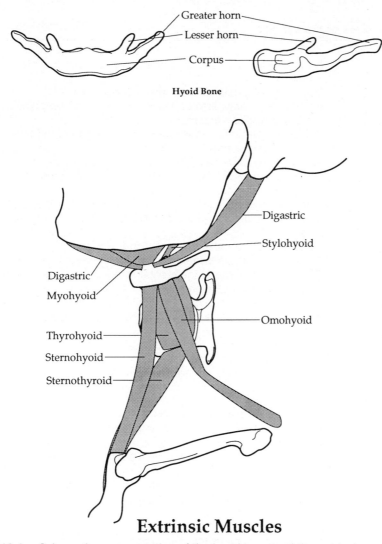

Figure 10.1. Schematic representation of the hyoid bone and the extrinsic muscles of the larynx. Part of the extrinsic muscle group forms a sling to support the hyoid bone and larynx from above. These muscles can move the hyoid and larynx upward, forward, or backward. The other group of extrinsic muscles can pull the hyoid and larynx down.

style of singing and the music (Shipp, 1975; Shipp and Izdebski, 1975). Speakers with voice problems may have a tendency to maintain higher than normal laryngeal position. This may be indicative of excessive muscle tension (Aronson, 1985; Morrison, Rammage, Belisle, Pullan, and Nichol, 1983) in the extrinsic muscles of the larynx.

Cartilages of the Larynx

The framework of the larynx is composed of hyaline cartilage. Cartilage is softer and more flexible than bone. Hyaline refers to the type of cells that make up the cartilage. (See Chapter 3 for more details.)

Table 10.1.
Extrinsic Muscles of the Larynx

Suprahyoid Muscles
Digastric	A two-part muscle consisting of a posterior belly and an anterior belly.
Origin	Posterior belly: originates on the mastoid process.
	Anterior belly: originates on the lower border of the mandible near the mandibular symphysis.
Insertion	Posterior belly: intermediate tendon connecting to the hyoid bone.
	Anterior belly: intermediate tendon.
Function	Anterior belly: pulls hyoid bone anteriorly and slightly upward.
	Posterior belly: pulls hyoid bone posteriorly and upward.
Mylohyoid	A thin muscle forming the floor of the mouth.
Origin	Along the mylohyoid line on the inner surface of the mandible.
Insertion	Most fibers meet with fibers of the opposite side at the midline raphe.
Function	Pulls hyoid bone anteriorly and slightly upward.
Geniohyoid	A cylindrical muscle located above the mylohyoid muscle.
Origin	On the mental spine at the mental symphysis of the mandible.
Insertion	Anterior surface of the corpus of the hyoid bone.
Function	Pulls hyoid bone anteriorly and slightly upward.
Stylohyoid	A long slender muscle located superficially to the posterior belly of the digastric.
Origin	On the styloid process of the temporal bone.
Insertion	On the body of the hyoid bone.
Function	Pulls hyoid bone posteriorly and upward.

Infrahyoid Muscles
Thyrohyoid	A thin muscle that lies deep to the omohyoid.
Origin	From the oblique line on the thyroid lamina.
Insertion	On the lower border of the greater horn of the hyoid bone.
Function	Decreases distance between thyroid and hyoid, especially anteriorly.
Sternothyroid	A long, thin muscle on the anterior side of the neck.
Origin	Posterior surface of the manubrium of the sternum and the first costal cartilage.
Insertion	On the oblique line of the thyroid.
Function	Pulls down on the thyroid cartilage.
Sternohyoid	A thin muscle lying on anterior side of the neck.
Origin	On the posterior surface of the manubrium of the sternum and end of the clavicle.
Insertion	On the lower border of the body of the hyoid bone.
Function	Pulls down on the hyoid bone.
Omohyoid	A long, narrow, two-part muscle on the anterior and lateral surfaces of the neck.
Origin	Inferior belly: along the upper surface of the scapula.
	Superior belly: intermediate tendon.
Insertion	Inferior belly: intermediate tendon.
	Superior belly: the border of the great horn of the hyoid bone.
Function	Both divisions pull down on the hyoid, although the superior belly has a more pronounced effect in this direction than the inferior belly.

The cartilages of the larynx are presented in Figure 10.2. The major cartilages are the thyroid, cricoid, and arytenoid. The other cartilages are much smaller and form parts of other structures. For example, the corniculates are small cartilages attached to the arytenoid at their apices. The cuneiforms are small cartilages embedded in the muscle tissue that connects the arytenoids to the epiglottis.

Thyroid Cartilage

The thyroid cartilage is the largest cartilage of the larynx. The most anterior angle of this cartilage, commonly referred to as the Adam's apple, is a very prominent feature in some men. It is shaped like a shield and can be thought of as shielding the structures inside. The thyroid is actually composed of two plates of cartilage, called lamina, joined at the midline to form an angle of about 80 degrees in men and about 90 degrees in women (Zemlin, 1988). The more acute angle of the thyroid together with laryngeal size accounts for the more pronounced outline of the larynx in the male neck.

Posteriorly, the thyroid cartilage has two horns or cornua. The superior horn connects the thyroid to the hyoid bone, and the inferior horn connects it to the cricoid cartilage below. Along the lateral surface of the thyroid lamina is a ridge identified as the oblique line. It is here that the thyrohyoid and sternothyroid muscles attach.

Cricoid Cartilage

The second largest laryngeal cartilage is the cricoid, which completely surrounds the trachea. Sometimes it is referred to as the uppermost tracheal ring, but it is quite different in configuration from the other tracheal rings. It is larger and higher posteriorly, while anteriorly it tapers to the cricoid arch. The thyroid cartilage articulates with the cricoid on its posterolateral surface. Two kinds of movements of the thyroid on the cricoid cartilage are permitted, as illustrated in Figure 10.3. The arytenoids articulate with the cricoid on its posterosuperior surface. The details of this articulation are important and will be discussed further in the next section.

Arytenoid Cartilages

There are two arytenoid cartilages, each positioned on either side of the midline on the supraposterior surface of the cricoid cartilage. The arytenoids are roughly pyramidal in shape and have four surfaces, three angles at the base, and, of course, a single point at the apex. The basal surface is important to consider because essential musculature attaches at two of its angles.

The most anterior angle of the base of the arytenoid is referred to as the vocal process. It is here that the true vocal folds attach. The more lateral angle, referred to as the muscle process, is the point of attachment for the posterior cricoarytenoid and the lateral cricoarytenoid muscles.

The surface of the arytenoid that articulates with the cricoid cartilage is concave in appearance. The surface of the cricoid that meets the arytenoid is convex. These surfaces help to determine how the arytenoid will move on the surface of the cricoid. Because of the shape of these surfaces, a rotating motion is not permitted, but a rocking motion can occur (von Leden and Moore, 1961a; Broad,1973). Broad has described the permitted motions by comparing them to the movement of two matching cylinders, as shown in Figure 10.4. Two kinds of motion are permitted, a gliding motion along an anteroposterior plane and a rocking motion in a mediolateral direction. When these two motions occur together, there is the appearance of a rocking motion either medially and anteriorly di-

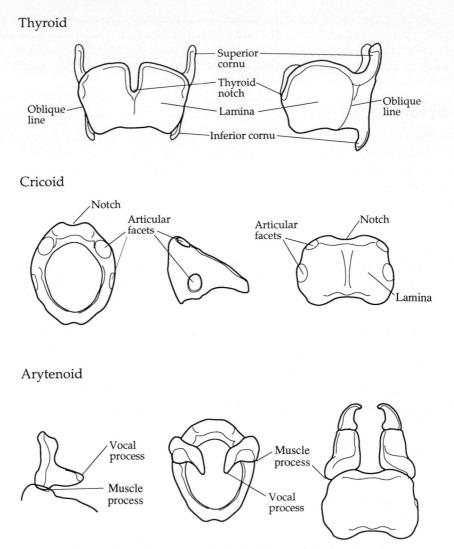

Figure 10.2.   Schematic of the cartilages of the larynx.

rected (if the arytenoids are moving in) or posteriorly (if the arytenoids are moving out). Depending on speed of medial movement relative to anterior movement of the arytenoids, it is possible for the vocal processes to be the first point of contact during adduction of the vocal folds.

Epiglottis

The epiglottis is a leaf-shaped cartilage attached on the mesial surface of the thyroid cartilage at the juncture of the two thyroid plates. The anterior surface of the epiglottis attaches to the hyoid bone via a ligament.

The epiglottis assists in directing food and liquids into the esophagus during swallowing. During phonation, it is usually out of the way of the egressive airstream. However, it moves considerably during the production of different vowels and consonants. In some cases, it will obscure the view of the vocal folds. However, tongue position in the production of vowels like /ee/ and /oo/ usually results in forward movement of the epiglottis, thereby allowing a good view of the vocal folds. There is no evidence to

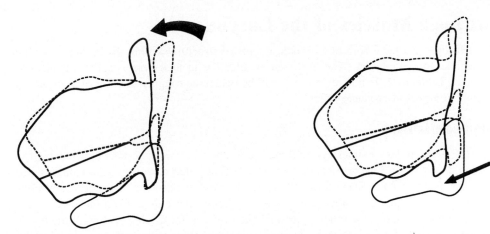

Figure 10.3. Movements permitted by the articulation of the thyroid and cricoid cartilages. A rocking motion of the thyroid on the cricoid is the major movement permitted (left panel). In addition, a slight anteroposterior movement is possible (right panel).

support the contention that the shape of the epiglottis will alter the voice. Certainly, pulling the epiglottis over the laryngeal opening will affect sound transmission and intensity level.

The epiglottis can vary considerably in shape and curvature. Usually it is slightly concave when viewed via a laryngeal mirror or fiberscope. Sometimes it may have a very pronounced omega shape. The so-called omega-shaped epiglottis appears to be found most often in immature larynges or children's larynges. However, it may also be simply a variation of normal human laryngeal anatomy.

Other Cartilages

The remaining cartilages are the corniculate and the cuneiform cartilages. The corniculates are small cone-shaped cartilages that form the apex of the arytenoid. The cuneiforms are small rod-shaped cartilages found within the aryepiglottic fold, a fold of tissue and muscle coursing from the arytenoids to the epiglottis.

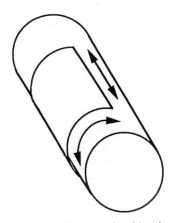

Figure 10.4. Type of movements permitted by the cricoarytenoid joint.

Intrinsic Muscles of the Larynx

Muscles that have both of their attachments to structures within the larynx are called intrinsic laryngeal muscles. The five muscles, along with their origins and insertions, are shown in Table 10.2. In this review they will be discussed roughly in order of their activation when a person produces voice.

Arytenoideus

The arytenoideus or interarytenoid muscle is a two-part muscle lying between the two arytenoid cartilages. One part consists of muscle fibers that course in a horizontal direction. The effect of these fibers is to pull the bases of the two arytenoids toward each other, thus adducting them. The other part consists of fibers that course from the base of one arytenoid to the apex of the other arytenoid. The effect of these fibers is to pull the tips of the arytenoids together. Together, the two parts adduct the arytenoids and close off the extreme posterior airway. Although the time when these muscles are activated depends on the speech task, in general, activity in the arytenoideus occurs anywhere from 0.5 to 0.3 seconds before sound is produced.

Lateral Cricoarytenoid

The lateral cricoarytenoid muscle is a paired muscle coursing from the sides and upper surface of the cricoid cartilage to the muscle process of the arytenoid. The effect of this muscle is to pull the muscle process anteriorly, rocking the arytenoid medially and adducting the vocal folds themselves. Time of activation may be about 0.1 second after activity in the arytenoideus.

These two muscles (arytenoideus and lateral cricoarytenoid) function together to adduct the vocal folds. It is not necessary to completely adduct the folds for phonation to commence. Rather, there need only be sufficient adduction to impose an obstruction to the flow of air coming from the lungs, for phonation to begin.

Posterior Cricoarytenoid

This is the only intrinsic muscle that abducts the vocal folds. From its origin on the posterior lamina of the cricoid, the muscle fibers converge to insert on the muscle process. Contraction of the muscle will pull the muscle process posteriorly, thus opening the vocal folds.

The posterior cricoarytenoid is active at the end of phonation in order to open the folds. However, it is also active during speech since there are many speech sounds that require an absence of vocal fold vibration (e.g., the stop consonants /p/, /t/, and /k/; the fricative consonants /s/ and /sh/, etc.). Thus, a short burst of activity in the posterior cricoarytenoid quickly abducts the vocal folds enough to stop their vibration.

Cricothyroid

The origin of the cricothyroid muscle is along the upper surface of the sides of the cricoid cartilage. Its insertion is along the lower border of the thyroid cartilage. It is considered to be the main muscle for pitch control and its major function is to raise vocal pitch. It does so by rocking the cricoid cartilage upward or the thyroid cartilage downward, thereby increasing the distance between the thyroid cartilage and the vocal processes of the arytenoids, which are situated on the rear surface of the cricoid. The vocal folds, which are attached anteriorly on the inner surface of the thyroid cartilage

Table 10.2.
Intrinsic Muscles of the Larynx

Arytenoideus	An unpaired muscle consisting of fibers oriented in two directions, oblique and transverse.
Origin	Oblique fibers originate at the base of one arytenoid and course to the apex of the other arytenoid. Transverse fibers originate along the lateral margin of one arytenoid and course to the lateral margin of the other arytenoid.
Insertion	Arytenoid of opposite side.
Function	Adducts arytenoids, thus closing the cartilaginous glottis.
Lateral Cricoarytenoid	A fan-shaped muscle lying along the upper surface of the cricoid cartilage.
Origin	On the upper border of the cricoid.
Insertion	Anterior surface of the muscular process of the arytenoid.
Function	Adducts the vocal processes of the arytenoids, thus closing the membranous glottis.
Posterior Cricoarytenoid	A fan-shaped muscle located on the posterior surface of the cricoid.
Origin	On the posterior lamina of the cricoid.
Insertion	Posterior surface of the muscular process of the arytenoid.
Function	Abducts the arytenoids, thus opening the glottis.
Cricothyroid	A fan-shaped muscle located between the cricoid and thyroid cartilages, consisting of two divisions, pars oblique and pars recta. These divisions refer to the different orientation of the fibers.
Origin	Arch of the cricoid.
Insertion	Inner inferior margin of the thyroid.
Function	Decreases the space between the thyroid and cricoid, thus increasing the distance between the thyroid and arytenoid cartilages; increasing the length of the vocal folds, decreasing their mass, and increasing their tension; and increasing vocal pitch.
Thyroarytenoid	A bundle of muscle fibers making up the true vocal folds.
Origin	Anteriorly, from the posterior surface of the thyroid.
Insertion	Along the lateral base of an arytenoid from the vocal process to the muscle process.
Function	Decreases the distance between the thyroid and arytenoid cartilages, shortening the vocal folds, increasing their mass, and decreasing their tension, and decreasing vocal pitch.

and posteriorly on the vocal processes of the arytenoids, are stretched and elongated by either of these actions. Stretching the vocal folds decreases their cross-sectional area and subjects the folds to greater longitudinal tension. The decrease of area and increase of tension permit the vocal folds to vibrate at higher frequencies and thus produce the perception of higher pitch.

Decreasing the level of activity in the cricothyroid will result in a decrease of tension, resulting in a slower vibratory rate and a decrease of fundamental frequency. However, the rate of decay of muscle activity in the cricothyroid may be too slow for speech purposes. That is, it may be necessary, for linguistic purposes, to lower pitch more rapidly than would be possible by waiting for the decay of cricothyroid activity. Thus, other physiological mechanisms of frequency change may be operating to actively lower vocal pitch during speech.

Thyroarytenoid

The thyroarytenoid muscle comprises the bulk of the vocal folds. Its contraction decreases the length of the vocal folds, increases their cross-sectional area, and decreases longitudinal tension. The action of this muscle represents one way to actively lower vocal pitch. Of course, contraction of this muscle also changes the configuration of the vocal folds themselves, thereby affecting how they will move within the vibratory cycle.

The thyroarytenoid may be divided into two muscle groups. The medial portion of the muscle is called the thyrovocalis muscle, and the more lateral portion is referred to as the thyromuscularis muscle. There is some controversy about whether or not the two parts are anatomically distinct (Dickson and Maue-Dickson, 1982). From a functional point of view, the medial portion of the thyroarytenoid (or thyrovocalis) is most active during the vibratory activity of the vocal folds and therefore may have a significant effect on phonation. The lateral (or thyromuscularis) portion may exhibit little movement during vibration, and thus its action may have minimal effect on the vibratory characteristics of the vocal folds.

Detailed Anatomy of the Vocal Folds: The Body Cover Model

Hirano (1974, 1981a) has proposed a model of the vocal folds that has considerable merit in explaining the variation of human voice production. Simply stated, the vocal folds consist of three layers: (*a*) the outer cover, consisting of epithelium; (*b*) a middle layer, the lamina propria; and (*c*) the body. A schematic diagram of the three layers is shown in Figure 10.5.

The cover of the vocal folds is composed of squamous cell epithelium. Mechanically, epithelium is very stiff, making this the layer much stiffer than its neighbor, the lamina propria (Kakita, Hirano, and Okmaru, 1981). It is this difference of stiffness that determines the manner in which the layers will respond to deformation during vibration. In some modes of vibration, the degree of coupling between the epithelium and the lamina propria is very small (as in low frequency speech activities). In other modes of vibration, the degree of coupling between the cover, the lamina propria, and the body may be very great (as may be the case in falsetto voice). Thus, the combination of the mechanical characteristics of the three layers will ultimately determine the mode of vocal fold vibration. (See Fujimura, 1981, for a good discussion of the relationships between biomechanical characteristics of the vocal folds and sound production.)

The lamina propria is actually a three-layered area lying between the cover and the body. Its superficial layer is very pliable, consisting of loose fibrous components. The intermediate layer consists primarily of elastic fibers. The deepest layer consists of collagenous fibers. Mechanically, each layer will exhibit different characteristics, and variation in the composition of each of the three layers of the lamina propria will alter the manner of vocal fold vibration.

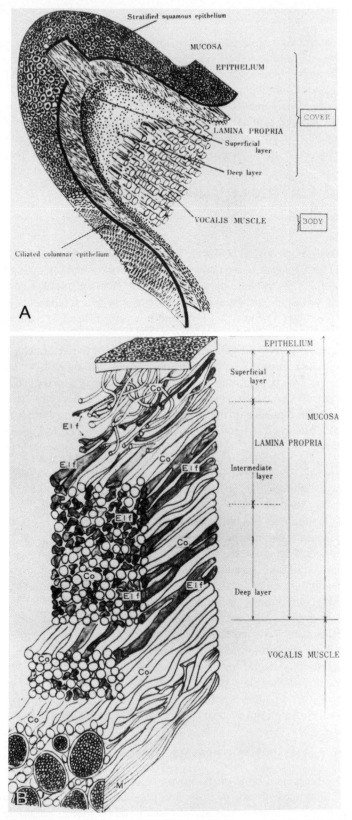

Figure 10.5. Schematic representation of the vocal folds as a body and cover. **A**, Cross-sectional representation. **B**, The kinds of fibers present in each layer. (From Hirano, 1981a.)

The body of the vocal fold is the vocalis muscle. Although muscle cells are the primary components of muscle, blood cells, collagen cells, and inorganic material are also present. Muscle fibers themselves exhibit different mechanical characteristics when they are in the process of contracting than when they are contracted or at rest (Colton, 1988). Thus, there can be considerable variation in the mechanical characteristics of the body, depending on the amount of muscle activation, the amount of collagenous or elastic fibers present, the amount of heat generated (Hill, 1938; Titze, 1981; Cooper and Titze, 1983), and other variations due to blood flow, oxygen consumption, and the like.

Folds and Cavities of the Larynx

Folds

The folds and cavities of the larynx are shown in Figure 10.6, a coronal cross-section of the larynx. The major folds of interest are, of course, the true vocal folds. Superior and lateral to the true vocal folds are the false or ventricular folds. The false vocal folds do not usually vibrate in normal voice production, except perhaps at very low fundamental frequencies (50 Hz or below). They have few muscle fibers, and it is very difficult to regulate their tension, mass, and length. Occasionally they are seen to adduct partially or almost completely and obscure the true vocal folds. Only infrequently is vibration of the ventricular folds observed.

The aryepiglottic folds comprise a ring of muscle and connective tissue extending from the tips of the arytenoids to the epiglottis. In effect, they form a sphincter enclosing the entrance to the larynx. During swallowing and protective acts, the aryepiglottic folds contract to reduce the diameter of the laryngeal entrance and thus protect the airway. We have occasionally observed sphincteric movement of these folds during phonation.

Cavities

The major cavities of the larynx are (*a*) the supraglottal cavity, (*b*) the subglottal cavity, and (*c*) the ventricles.

The supraglottal cavity lies above the glottis or the opening between the vocal folds. Its superior boundary is the aryepiglottic sphincter. This cavity could potentially act as a resonator of the sound produced by the vibrating vocal folds. Sundberg (1974) has shown that under certain conditions, it could resonate frequencies in the vicinity of 2800 Hz. In most speech conditions, however, its resonant effect on sound is minimal.

The subglottal cavity lies beneath the true vocal folds. Its lower boundary is the first tracheal ring. It is in this cavity that pressure increases beneath the closed vocal folds until it becomes sufficient to force the vocal folds open and begin phonation.

The ventricles, often referred to as the ventricles of Morgagni, are paired cavities lying above and slightly lateral to the true vocal folds. The opening of these cavities is usually very small, and thus they seem to have little effect on the sound produced at the vocal folds. However, in some conditions encountered in singing, the opening may be sufficient to permit meaningful resonance and thus add to the glottal tone.

Laryngographic/Fiberoptic Anatomy of the Larynx

Figure 10.7 presents a view of the larynx typically seen when observing the larynx either through a laryngeal mirror or a flexible fiberoptic (or solid) laryngoscope. It is a common view to most otolaryngologists and should be to speech pathologists and voice scientists. The various structures that can be viewed are identified in this figure. Study of

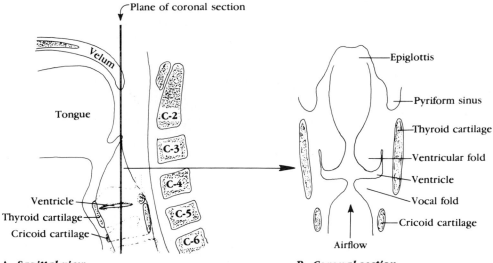

Figure 10.6. Cross-sectional representation of the larynx. (From Dickson and Maue-Dickson, 1982.)

these landmarks should be made if one expects to properly interpret pictures or video images of the larynx. A good knowledge of normal anatomy and its variations is needed in order to correctly identify laryngeal pathology. It is important to recognize that there is much variability in normal anatomic structures. Examples of this variability as seen fiberscopically were discussed by Casper, Brewer, and Colton (1987a).

Summary

A brief review of the anatomy of the larynx and the vocal folds is presented. The extrinsic muscles of the larynx help to support and adjust the position of the larynx. The intrinsic muscles of the larynx attach to the various cartilages of the larynx (thyroid, cricoid, arytenoid) and serve to adjust the length, tension, and mass of the vocal folds, as well as to adduct them. A brief discussion of the cavities and folds of the larynx is presented, concluding with a presentation of laryngeal anatomy as viewed through a fiberscope.

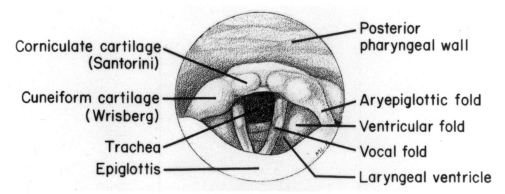

Figure 10.7. Laryngoscopic view of the larynx. This is a view typically seen during indirect mirror, fiberoptic, or stroboscopic examination of the larynx.

11

Phonatory Physiology

The vibrating vocal folds are the major source of periodic sound for speech. There are other periodic sound sources (e.g., flapping lips), but these are minor compared to the sound required from the vocal folds. In addition, there are aperiodic sound sources used for the production of voiceless consonants. The vocal folds may also produce aperiodic sound, as, for example, in the consonant /h/.

In this chapter, we will review the basic concepts of phonatory physiology. First, the conditions that must exist before sound can be produced will be presented, followed by discussion of the mechanisms necessary for initiating and sustaining sound. The third and fourth sections will be brief outlines of the physiological mechanisms for control of vocal pitch and intensity control by the vocal folds, respectively. Finally, a review of some of the mechanisms for control of voice quality will be presented.

Glottal Tone Initiation

Before sound can be produced from the vocal folds, several conditions must be established. First, the vocal folds must be approximated or at least brought to the phonatory position. This position, in comparison to the inspiratory position of the vocal folds (Fig. 11.1A), is shown in Figure 11.1B. Phonation may also be initiated after completely closing the vocal folds.

It is also necessary to properly tense and elongate the vocal folds prior to actually producing sound. Length and tension are important determinants of the fundamental vibrating rate of the vocal folds, in ways that will be discussed under "Mechanism of Vocal Frequency Change."

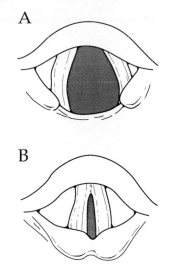

Figure 11.1. Schematic representation of the stages of vocal fold adduction. **A,** During inspiration. **B,** At start of phonation.

Finally, there must be airflow from the lungs. In order to be able to produce the required flow of air from the lungs, there must be a sufficient quantity of air in the lungs. A speaker may find it necessary to inspire before being able to produce a sound.

Once these initial conditions have been established, phonation can start. When the vocal folds are in the slightly open phonatory position, it is necessary to close them in order to start vibration. If one starts with the vocal folds fully closed, it is necessary to open them in order to start vibration. Whatever the starting point, the process thereafter is similar and is simply described as a series of alternate openings and closings of the vocal folds. The opening and closing is regulated by the degree of tension in the vocal folds and two aerodynamic events.

The aerodynamic event important for closing the vocal folds is called the Bernoulli effect, named after a famous 18th-century French physicist. Bernoulli was most interested in fluid flows, but his principles hold for gas flows as well. Simply stated, Bernoulli's second law of fluid mechanics states that the sum of the static pressures and the kinetic pressures in a gas are always equal to a constant. The constant may vary according to the temperature, pressure, or molecular structure of the gas. But within these conditions, when motion of the molecules changes, there is a change in the static pressure exerted by the molecules. Stating the principle another way, when there is increased motion of gas molecules, there will be decreased pressure.

The Bernoulli effect is often evoked to explain how airplanes rise in the air. The undersurface of the wing of an airplane is rather flat, whereas the upper surface is markedly convex in shape. This curvature on the upper wing surface means that the air molecules passing over the top of the wing have a greater distance to travel to pass over the wing than those molecules that pass under the wing. The velocity of the molecules traveling along the surface of the upper wing must increase in order to travel the distance in the same time as the lower wing molecules. In short, their kinetic "pressure" has been increased. According to Bernoulli's principle, when the kinetic pressure increases, the static pressure must decrease. Thus, there is less pressure along the upper surface of the wing. By the same token, there is greater pressure below the wing, and this greater pressure will lift the wing (and the airplane) into the sky.

The same principle holds for the vocal folds. The vocal folds impose a partial obstruction to the flow of air. The molecules traveling along the sides of the trachea, when meeting the vocal folds, must travel a greater distance around the fold to meet the molecules traveling up the center of the trachea. The molecules along the surface of the vocal folds must increase their velocity and kinetic pressure. Again, static pressure on the surface of the vocal folds will be decreased. The vocal folds, being pliable and movable, will begin to move toward the center of the trachea because of this pressure differential. Eventually, the two vocal folds will meet at the midline, and airflow will cease.

During the closed phase of the vibratory cycle, there continues to be a flow of air from the lungs, or least there is an attempt to continue airflow. With the complete obstruction, however, the attempts by the thorax/abdomen system to produce airflow creates a buildup of air pressure beneath the vocal folds. Eventually, the pressure below the vocal folds will reach a magnitude that results in a blowing open of the vocal folds. This completes one cycle of vibration, and the Bernoulli process can start again. In order to maintain vibration, airflow must continue, and the proper tension in the vocal folds must be maintained. Maintenance of appropriate tension requires activity in the various intrinsic and perhaps extrinsic muscles of the larynx.

We should mention that an alternative explanation for the opening of the vocal folds during phonation has been proposed by Conrad (1984). This model involves a collapsible tube analogy of the vocal folds, in which supraglottal resistance creates a negative resistance, causing vocal fold closure. Although this model has not been extensively tested, it appears to have some merit in explaining the phenomenon of phonation.

Mechanisms of Vocal Frequency Change

The human vocal mechanism is capable of producing a wide range of frequencies, sometimes in excess of 3 octaves. In this section, we will review some of the physiological mechanisms that determine the fundamental vibrating rate of the vocal folds.

Early in the study of phonation, individuals compared the vocal folds to vibrating strings. After all, both the vocal folds and strings had a length and a mass and were under tension. Furthermore, much was known about the determinants of frequency in strings, and the analogy appeared to be a good one.

As voice physiology research progressed, evidence accumulated that prompted a reevaluation of the analogy between the mechanism of frequency variation by the vocal folds and by a string. However, there seemed to be some merit in comparing other properties of a string also known to affect its frequency to the control of fundamental frequency by the vocal folds. Subsequent research has continued to focus on these properties of strings and how they relate to the control of frequency by the vocal folds. These will be discussed in the next three sections.

The vibratory frequency of a string is determined by its length, tension, and mass. Actually, it is not the total mass that is significant but rather the mass per unit length of the string. Another way of looking at this parameter is to consider the cross-sectional area of the string (or vocal folds) very important in determining the frequency that will be produced.

Vocal Fold Length and Fundamental Frequency

A convenient way of understanding the relationships between length, mass, and tension in a string and in the vocal folds is by graphing the parameters as a function of frequency. A schematic plot of string length versus frequency, as shown in Figure 11.2, demonstrates that as length increases, frequency decreases. Also shown in Figure 11.2 is an idealized schematic of the length-frequency relationships for the vocal folds. As the length of the vocal folds increases, frequency increases, a relationship clearly opposite that for strings. This result, showing opposite effects, is why the string analogy was thought by some to be inappropriate for the control of fundamental frequency by the vocal folds.

Vocal Fold Mass and Fundamental Frequency

Before we agree with this conclusion, let's look at the relationships for mass and tension. Figure 11.3 shows the idealized relationship between mass and frequency for a string in which it is seen that as mass increases, frequency decreases. Also shown in the figure are the experimental results of studies in which the mass of the vocal folds was measured as fundamental frequency of phonation was varied (Hollien, 1962; Hollien and Colton, 1969). Note that for the vocal folds, as mass increases, vocal frequency decreases, a relationship similar to that for a vibrating string.

Vocal Fold Tension and Fundamental Frequency

The idealized relationship between tension and frequency for a string is shown in Figure 11.4. As tension increases, so too does frequency. Also shown in this figure are experimental results in which tension was varied in excised larynges, and the fundamental frequency of phonation was recorded (van den Berg and Tan, 1959). In general, tension variation produces similar variation of fundamental frequency in the vocal folds as in strings.

It is very difficult to measure tension directly in the living human vocal fold. Indirect evidence must be obtained from recordings of muscle activity or measurements made on dog or excised human larynges (Perlman, Titze, and Cooper, 1984; Perlman and Titze, 1988). Moreover, the variations of tension produced by muscle contraction must also be considered (Colton, 1988) when trying to understand how tension determines the fundamental frequency of phonation.

Tension becomes more important in the determination of fundamental frequency at certain areas of an individual's total phonational range. Van den Berg and Tan (1959) have shown that the largest variation of tension occurs at upper frequencies, most often produced in the falsetto register. Only a small amount of tension variation occurs at frequencies typically heard in speech. Thus, although tension is an important determinant of fundamental frequency variation, it is not the only determinant. As has been shown, the mass of the vocal folds (or more accurately, their mass per unit length) has a pronounced influence on the fundamental frequency of the vibration.

It is clear that there may be various mechanisms determining fundamental frequency in the human voice. At some frequencies, overall mass may be the most important determinant (Allen and Hollien, 1973), whereas at other frequencies, tension may be the predominant factor. It is the combination of these factors that ultimately determines the fundamental frequency of vocal fold vibration.

The data from van den Berg and Tan also show that the relationship between tension and fundamental frequency differs as airflow rates differ. Thus, airflow appears to be another contributing factor in the physiological mechanisms of vocal frequency control. In some cases, airflow may be the major determinant of frequency, much as it is for aeolian tones. You may have walked through an open field in which telephone or electrical wires passed overhead and heard the sound the wind makes when striking the wires. This is an example of an aeolian tone. The frequency of an aeolian tone is determined by the speed of

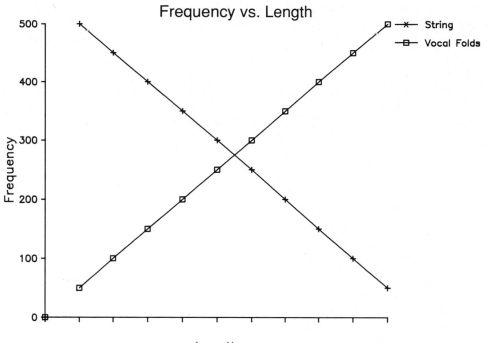

Figure 11.2.   Schematic representation of fundamental frequency versus length, for strings and the vocal folds.

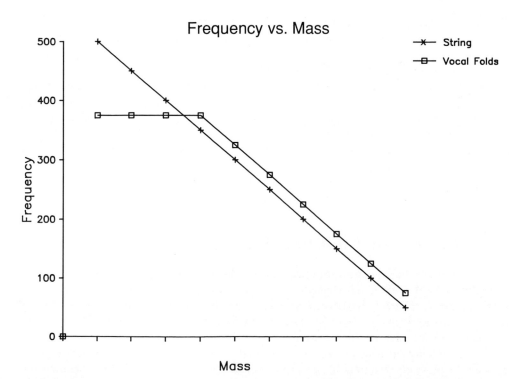

Figure 11.3.   Schematic representation of fundamental frequency versus mass, for strings and the vocal folds.

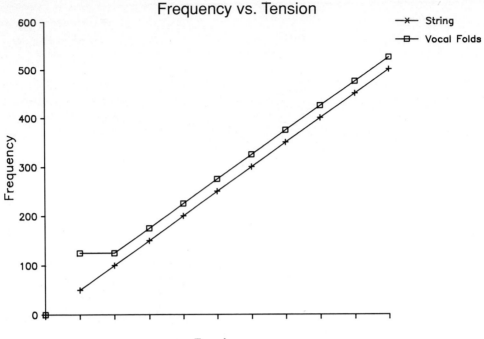

Figure 11.4. Schematic representation of fundamental frequency versus tension, for strings and the vocal folds.

the airflow rushing across the wire. In many patients with phonatory disorders, there is excessive airflow. Although the speed of the airflow may not directly affect the fundamental frequency of the vocal folds, as in an aeolian tone, it may be a sign of an inefficient mechanism being used for the variation of vocal pitch. Or it may be that the patient is using combinations of tension, mass, and airflow that cause or contribute to the voice problem. These possibilities point to the need for information about all of these parameters with voice patients. The availability of such information may help in understanding the bases for the patient's vocal problem.

As in a string, the fundamental frequency of the vocal folds is determined by a complex interaction between length, mass, and tension. There may be various combinations of these parameters that produce the same fundamental frequency. However, not all combinations of length, mass, and tension may be efficient for the production of voice.

Mechanisms of Loudness Change

The human voice is capable of producing a wide range of vocal intensities, sometimes exceeding 60 dB. Additional changes of intensity result from variation in the size and shape of the vocal tract, which acts as a resonator of sound. The mechanisms for the control of vocal intensity, much as those of pitch control, involve muscular activity in combination with airflows and pressures.

Vocal intensity is usually reported in decibels of sound pressure level. Since sound is basically a pressure disturbance, we would expect that increased pressures beneath the vocal folds, when released by the folds, would produce a greater intensity, and indeed, experimental evidence supports this expectation (Ladefoged and McKinney, 1963). As shown in Figure 11.5, when the subglottal air pressure increases, intensity increases, although the exact relationship will vary for different vowels and voice qualities.

However, the controlling mechanism of vocal intensity is not subglottal air pressure. Rather, the controlling mechanism is the degree and time of closure of the vocal folds themselves. That is, by maintaining closure of the vocal folds, there is more time to build up pressure beneath them. More intense sound results when the subglottal air pressure is sufficient to overcome the resistance of the vocal folds. Resistance is the important factor in intensity control. The more vocal fold resistance there is to opening, the greater the pressure disturbance when the resistance is overcome and the folds are forced to open. Thus, intensity is most often controlled by the vocal folds through variations of glottal resistance. Glottal resistance is defined as the ratio of the pressure divided by the flow. Measuring these two quantities will allow the calculation of resistance.

Isshiki (1964, 1965) has shown that glottal resistance is a major controlling mechanism of vocal intensities for low fundamental frequencies, that is, fundamental frequencies produced in the lower part of an individual's phonational range or in the modal register. At higher frequencies, especially frequencies produced in falsetto, glottal resistance is no longer the major factor. Rather, it appears that airflow becomes the dominant variable in intensity variation at these high fundamental frequencies. Furthermore, the range of intensities an individual can produce in the falsetto register is much smaller than can be produced in the modal register (Colton, 1973). This finding would suggest, or at least be in consonance with, the existence of a different controlling mechanism for intensity control in falsetto.

For a variety of reasons, some patients have difficulty in completely closing their vocal folds. In an attempt to speak at a normal vocal intensity, these patients increase air pressure by increasing the expiratory force from the thorax/abdomen system. The patient may also attempt to increase glottal closure in an effort to increase glottal resistance and to maintain an adequate level of tension in the vocal folds. As a result of this effortful vocal behavior, greater than normal subglottal pressures are developed, and there is increased tension in the vocal folds. Because greater than normal muscle activity is involved, these conditions may create vocal fatigue as well as excessive air rushing across the vocal folds. The latter creates greater noise levels in the voice. A vicious cycle ensues, as the vocal fatigue may result in even poorer vocal fold adduction and the need for even greater effort on the patient's part, leading cyclically to poorer voice.

There is another factor that will affect the sound pressure level (SPL) of phonation. That factor is the spectral characteristics of the tone produced by the vocal folds. It is well known that variation of the frequency composition of a tone will vary its intensity. Adding frequencies or varying the amplitude of the components of the tone will affect the intensity of the complex tone. Similarly, the spectrum of the vocal folds can be varied within limits and thus alter the overall intensity of the vocal fold tone. Consequently, the vocal folds can affect the intensity of the tone by variation of the frequency components in the tone.

In some patients with phonatory disorders, the spectral characteristics of the tone produced are markedly different from normal. Usually, but not always, the number of frequency components in the pathological voice is much smaller than in the normal voice. When that is the case, then lower intensities would be expected. In order to compensate for the different spectral characteristics and their effect on intensity, a patient may try to increase subglottal pressures or adductory forces, resulting in increased strain and subsequent abuse of the vocal folds.

Loudness is the perceptual correlate of intensity, but intensity is not the only physical factor that affects loudness. The pitch of the voice and its spectral composition may also affect its perceived loudness. Of course, factors such as the distance from the speaker,

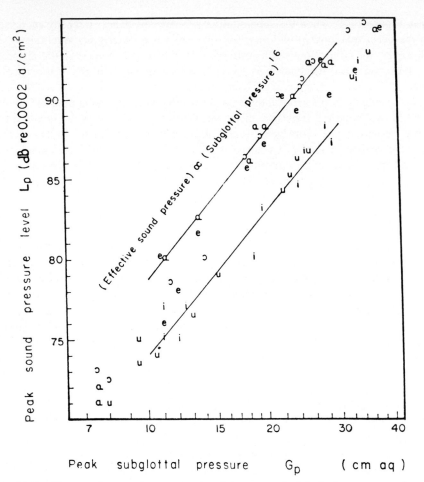

Figure 11.5. The peak sound pressure level versus subglottal air pressure, for vowels within words spoken by a British speaker. (From Ladefoged and McKinney, 1963.)

room acoustics, diffraction, and interference may also affect the loudness of a voice as perceived by a listener.

Mechanisms of Quality Variation

Voice quality is an important attribute of normal and abnormal voices. Voice quality identifies the individual and sets him or her apart from another. A change of voice quality may signal the presence of a benign problem or one that could be life threatening. But defining voice quality can be difficult and imprecise.

Many adjectives are used to describe voice quality: pleasant and unpleasant, normal and pathological. Singers, actors, professional speakers, and those who work with the voice use many jargon terms to decribe the variation of normal voice quality. Quantification of these terms either acoustically or physiologically has proven to be very difficult.

Acoustically, the important parameter concerned with voice quality is spectrum. Spectrum refers to the number and amplitude of the frequencies present in a complex tone, such as the vocal fold tone. Figure 11.6 presents the spectrum of a typical vocal fold tone produced during speech. However, the vocal folds can produce many different voice qualities, each with its own spectral characteristics (Fig. 11.7).

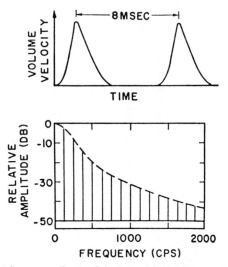

Figure 11.6.   A typical airflow waveform of the vocal folds (top panel) and its corresponding frequency spectrum (bottom panel). (From Stevens and House, 1961.)

Other factors may be important in describing a voice quality acoustically. Although pitch would be expected to be one such factor, it is interesting to note that it apparently is not used in distinguishing one voice quality from another (Colton, 1987). This finding is similar to the influence of pitch in the perception of nonphonatory sounds like complex sounds (Plomp, 1976) and noise bands (Chipman and Carey, 1975). Varying the pitch level may alter some of the details of a voice, but not its basic voice quality.

Voice quality is not solely determined by the vibratory characteristics of the vocal folds. The shape and configuration of the vocal tract are also determinants of voice quality. For example, females have slightly different vocal tract configurations than males, and as a result, female voices can still be recognized as female even when the obvious pitch difference is removed (Coleman, 1971, 1973, 1976). The overall characteristics of an individual's vocal tract, such as the length, cross-sectional area, ratio of oral to pharyngeal cavity size, and so on, would also determine that individual's voice quality.

Physiological change in laryngeal and vocal tract configurations and characteristics have been observed in individuals as they produced various voice qualities (Colton and Estill, 1981; Painter, 1986). For example, in some voice qualities, the size of the pharyngeal cavity is much larger than in other voice qualities. Many of these differences appear to occur in the larynx itself, as well as in the pharynx. We have little information about the vocal tract characteristics of patients with voice disorders. However, it is possible that differences might be found in the shape and configuration of the vocal tracts of patients with voice disorders when compared to those of normal speakers.

Summary

In this chapter, a brief review of the mechanisms for voice production, frequency control, intensity variation, and the generation of voice quality have been reviewed. The tone produced by the vocal folds results from the complex interaction of airflow, air pressure, and muscular activity, which regulate the length, mass, and tension of the vocal folds. Variation in these parameters will affect the fundamental frequency of the voice, as well as its intensity and voice quality. Measurement of these acoustic parameters of the voice will assist in the quantification of the vocal behavior and help to determine the

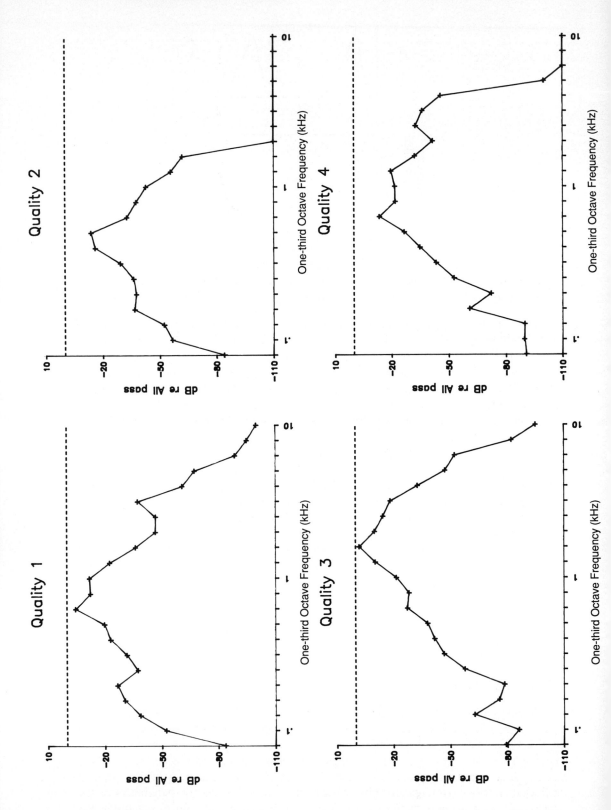

nature of the problem. Accurate measurement of all parameters, acoustic, perceptual or physiological, is important in the preparation of a treatment plan for the patient and in documentation of treatment efficacy.

Figure 11.7 *(opposite).*   Some spectra of different voice qualities. The top left panel is for a quality typically heard during speech. The top right panel presents the spectrum for a sound heard during sobbing or during the singing of a lullaby. The bottom left panel is the spectrum of a sound typically heard in country Western singing. The bottom right panel is the spectrum of sound heard in operatic singing. (Based on data reported in Colton, Estill, and Gertsman, 1981.)

12

Neuroanatomy of the Vocal Mechanism

Volitional control of the muscles of the larynx resides in the brain. However, there are many connecting points or stations within the brain, including the cortex, subcortical areas, midbrain, and medulla, that play an important role in the ultimate control of phonation. Thus, saying that phonation is controlled by the brain is much too simplistic and underemphasizes the roles various structures play in integrating information and coordinating the activity of the muscles active in phonation. In this chapter, a brief review of the neuroanatomy and neurophysiology of phonation will be presented. A further and more detailed review of brain mechanisms controlling vocalization may be found in Larson (1988).

Cortical Mechanisms of Phonatory Control

The cerebral cortex is that portion of the brain responsible for the conceptualization, planning, and execution of the speech act, including phonation. Some areas of the cortex may be responsible for creating the act, others for its linguistic characteristics, and still others for the emotionality of the act. Penfield and Roberts (1959) have identified three major areas of the cortex directly responsible for vocalization. These are, in decreasing order of importance, (*a*) the precentral and postcentral gyrus (Rolandic area), (*b*) the anterior (or Broca's) area, and (*c*) the supplementary motor area. These areas are shown in Figure 12.1. Experiments have demonstrated that vocalization occurs when certain spots within these areas are stimulated in both the dominant and nondominant hemispheres (Fig.

12.2). Within these areas, depending on the specific spot stimulated, it has been shown that vocalization can be initiated or stopped and speech can be slurred or distorted. These behaviors occur as the result of stimulation in either the dominant or the nondominant hemisphere. Speech and phonation are complex motor acts involving simultaneous activation and control of many muscles. Although the control of these motor acts occurs primarily in the cortex, control of individual muscles seems to occur at a much lower level in the brain. There is no evidence to suggest that cortical stimulation produces a response in a single solitary muscle. Higher brain function is concerned with idealization of the event, integration of sensory information, feedback control, and coordination of various muscles required for the motor act.

Subcortical Mechanisms

The motor cortex has numerous connections to the thalamus, a major portion of the diencephalon or interbrain. Other parts of the diencephalon include the hypothalamus, metathalamus, epithalamus, and subthalamus (Riklan and Levita, 1969). The third ventricle is also part of the diencephalon (Gardner, 1963). The thalamus has major pathways to the motor cortex and Broca's area (Penfield and Roberts, 1959). In addition, the thalamus has numerous connections to the cerebellum, midbrain, and other structures in the diencephalon (Fig. 12.3). There are various nuclei in the thalamus that project to parts of the cerebral cortex. These are shown in Figure 12.4. Note that the motor area (precentral gyrus) located anterior to the central sulcus receives much of its projection from the ventrolateral nucleus of the thalamus. Botez and Barbeau (1971) concluded that the ventrolateral nucleus was responsible for the initiation of speech movements as well as control of loudness, pitch, rate, and articulation. Broca's area receives connections from the dorsomedian and centromedian nuclei of the thalamus.

The thalamus is a most fascinating structure in the diencephalon since it appears to act both as a relay for impulses occurring in lower areas of the brain and as an integrator of information (Riklan and Levita, 1969). Furthermore, the thalamus is involved in the maintenance of consciousness, alertness, and attention and may also integrate emotion into a complex motor act. Some of the thalamic nuclei are nonspecific and project to many areas on the cortex (Fig. 12.5). Thus, insofar as speech and voice are concerned, the thalamus plays a major role in integrating incoming sensory information, coordinating outgoing information from the cortex and other areas of the brain, and, perhaps, adding emotionality to speech and voice.

Midbrain Structures

The midbrain or mesencephalon lies beneath the thalamus (House and Pansky, 1967). On the anterior surface of the midbrain are the cerebral peduncles that connect the cerebrum with the brainstem and spinal cord. On its posterior surface, there are four rounded areas called the colliculi. The superior colliculi are concerned with visual function, whereas the inferior colliculi are concerned with audition. Within the midbrain there is a cavity called the cerebral aqueduct of Sylvius, which is surrounded by a thick zone of gray matter. An important area of this gray matter, dorsal to the aqueduct, is called the periaqueductal gray.

Several investigators have shown that stimulation of the dorsal and ventrolateral areas of the periaqueductal gray produces activity in some laryngeal muscles (Larson, 1985;

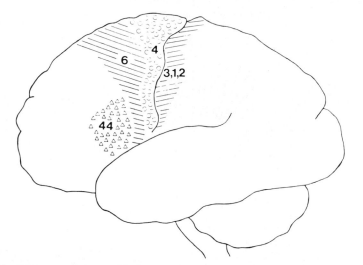

Figure 12.1. Diagram of the cortical areas involved in speech movement control. Area 4 (primary motor cortex), areas 3, 1, and 2 (somatosensory cortex), area 44 (Broca's area), and area 6 (premotor cortex and supplementary motor area). (From McClean, 1988.)

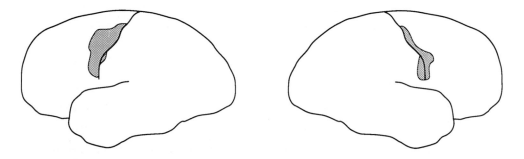

Left Hemisphere   Right Hemisphere

Figure 12.2. Areas on the left and right hemispheres that produce vocalization when stimulated. (Based on data presented by Penfield and Roberts, 1959.)

Larson and Kistler, 1986; Ortega, DeRosier, Park, and Larson, 1988). Larson (1985) has reported that some cells in the ventrolateral area stimulate muscle activity, whereas other cells suppress activity. He suggested that the periaqueductal gray may be an intermediate area between the recognition of a stimulus or event and the subsequent production of the motor act. Other areas, such as the hypothalamus, amygdala, and anterior cingulate gyrus, are responsible for vocalizations but of a kind that Larson (1985) notes are species spe-

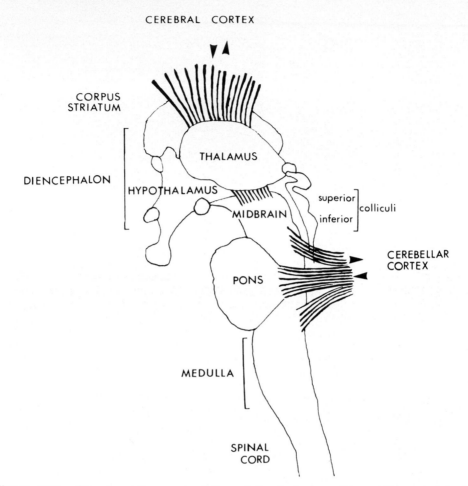

CEREBRAL CORTEX

CORPUS
STRIATUM

DIENCEPHALON

THALAMUS

HYPOTHALAMUS

MIDBRAIN

superior

inferior

colliculi

CEREBELLAR
CORTEX

PONS

MEDULLA

SPINAL
CORD

Figure 12.3. Diagrammatic representation of the brainstem. (From Riklan and Levita, 1969.)

cific. Botez and Barbeau (1971) also implicated the periaqueductal gray in disorders involving mutism.

Brainstem

The major bilateral structures in the brainstem implicated in the neural control of phonation include the nucleus ambiguus, nucleus tractus solitarii, and nucleus parabrachialis. Yoshida, Mitsumasu, Hirano, Morimoto, and Kanaseki (1987) performed an elegant study in which they traced the connections among these structures. When they injected a tracer chemical into one nucleus ambiguus, they found evidence of the tracer throughout the contralateral nuclei, in the nuclei tractus solitarii bilaterally, in the nuclei parabrachialis, and bilaterally in the lateral and ventrolateral parts of the periaqueductal gray area, with a predominance ipsilaterally. Injection of the tracer into the nucleus tractus solitarii resulted in labeled cells throughout the nucleus itself, as well as in the dorsal motor nucleus of the vagus, part of the hypoglossal nucleus, the medial portion of the nucleus gracilis, and the dorsal part of the reticular formation. Clearly, there are many interconnections bilaterally among the nucleus ambiguus, nucleus tractus

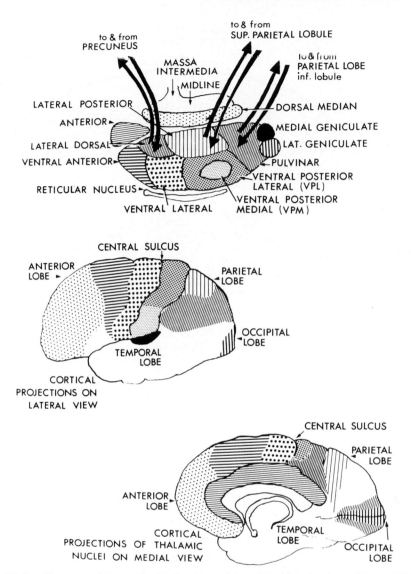

Figure 12.4. Diagram of the major thalamic nuclei and their projections. (From Riklan and Levita, 1969.)

solitarii, reticular formation around the nucleus ambiguus, motor roots of the vagus, and periaqueductal gray area.

Cerebellum

The cerebellum, a structure lying immediately posterior to the midbrain area, is strongly implicated in the control of movement. Its location is shown in Figure 12.6A. Figure 12.6B shows the cerebellum from a superior view after the cerebrum has been removed. The three main portions of the cerebellum are seen in this diagram: the vermis (V), the pars intermedia (PI), and the hemispheres (H). The cerebellum consists of many transverse folia, shown in Figure 12.6C, whose complex infolding vastly increases the

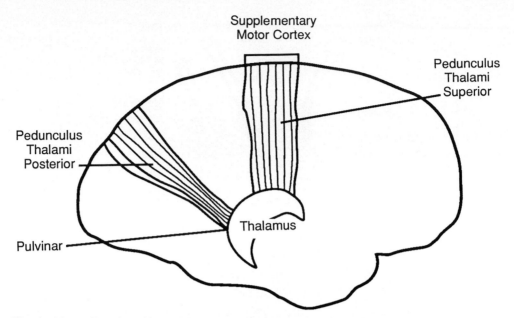

Figure 12.5. Drawing showing the connections between the pulvinar nuclei of the thalamus and the posterior speech area of the cortex. Diagram also shows the pathway between the thalamus and the superior speech cortex (supplementary motor area). (Based on data presented by Penfield and Roberts, 1959.)

surface area of the cerebellum in much the same way as is seen in the cerebrum. The fissura prima (FP) is a deep fissure separating the anterior and posterior lobes.

Two major areas of the cerebellum are instrumental in the control of movement (McClean, 1988). The first, the pars intermedia, has many direct connections via midbrain nuclei with the cerebrum (Fig. 12.7A). Impulses from the motor cortex are quickly relayed from the pyramidal tracts (PT) to the pars intermedia via the nuclei pontis, lateral reticular nucleus, and inferior olive. The pars intermedia analyzes the movement patterns and quickly returns the results of its analysis to the cerebral cortex via connections through the interpositus nucleus, the ventrolateral nuclei of the thalamus, and the red nucleus. As such, the pars intermedia acts like a computer controlling a missile. It may not have given the original command to fire, but it constantly monitors the missile, taking small corrective actions whenever the missile deviates from its intended flight plan (Eccles, 1977).

The cerebellar hemispheres seem to play a different role in movement control, more akin to the planning stages of a movement pattern. As shown in Fig. 12.7B, there are few direct connections to tracts that lead to lower motoneurons, as was the case for the connections between the cerebrum and pars intermedia of the cerbellum. Rather, the connections from the motor cortex pass through the nuclei pontis and inferior olive directly to cells within the cerebellar hemispheres, and impulses from the cerebellar hemispheres pass through the nucleus dentatus to the ventrolateral nuclei of the thalamus and red nucleus back to the cerebral hemispheres, where movement is initiated. It appears that the command center, after drafting a movement plan, sends it on to the cerebellar hemispheres for revision and refinement before adopting it. According to Eccles (1977), the cerebellar

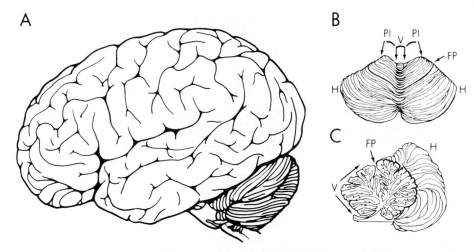

Figure 12.6. **A,** Human cerebrum and cerebellum. **B,** The cerebellum from its dorsal aspect. **C,** Midline view after sagittal section. *H,* hemispheres; *V,* vermis; *Pl,* the pars intermedia; *FP,* transverse folia. (From Eccles, 1977.)

hemispheres are concerned with anticipatory planning based on learning, experience, and sensory information they receive from other brain centers.

The importance of the cerebellum in the control of speech movement cannot be emphasized enough. Kornhuber (1977) believes that without it (and other midbrain areas) the cerebral cortex could not function and would be ineffective in the generation of movements. The cerebellum acts to regulate motor movement continuously and quickly, requir-

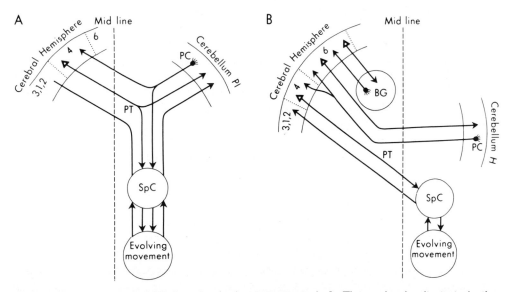

Figure 12.7. Cerebrocerebellar circuits in motor control. **A,** The main circuit starts in the motor cortex (4) and travels down the pyramidal tract (*PT*) to the spinal cord, with side branches via the pars intermedia (*PI*) to the cerebellum. Impulses from Purkinje cells (*PC*) in the cerebellum communicate with the motor cortex and down to the spinal cord. **B,** Circuits from area 6 in the cerebrum to the cerebellar hemispheres (*H*). A return circuit from the Purkinje cells (*PC*) back to areas 4 and 6 is shown. Also shown is a circuit from area 6 to the basal ganglia (*BG*) and its return to the cerebrum. (From Eccles, 1977.)

ing some degree of preprogramming and adjustment by learning. Certainly, coordination of muscles within the larynx is necessary for phonation, as is coordination with other systems involved in speech production.

Peripheral Connections: The Vagus Nerve

The vagus nerve is the major nerve that supplies the larynx (and other parts of the body as well). The vagus provides sensory fibers within the larynx, as well as fibers that control all the muscles of the larynx. The cell bodies of the vagus are located in the nucleus ambiguus. Laryngeal muscles are controlled by cells in the more caudal portions of the nucleus. The vagus emerges from the surface of the medulla between the cerebellar peduncle and the inferior olives in the midbrain. It exits the skull through the jugular foramen.

After exiting the skull, the vagus divides into many branches that serve the head, neck, thorax, and abdomen. These are shown schematically in Figure 12.8. Shortly after exiting the jugular foramen, a small filament (the meningeal filament) exits the nerve to serve the dura mater on the posterior fossa of the base of the skull. The auricular branch provides sensory fibers to the skin behind the pinna and to the posterior part of the external auditory meatus. The pharyngeal branch provides motor fibers to the muscles of the pharynx and soft palate.

The major portions of the vagus serving the larynx are the superior laryngeal and the recurrent laryngeal nerves. The superior laryngeal is the primary sensory nerve for the larynx. It arises from the inferior ganglion of the vagus and descends along the side of the pharynx behind the internal carotid artery, where it sends off two branches. The external branch descends along the side of the larynx to serve the cricothyroid muscle. The internal branch descends to an opening in the thyrohyoid membrane and enters the larynx to serve the mucous membrane of the larynx down to the true vocal folds. The recurrent laryngeal nerve follows a different course on either side of the body. On the right side, the recurrent descends in the neck to loop around the subclavian artery (just below the clavicle) and then ascends alongside the trachea to serve the remaining intrinsic muscles of the larynx. On the left side, the recurrent laryngeal nerve takes a much more circuitous route, descending into the thorax, looping around the aorta, and then ascending alongside the trachea until it reaches the larynx. It also provides motor fibers to the remaining intrinsic laryngeal muscles.

There are other branches of the vagus nerve in the neck, thorax, and abdomen that provide sensory innervation to various structures within these areas. These branches of the vagus are shown in Table 12.1.

The extrinsic laryngeal muscles are innervated by several nerves. The anterior belly of the digastric muscle receives its innervation from the mylohyoid branch of the inferior alveolar nerve, whereas the posterior belly is innervated by the 7th cranial (or facial) nerve. The mylohyoid muscle is innervated by the mylohyoid branch of the inferior alveolar nerve, and the geniohyoid, sternohyoid, sternothyroid, and omohyoid muscles by the ansa cervicalis (C1). The thyrohyoid is innervated by ansa cervicalis (C1) via the hypoglossal nerve.

There are numerous protective mechanisms within the respiratory tract, but the most vigorous exist in the larynx. Some are mechanical and act to close off the airway; others are expulsive and serve to force foreign substances from the airway. All are reflexive and operate under involuntary control.

There are many sensory endings within the larynx that collect information about the state of the larynx and respiratory tract and transmit this information via several reflex arcs

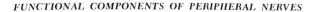

FUNCTIONAL COMPONENTS OF PERIPHERAL NERVES

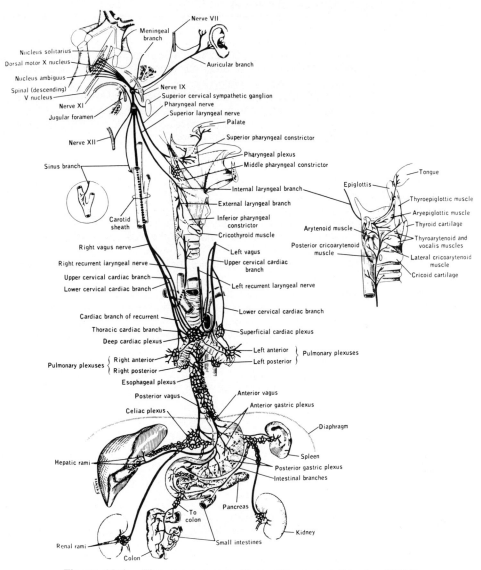

Figure 12.8.   The vagus nerve. (From House and Pansky, 1967.)

as well as directly to the central nervous system. Wyke (1967,1969) has written extensively about these reflex control mechanisms. The complexity of these control systems and their interactions with the respiratory and other body systems makes this a fascinating area of study. For example, sensory endings exist in the mucosa or lining of the larynx that respond to mechanical forces or air pressure changes within the tract. These nerve endings are capable of sending information to the central nervous system about the mechanical state of the lining of the respiratory tract. Furthermore, reflex endings exist within the joints of the various cartilages of the larynx that discharge when these joints are moved. These discharges have been shown to affect the ongoing electrical activity of some intrinsic laryngeal muscles (Wyke, 1967). Finally, the intrinsic laryngeal muscles contain specialized stretch receptors that discharge when the muscle is stretched or contracted (Wyke,

Table 12.1.
Branches of the Vagus (10th Cranial Nerve)

In the jugular fossa

Meningeal	Serves dura mater in posterior fossa at the base of the skull.
Auricular	Serves skin on back of outer ear (auricle) and posterior part of the external acoustic meatus.
Pharyngeal	Joins with glossopharyngeal, sympathetic, and external laryngeal nerves to form pharyngeal plexus, which serves the muscles and membranes of the pharynx and muscles of the soft palate, with the exception of the tensor.

In the neck

Superior laryngeal	(2 branches)
External	Supplies cricothyroid.
Internal	Pierces the hyothyroid membrane to supply the mucous membrane of the larynx down to the true vocal folds.
Recurrent	
Right side	Arises in front of the subclavian artery to travel upward along the trachea.
Left side	Arises on the left side of the arch of the aorta.
Both	Enter the larynx behind the articulation of the inferior cornu of the thyroid with the cricoid.
	Serve all intrinsic muscles with the exception of the cricothyroid.
Superior cardiac	Serves cardiac plexus.
Inferior cardiac	Serves cardiac plexus.

In the thorax

Anterior bronchial	Sensory to the lung.
Posterior bronchial	Sensory to the lung.
Esophageal	Sensory to the esophagus.

In the abdomen

Gastric	Sensory to the stomach.
Celiac	Sensory to the pancreas, spleen, kidneys, suprarenal bodies, and intestine.
Hepatic	Sensory to the liver.

1969). The various levels of reflex mechanisms within the larynx suggest that elaborate precautions are in place to protect the airway and maintain life. From our perspective in voice pathology and its treatment, they are important to consider when trying to understand the physiology of normal and aberrant human phonation. Wyke (1969) hypothesizes that some types of stuttering may be related to disorders of the various reflex mechanisms within the larynx.

Summary

Proper control of the muscles of the larynx is critical in the production of voice. The levels of control within the central nervous system are multiple and complex. Lesions in some parts of the system, especially in the cortex and thalamus (and related structures) would be expected to have profound effects on speech and voice production. However, the fact that cortical and some subcortical controls are present bilaterally provides some measure of safety when lesions are unilateral. Indeed, cases have been reported wherein portions of the cerebral cortex were surgically removed with little lasting effect on speech and phonation (Penfield and Roberts, 1959). Lesions further down in the brain might be expected to have a more singular effect on a specific muscle or set of muscles. However, innervation is still bilateral and redundant in some lower level brain areas, thus affording considerable protection of the systems involved in speech production. Once the nerves exit the skull, lesions of a nerve will have more specific effects involving, perhaps, a single muscle or small number of muscles bilaterally or unilaterally.

13

Some Normative Data on the Voice

Introduction

In this chapter some normative data on the voice are presented. Our purpose is not to present all the available data, much of which is incomplete and confusing, but rather to provide the most meaningful data against which patient data may be compared clinically. The data reported here were gathered from a variety of sources, all of which are referenced for those seeking further information. An invaluable source for more complete data is Baken's book, *Clinical Measurement of Speech and Voice* (1987). The sources of the data in the tables in this chapter are indicated by numbers in the body of the table, keyed to references below the table. The full citation for these sources appears in the reference list at the end of the book. Additional information about these measures and how they are obtained can be found in Chapter 7.

Fundamental Frequency

The measure of fundamental frequency, reflecting the vibratory rate of the vocal folds, is useful for comparing intra- and intersubject pitch levels. Fundamental frequency can be measured during production of sustained vowels or during a reading passage. It is important to note, however, that fundamental frequency will vary depending on the type of speech material used. There are considerable data on fundamental frequency, covering ages from birth to death. At many ages, however, fundamental frequency plateaus and may not change for many years. The data in Table 13.1 represent a summary of fundamen-

Table 13.1.
Fundamental Frequencies

Age Range	Mean f_o	SD (ST)[a]	Range	Reference[b]
	Males Reading			
7	294	2.2		1
8	297	2.0		1
10	270	2.4		1
11	227	1.5	192–268	2
14	242	3.4		1
19	117	2.1	85–155	3
Adult	132	3.3		4
20–29	120			5
30–39	112			5
40–49	107			5
50–59	118			5
60–69	112			5
70–79	132			5
80–89	146			5
	Females Reading			
7	281	2.0		6
8	288	2.8		6
11	238	1.5	198–271	2
19	217	1.7	165–255	3
20–29	224	3.8	192–275	7
30–40	196	2.5	171–222	8
40–50	189	2.8	168–208	8
60–69	200	4.3	143–235	7
70–?	202	4.7	170–249	7
80–94	200	2.7	183–225	9

[a]Standard deviation (SD) is expressed in semitones.
[b]Reference key:
1. Fairbanks, Wiley, and Lassman, 1949.
2. Horii, 1983.
3. Fitch and Holbrook, 1970.
4. Snidecor, 1943.
5. Hollien and Shipp, 1972; Shipp and Hollien, 1969.
6. Fairbanks, Herbert, and Hammond, 1949.
7. Stoicheff, 1981.
8. Saxman and Burk, 1967.
9. McGlone and Hollien, 1963.

tal frequencies. There have been several studies reported of fundamental frequency at certain ages or within certain age ranges. The data in Table 13.1 represent the average of these studies.

Fundamental Frequency Variation

The standard deviations of fundamental frequency, often referred to as the variability of fundamental frequency or pitch sigma, are also shown in Table 13.1. Variability is much smaller for sustained vowels than for reading passages. Fundamental frequency variability or lack thereof may be a physical measure that relates to the perception of voice monotone, a perceptual sign noted in some voice disorders.

Frequency Perturbation

Frequency perturbation or jitter refers to the variation of fundamental frequency present in all speakers to some degree and detected when the subject is attempting to produce a steady, sustained vowel. The frequency variations are the result of instability of the vocal folds during vibration. As such, perturbation reflects the biomechanical characteristics of the vocal folds, as well as variations of neuromuscular control. Normal speakers have a small amount of frequency perturbation, which may vary according to age, physical condition, and in and in some cases sex. These variables are included in Table 13.2, obtained from data reported by Casper in 1983.

Maximum Phonational Range

Maximum phonational range refers to the range of frequencies, from lowest to highest, that an individual can produce. The intensity of the tone is usually not controlled, and the person may be asked to sustain the tone for about 1 second. Placing further demands on the production of the sound (i.e., production at a specific intensity or for a longer duration) may be expected to alter the magnitude of the range obtained. The data reported in Table 13.3 were obtained from many sources and represent the means of several studies. Note that there are no data for children.

Vocal Intensity

Amplitude Perturbation

During sustained vibration, the vocal folds will exhibit slight variation of amplitude from one cycle to the next. This is called amplitude perturbation or shimmer. Normal speakers will present a small amount of shimmer, which depends both on the vowel used and the sex of the person. Some typical shimmer values are shown in Table 13.4.

Table 13.2.
Frequency Perturbation Data[a]

Age Range	Measure	Jitter Factor		Directional Perturbation Factor		Pitch Perturbation Quotient	
		/ee/	/oo/	/ee/	/oo/	/ee/	/oo/
		Males					
20–29	Mean	0.7817	0.7162	70.7341	69.4775	0.6477	0.5681
	SD	0.3980	0.3558	11.2467	14.8667	0.3030	0.2592
40–49	Mean	0.9862	0.8704	74.3651	72.4934	0.7678	0.6959
	SD	0.6141	0.5085	10.8633	14.8367	0.3789	0.3244
60–69	Mean	0.9070	0.8717	67.7711	69.4312	0.7702	0.7420
	SD	0.6296	0.5649	15.4633	14.5467	0.5029	0.4347
		Females					
20–29	Mean	0.5475	0.5630	46.3029	47.8344	0.5570	0.5681
	SD	0.4124	0.4061	19.6733	19.6800	0.3940	0.3731
40–49	Mean	0.6329	0.6144	53.0622	51.6690	0.6469	0.6088
	SD	0.4029	0.4215	16.5700	19.7600	0.4147	0.3983
60–69	Mean	0.6619	0.6989	49.9148	48.8757	0.6508	0.6876
	SD	0.5197	0.5877	19.1033	18.6420	0.4928	0.5594

[a]All data are from Casper, 1983.

Table 13.3.
Maximum Phonational Range

Age Range	Low Frequency	High Frequency	Range	Reference[a]
		Males		
17–26	80	764	39.06	1
18–36	80	675	36.92	2
35–75	80	260	20.40	3
40–65	83	443	28.99	5
68–89	85	394	26.55	4
		Females		
18–38	140	1122	36.03	2
66–93	134	571	25.09	4
35–70	136	803	30.75	5

[a]Reference key:
1. Hollien and Jackson, 1973.
2. Hollien, Dew, and Phillips, 1971.
3. Canter, 1965.
4. Ptacek, Sander, Maloney, and Jackson, 1966.
5. Colton, 1982.

Maximum Intensity Level

Patients may vary considerably in their ability to produce loud tones. This may be a helpful diagnostic sign or a measure of change following treatment. Thus, it may be useful to measure maximum intensity output. Normal speakers can usually produce maximum outputs in excess of 110 dB; this is somewhat dependent upon sex, age, the frequency at which the phonation is produced, and the measurement procedure. Table 13.5 presents a summary of maximum intensity levels for different ages and both sexes.

S/Z Ratio

The s/z ratio is a simple measure designed to examine the effect of pathology on phonation. Although there is some variation among normal speakers, generally ratios

Table 13.4.
Amplitude Perturbation Data[a]

Vowel	Mean	SD
	Males	
/ah/	0.47	0.34
/ee/	0.37	0.28
/oo/	0.33	0.31
Mean	0.33	0.31
	Females	
/ah/	0.33	0.22
/ee/	0.23	0.08
/oo/	0.19	0.04
Mean	0.25	0.11

[a]Adapted from Baken, 1987, p. 117.

Table 13.5.
Maximum Intensity Levels

Age Range	Mean	SD	Range	Reference[a]
		Males		
18–39	106	5.1	92–116	1
45–65	110	7.1	99–129	2
68–89	101	5.9	88–110	1
		Females		
18–38	106	3.0	99–112	1
40–70	101	18.2	93–115	2
66–93	99	4.5	90–104	1

[a]Reference key:
1. Ptacek, Sander, Maloney, and Jackson, 1966.
2. Colton, Reed, Sagerman, and Chung, 1982.

greater than 1.4 are considered abnormal. Ratios around 1 are normal and expected for both children and adults of different ages (Table 13.6).

Maximum Phonation Duration

Maximum phonation duration is the maximum time a person can sustain a tone on one continuous expiratory breath. It supposedly is a measure of phonatory control and respiratory "support." As Kent, Kent, and Rosenbek (1987) have pointed out, maximum phonation duration can be influenced by variables that have little to do with phonatory control. Important variables include age, sex, and, of course, the physical characteristics of the respiratory system. Table 13.7 presents a summary of the data reported on maximum phonation duration from many studies. This measure should be used with care because of uncertainty about its validity and stability on repeat trials (Kent et al., 1987).

Table 13.6.
S/Z Ratios

Age	Mean	Range	Reference[a]
		Males	
5	0.92	0.82–1.08	1
7	0.70	0.52–0.97	1
9	0.92	0.66–1.5	1
		Females	
5	0.83	0.50–1.14	1
7	0.78	0.51–1.10	1
9	0.91	0.75–1.26	1
Adults	0.99	0.41–2.67	2
Aged	0.76		3
	0.82		3

[a]Reference key:
1. Tait, Michel, and Carpenter, 1980.
2. Eckel and Boone, 1981.
3. Young, Bless, McNeil, and Braun, 1983.

Table 13.7.
Maximum Phonation Duration[a]

Age	Mean	Standard Deviation
Males		
Young children	8.95	2.16
Children	17.74	4.14
Adults	25.89	7.41
Aged	14.68	6.25
Females		
Young children	7.50	1.80
Children	14.97	3.87
Adults	21.34	5.66
Aged	13.55	5.70

[a]Adapted from Table 2 in Kent, Kent, and Rosenbek, 1987. Data represent the means of the means reported by several studies in which maximum phonation duration was measured and grouped into different age groups depending on the results. Young children are 3 to 4 years old, children are aged 5 to 12 years old, and adults include the ages from 13 to about 65 years. The aged are over 65 years old.

Airflow

Average Airflow Rates

Measurements of physiological parameters such as airflow and air pressure have some face validity in that vocal pathology will affect their magnitude. Both airflow and air pressure are dependent on a number of factors, however, including respiratory drive, vocal fold valving, frequency, and intensity. Thus, the conditions under which these measurements are obtained must be understood and controlled in order to be properly interpreted.

Table 13.8.
Average Flow Rates (ml/sec)

Age	Task	Mean	Range	N	Reference[a]
Males					
7	/ah/	96	51–128	10	3
Adult	/ah/	119	96–141	5–36	1
	/ee/	144	89–136	30	4
	Reading	177	141–218	4	2
Females					
7	/ah/	72	45–115	10	3
Adult	/ah/	112	89–136	5–36	1
	/ee/	177		30	4
	Reading	159	152–170	4	2

[a]Reference key:
  1. Based on data presented in Table 3.1 of Hirano, 1981a.
  2. Horii and Cooke, 1978.
  3. Beckett, Thoelke, and Cowan, 1971.
  4. Woo, Colton, and Shangold, 1987.

Table 13.9.
Vibratory Airflows Based on Inverse Filtering of Oral Airflow Data (ml/sec)

Age Range	N	Condition[a]	AC Flow	Min. Flow	Reference[b]
		Males			
17–30	25	Normal	234	101	1
		Soft	193	152	1
		Loud	461	103	1
21–30	8	Normal	303	68	2
		Females			
17–30	25	Normal	141	76	1
		Soft	232	109	1
		Loud	271	75	1
21–30	8	Normal	189	75	2

[a]Normal, soft, and loud refer to the loudness level at which the speakers were asked to produce the phonation.
[b]Reference key:
 1. Holmberg, Hillman, and Perkell, 1988.
 2. Brodie, Colton, and Swisher, 1988.

Average airflow measures are shown in Table 13.8. Average airflow is reported in cubic centimeters per second or milliliters per second. Many researchers and clinicians have reported data on airflow for both normal speakers and those with vocal pathology. Some of the data for normal-speaking subjects are reported in Table 13.8. There is some variation depending on the task the subject performs, and there is some suggestion that children have much smaller flows than adults. Females tend to have slightly lower flows than males.

Vibratory Airflow

Vibratory airflow refers to the variations of airflow during a cycle of vibration. Two major aspects of vibratory flow have been measured and are reported in Table 13.9. The first, AC flow, refers to the peak airflow during vibration. The second, minimum or DC flow, refers to any airflow that occurs when the vocal folds are supposedly closed. Both appear to be correlated with breathiness in the voice. AC flow varies both as a function of sex and of the intensity level at which the phonation is produced. Females have much lower AC flows than males, and there is a tendency for minimum or DC flow to be lower for female speakers also. As intensity levels increase, so too does airflow.

Air Pressure

The amount of air pressure used in producing phonation will, in large measure, determine the intensity of the voice. In normal speakers, air pressure ranges between 4 and 5 cm/H_2O for normal conversational or moderate level phonations (Table 13.10). Air pressure will also affect the magnitude of airflow; thus, it is important to know at what pressures airflow measures have been collected. These data were derived from measurement of intra-oral air pressure according to techniques described by Rothenberg (1968), Smitheran, and Hixon (1981), and Rothenberg (1982).

Table 13.10.
Air Pressure Measurements Based on Intraoral Pressure Estimates (cm/H$_2$O)

Age Range	N	Condition[a]	Pressure	SD	Reference[b]
		Males			
17–30	25	Normal	5.91		1
		Soft	4.79		1
		Loud	8.39		1
21–30	8	Normal	4.12	1.00	2
		Females			
17–30	25	Normal	6.09		1
		Soft	4.79		1
		Loud	8.46		1
21–30	8	Normal	4.28	0.88	2

[a]Condition refers to the loudness level at which the phonation was produced.
[b]Reference key:
 1. Holmberg, Hillman, and Perkell, 1988.
 2. Brodie, Colton, and Swisher, 1988.

APPENDIX

Forms Used in Voice Evaluation Laboratory and Communication Disorder Unit

VOICE EVALUATION LABORATORY
Department of Otolaryngology and Communication Sciences
SUNY Health Science Center at Syracuse
Syracuse, New York 13210
(315) 464-5573 or 464-4678

TELEPHONE CONTACT SHEET

Name _____ Age_____

Telephone _____

Address _____

Referred by _____

        M.D. _____ Speech Path. _____ Voice Coach _____ Other (who?) _____

Referring Complaint:
        Hoarseness _____   Pain in Throat _____
        Loss of Voice _____   Difficulty Singing _____
        Other _____

Services Desired (check appropriate items)

      _____ Complete Evaluation & Diagnosis*   _____ Pre-op Documentation
      _____ Second Opinion/Consult   _____ Post-op Documentation
      _____ Diagnosis and Treatment   _____ Voice Recording Only

* (Complete evaluation includes: ENT examination, fiberoptic study, speech pathology consult, air flow studies, EGG, and voice recording)

If medical referral: pertinent history, treatment and physical findings:

If not medical referral: Name of doctor: _____

Are records available?_____

– –

Appt. Date _____   History form mailed _____
                                                   (date)

Appt. Time _____   Appointment card mailed_____
                                                   (date)

VOICE EVALUATION LABORATORY
Department of Otolaryngology and Communication Sciences
SUNY Health Science Center at Syracuse
Syracuse, New York 13210
(315) 464-5573 or 464-4678

REFERRAL FORM

Patient's Name_____   Age _____   Date of Referral_____

Address _____   Tel. (___) _____

Chief Complaint: _____

SERVICES DESIRED (check appropriate items)

_____ COMPLETE EVAL & DIAGNOSIS*   _____ Pre-op Documentation
_____ Second Opinion   _____ Post-op Documentation
_____ Dx and Treatment   _____ Voice Recording Only

*Complete evaluation includes: ENT Examination, Videotaped Fiberoptic Study, Speech Pathology Consult, Air Flow Studies, Electroglottography, Voice Recording.

PERTINENT HISTORY (physical findings, previous treatment, surgery, etc.)

_____

_____

_____

_____

(Please submit copies of pertinent reports, operative notes, etc.)

Report sent to: ___ You; ___ School; ____ Other: _____

If other examinations are indicated, (e.g., Neurological, Psychiatric) should patient be informed?
___Yes ___No

Do you wish to discuss our findings and recommendations with the patient?
_____ Yes _____ No

___Patient will call for appointment.
___Please contact patient for appointment.

FOR APPOINTMENT CALL: (315) 464-5573

_____
referral source-print

_____
address

_____
telephone number

VOICE EVALUATION LABORATORY
Department of Otolaryngology and Communication Sciences
SUNY Health Science Center at Syracuse
Syracuse, New York 13210
(315) 464-5573 or 464-4678

VOICE HISTORY

Date of
Name _____ Birth _____ Age ____ Date _____

Complaint (please state the main concern in your own words)
_____
_____

When did you first notice a problem with your voice?_____

Please describe the course of the problem, the treatment you have had, where, and who treated you.
_____
_____
_____

Please describe any feelings you have in your throat (such as tickle, lump, pain, difficulty swallowing, strain, fatigue, etc.) _____
_____

Does your voice get better, worse, stay the same?_____
    When is it better? _____
    When is it worse? _____

Do you have any of the following?

    ——— Allergies   ——— Neurological Problems
    ——— Respiratory Problems   ——— Endocrine/Hormone Problems

Have you had any of the following?

    ——— Surgery on your larynx? When _____
    ——— Heart Surgery? When_____
    ——— Chest Surgery? When_____
    ——— Thyroid Surgery? When_____
    ——— Stroke? When_____
    ——— Injury to the Neck? When _____
    ——— Chemical or Inhalation Exposure? When _____

Do You:
    ——— Smoke? (Tobacco or other substances)
        How much?_____
    ——— Drink? (Beer, wine, other alcoholic substances)
        How much?_____
    ——— Take any medication regularly? (Include aspirin)
        What?_____
    ——— Talk above noise? What noise?_____
        How much?_____
    ——— Talk loud, scream, yell? How much?_____
    ——— Sing: ____Choir, ____ Solo, ____with musical group

Are you employed? ____ Yes ____ No
What kind of work do you do?_____

Is talking required for your job? ——— Yes ——— No

Please add any other information which you think may be pertinent.

VOICE EVALUATION LABORATORY

EXAMINATION RECORD

Date _____

Name _____ DOB _____ Age _____

Address _____

Insurance Co. _____ Policy # _____

Medicare: Yes _____ No _____ Policy # _____

Medicaid: Yes _____ No _____

Referred by: _____

Referral Diagnosis: _____

PT.'S Complaint: _____
_____
_____

Duration of Problem: _____

Hx. of Present Illness _____
_____

Findings:

   ENT Exam:

   Fiberoptic Video: Cassette # _____ Footage # _____ To _____

   Videofluoroscopy: Cassette # _____ Footage # _____ To _____

   Vibratory Characteristics:

   Perceptual Characteristics:

   Response to Intervention:

Diagnosis:

Suggested Follow-up:

Return to Care of:

Examiners:

VOICE EVALUATION LABORATORY
Department of Otolaryngology and Communication Sciences
SUNY Health Science Center at Syracuse
Syracuse, New York 13210
(315) 464-5573

Patient Number_____   Recorded on _____

Last Name _____   First Name _____

Address _____

City_____   State_____   Zip_____

Phone (____)_____   Occupation _____

Date of Birth _____   Sex _____   SS# _____

Hospital Number_____   Smoker_____   Drinker_____

Video Tape Number_____   Counter_____   Additional Videos?_____

Problem_____
_____
_____
_____

Major Category_____   Minor Category_____

Referred by_____   Examined by _____

ENT Exam_____
_____
_____
_____

Acoustic Data?_____   Strobe Data_____   Air Flow Data _____

Comments:

November 1988

COMMUNICATION DISORDER UNIT
SUNY Health Science Center
Syracuse, New York

VOICE HISTORY AND EVALUATION

Patient's name:_____ DOB:_____ Age:_____ Date of Eval:_____

Referred by:_____ Medical Dx _____

Complaint as stated by patient:_____

HISTORY OF PROBLEM: [onset, duration, prior episodes, treatment, effect]

I. VOICE SYMPTOM HISTORY:
  A. Variability/Consistency [use related, situational, physical well-being, time of day]:

  B. Associated Symptoms and Sensations [pain, dryness, tickle, lump, strain, fatigue, dysphagia, weight loss, heartburns slurred speech]:

— —

  CLINICAL OBSERVATIONS AND PHYSIOLOGICAL IMPLICATIONS:
    1. Perceptual Observations: Physiological Correlates:

    2. Behavioral Observations: Physiological Correlates:

— —

II. VOICE USE HISTORY:
  A. Talking [how much, where, how, to whom]

  B. Other voice use [singing, acting, sound effects, throat clear]

III. HEALTH HISTORY:
  A. Present health [neurological, respiratory, allergy, psychiatric, gastrointestinal, endocrine/hormonal, chronic conditions]:

  B. Past health [relevant to present problems]:

  C. Surgery [laryngeal, thyroid, cardiac, thoracic, intubation]:

  D. Trauma/Substance or Environmental Exposure [accident, assault, chemical ingestion, smoke, noxious gasses, burn, inhalation, noise]:

E. Substance Use [tobacco, alcohol, medications, illicit durgs]:

— —

CLINICAL OBSERVATIONS:
    IMPRESSIONS OF GENERAL HEALTH   PHYSIOLOGICAL IMPLICATIONS

— —

IV. SOCIAL, OCCUPATION, RECREATION HISTORY [family constellation, living arrangements, life style, job description, exercise programs, hobbies]

V. VOCAL FUNCTION TESTING:
    A. Phonational Range: low: _____ Hz   high: _____ Hz
    B. Speaking Fundamental Frequency: _____ Hz
    C. Dynamic Range: low: _____ dB   high _____ dB
    D. S/Z Ratio   [3x each]

         s ___ sec.   z ___ sec.   Mean s = ___ sec.
         s ___ sec.   z ___ sec.   Mean z = ___ sec.
         s ___ sec.   z ___ sec.   S/Z ratio = ___ sec.

    E. Sustained /a/ [3x]

         1. ___ sec   2. ___ sec   3. ___ sec   Mean = ___ sec
         steady ___   interrupted ___   tremor ___

    F. Frequency Perturbation [jitter]:
    G. Amplitude Perturbation [shimmer]:
    H. Lab Studies:
         1. Airflow data

         2. EGG

         3. Spectrography

         4. Fiberoptic, Stroboscopic etc.

VI. AUDIOLOGICAL EVALUATION [attach report or summarize]

VII. PERCEPTUAL CHARACTERISTICS:
    A. Quality:

    B. Pitch:

    C. Inflection:

    D. Rate:

VIII. ABILITY TO MODIFY VOCAL BEHAVIOR [pitch and loudness variability, easy onset, reflexive acts, etc.]

IX. DIAGNOSTIC IMPRESSIONS:

X. RECOMMENDATIONS:

XI. PROGNOSTIC CONSIDERATIONS

REPORTS TO:

_____

SPEECH PATHOLOGIST

SUNY HEALTH SCIENCE CENTER
Dept. of Otolaryngology
and Communication Sciences
Voice Evaluation Laboratory

STANDARD PROTOCOL - FIBEROPTIC ASSESSMENT

1. Observe larynx at rest.
   Instructions to patient.   Just sit quietly for a moment.

2. Observe deep inspiration.
   Instruction to patient: I want you to take a deep breath, and release it. Then do it two more
   times.

3. Observe sustained vowel phonation at comfortable (modal) pitch (3x) Repetitions.
   Instruction to patient: I'd like you to say /ee/ at a pitch that is comfortable for you and hold
   on to it for a few seconds. (Can be modelled.) (may be repeated
   using /oo/)

4. Observe sustained vowel phonation at elevated pitch (3x) Repetitions.
   Instruction to patient: Now I'd like you to do the same thing, hold on to that /ee/ but at a
   high pitch. (Can be modelled) (may be repeated using /oo/.)
   Alternate instruction: If patient does not elevate pitch, request the sound of a baby kitten,
   the squeal of a mouse, etc. It may be helpful to model these sounds.

5. Observe dynamics of pitch change.
   Instruction to patient: I want you to start with that high sound and let your voice glide down
   to a deep sound, like this: model a downward glissando. (3x) Repetitions
   Now let's start at the bottom low note and let your voice glide upward,
   like this: model an upward glide. (3x) Repetitions
   Alternate instruction: If patient has difficulty with this task, request a wolf howl sound that starts
   on a low /ah/ and glides up on an /oo/. It is helpful to model.

6. Observe speech.
   Instruction to patient: Please repeat each of these sentences twice.
   a. See the busy bees.
   b. We eat green beans.
   c. Do queens eat honey?
   d. Who hoots at the moon?
   e. Do you chew your food?

7. Observe non-phonatory laryngeal behavior.
   Instruction to patient: I'd like you to whistle for me like this: (model a few short interrupted
   bursts of whistle)
   Now I'd like you to whistle a little bit of Happy Birthday.
   If patient cannot whistle, a "pretend" whistle is acceptable.

8. Period of diagnostic therapy.
   The instructions to the patient will depend on the vocal maneuvers you wish to elicit. It is appropriate
   at this time to follow-up on any of the above activities if behaviors of interest were noted, or if you
   wish to make another attempt to teach a task. If a particular type of voice usage is of concern, for
   example, the high notes in singing or during lecturing, it is helpful to obtain a sample of that behavior.

SUNY Health Science Center
Department of Otolaryngology &
    Communication Sciences
Voice Evaluation Laboratory

Chart no._____
Date:_____
Tape no._____

STROBOSCOPIC ASSESSMENT

Name:_____ (M or F)   Age: _____

Clinical Diagnosis_____

	Smooth Straight				Rough Irregular	**COMMENTS**
						FO _____ SPL:_____
Voice Fold R	1	2	3	4	5	Voice quality_____
Edge L	1	2	3	4	5	_____

	Complete	Ant. Chink	Irreg.	Bowing	Post. Chink	Hour-glass	In-complete
Glottic Closure							

Phase Closure	Open phase predominates (whisper) 1	2	Normal 3	4	Closed phase predominates (hyperadduction) 5

Vertical level vf approx.	Equal 1	R. lower 2	L. lower 3	Questionable 4

		Normal	Slightly Decreased	Moderately Decreased	Severely Decreased	No Visible Movement
Amplitude R		1	2	3	4	5
L		1	2	3	4	5

		Normal	Slightly Decreased	Moderately Decreased	Severely Decreased	Absent
Mucosal Wave R		1	2	3	4	5
L		1	2	3	4	5

	Always fully present	Partial absence sometimes	Partial absence always	Complete absence sometimes	Complete absence always
Vibratory Behavior R	1	2	3	4	5
L	1	2	3	4	5

Phase Symmetry	Regular 1	Sometimes Irregular 2	Mostly Irregular 3	Always Irregular 4

Periodicity (regularity)	Regular 1	Sometimes Irregular 2	Mostly Irregular 3	Always Irregular 4

Ventricular Folds: Symmetry of movement: 1. R>L   2. L>R   3. Equal

Movement:	Normal	Sl. Compress	Mod. Compress	Full Compress
	1	2	3	4

Arytenoids: Symmetry of movement: 1. R>L   2. L>R   3. Equal

Movement:	Normal	Fair	Poor
	1	2	3

Hyperfunction: 1. not present   2. sometimes present   3. always present

Based on a form developed at the University of Wisconsin Voice Clinic, Madison, WS, Diane Bless, Ph.D., Director.

REFERENCES

Adran GM, Demp FH, Marland PM, (1954), Laryngeal palsy. Br J Radiol, 27:201–209.

Alberti PW, (1978), The diagnostic role of laryngeal stroboscopy. Otolaryngol Clin North Am, 11:347–354.

Allen EL, Hollien H, (1973), A laminagraphic study of pulse (vocal fry) register phonation. Folia Phoniatr, 25:241–250.

American Joint Committee for Cancer Staging and End Results Reporting, (1983), (2nd ed.), Philadelphia: JB Lippincott.

American Psychiatric Association, (1987). Diagnostic and Statistical Manual of Mental Disorders: DSM-III-R (3rd ed.), Washington, DC: American Psychiatric Association.

Aminoff MJ, Dedo HH, Izdebski K, (1978), Clinical aspects of spasmodic dysphonia. J Neurosurg Psychiatr, 41:361–365.

Ardran G, Kinsbourne M, Rushworth G, (1966), Dysphonia due to tremor. J Neurol Neurosurg Psychiatr, 29:219–223.

Aring CD, (1965), Supranuclear (pseudobulbar) palsy. Arch Int Med, 115:19.

Arnold GE, (1962), Vocal nodules and polyps: Laryngeal tissue reaction to habitual hyperkinetic dysphonia. J Speech Hear Disord, 27:205–217.

Arnold GE, (1959), Spastic dysphonia I: Changing interpretation of a persistent affliction. Logos, 2:3–14.

Arnold GE, (1973), Disorders of laryngeal function. In: Otolaryngology (Vol. 3), Paparella MM, Shumrick DA (eds.), Philadelphia: WB Saunders, pp. 631–648.

Arnold GE, (1980), Disorders of laryngeal function. In: Otolaryngology (Vol. 3), Paparella MM, Shumrick DA (eds.), Philadelphia: WB Saunders, pp. 2470–2488.

Arnold J, (1894), Myelocyste, transposition von Gewebskeimen und Sympodie. Bietr path Anat, 16:1–28.

Arnold KS, Emanuel FW, (1979), Spectral noise levels and roughness severity ratings for vowels produced by male children. J Speech Hear Res, 22:613–626.

Aronson AE, Peterson HW, Litin EM, (1966), Psychiatric symptomatology in functional dysphonia and aphonia. J Speech Hear Disord, 31:115–127.

Aronson AE, Brown JR, Litin EM, Pearson JS, (1968a), Spastic dysphonia I. Voice, neurologic, and psychiatric aspects. J Speech Hear Disord, 33:203–218.

Aronson AE, Brown JR, Litin EM, Pearson JS, (1968b), Spastic dysphonia II. Comparison with essential (voice) tremor and other neurologic and psychogenic dysphonias. J Speech Hear Disord, 33:220–231.

Aronson AE, (1973), Psychogenic Voice Disorders, Philadelphia: WB Saunders.

Aronson AE, DeSanto LW, (1981), Adductor spastic dysphonia: 1 1/2 years after recurrent laryngeal nerve resection. Ann Otol Rhinol Laryngol, 90:1–6.

Aronson AE, Hartman DE, (1981), Adductor spastic dysphonia as a sign of essential (voice) tremor. J Speech Hear Disord, 33:52–58.

Aronson AE, DeSanto LW, (1983), Adductor spastic dysphonia: Three years after recurrent laryngeal nerve resection. Laryngoscope, 93:1–8.

Aronson AE, (1985), Clinical Voice Disorders: An Interdisciplinary Approach, New York: Brian C. Decker.

Baer T, (1979), Vocal jitter: A neuromuscular explanation. In: Transcripts of the Eighth Symposium: Care of the Professional Voice (Part II), Lawrence V (ed.), New York: The Voice Foundation, pp. 19–22.

Baer T, Lofqvist A, McGarr N, (1983), Laryngeal vibrations: A comparison between high-speed filming and glottographic techniques. J Acoust Soc Am, 73:1304–1308.

Baken RJ, (1977), Estimation of lung volume change from torso hemicircumferences. J Speech Hear Res, 20:808–812.

Baken RJ, (1987), Clinical Measurement of Speech and Voice. Boston: College Hill Press.

Baker AB, (ed.), (1958), An Outline of Clinical Neurology, Dubuque, IA: William Brown & Co.

Balestrieri F, Watson C, (1982), Intubation granuloma. Otolaryngol Clin North Am, 15:567–579.

Ball J, Lloyd J, (1971), Myasthenia gravis as hysteria or the sounds of silence. Med J Australia, 1:1018–1020.

Ballantyne J, (1971), Occupational disorders of the larynx. In: Scott-Brown's Diseases of the Ear, Nose and Throat (Vol. 4), Ballantyne J, Groves J (eds.), Philadelphia: JB Lippincott, pp. 541–557.

Ballantyne JC, Groves J, (1978), A Synopsis of Otolaryngology (3rd ed.), Bristol: John Wright and Sons.

Ballenger JJ, (1985), Diseases of the Nose, Throat, Ear, Head and Neck (13th ed.), Philadelphia: Lea & Febiger.

Barker KD, Wilson FB, (1967), Comparative study of vocal utilization of children with hoarseness and normal voice. Paper presented at the convention of the American Speech Language Hearing Association, Chicago.

Barlow SM, Netsell R, Hunker CJ, (1986), Phonatory disorders associated with CNS lesions. In: Otolaryngology—Head Neck Surgery (Vol. 3), Cummings C, Fredrickson J, Harker L, Krause C, Schuller D (eds.), St. Louis: CV Mosby, pp. 2087–2093.

Barton RT, (1979), Treatment of spastic dysphonia by recurrent laryngeal nerve section. Laryngoscope, 89:244–249.

Basmajian JV, (1979), Muscles Alive: Their Functions Revealed by Electromyography, Baltimore: Williams & Wilkins.

Bassich CJ, Ludlow CL, (1986), The use of perceptual methods by new clinicians for assessing voice quality. J Speech Hear Disord, 51:125–133.

Bastian RW, (1985), Laryngeal biofeedback for voice modification. In: Transcripts of the Fourteenth Symposium: Care of the Professional Voice, Lawrence V, (ed.), New York: The Voice Foundation, pp. 330–333.

Bastian RW, (1986), Benign mucosal disorders, saccular disorders and neoplasms. In: Otolaryngology—Head Neck Surgery (Vol. 3), Cummings C, Fredrickson J, Harker L, Krause C, Schuller D (eds.), St. Louis: CV Mosby, pp. 1965–1987.

Bastian RW, (1987), Laryngeal image feedback for voice disorder patients. J Voice, 1:279–282.

Bauer H, Kent R, (1987), Acoustic analysis of infant structure fricative and trill vocalization. J Acoust Soc Am, 81:505–511.

Beasley D, Davis G, (eds.), (1981), Aging Communication Processes and Disorders, New York: Grune & Stratton, pp. 22–45.

Beck C, Richstein A, (1982), Medianverlagerung einer paretischen Stimmlippe durch partielle Schildknorpelimpression. Laryngol Rhinol Otol (Stuttg), 61:251.

Beckett RL, Thoelke W, Cowan L, (1971), A normative study of air flow in children. Br J Disord Commun, 6:13–17.

Belmont JR, Grundfast K, (1984), Congenital laryngeal stridor (laryngomalacia): Etiologic factors and associated disorders. Ann Otol Rhinol Laryngol, 93:430–437.

Benjamin B, Croxson G, (1985), Vocal cord granulomas. Ann Otol Rhinol Laryngol, 94:538–541.

Benjamin BN, Gatenby PA, Kitchen R, Harrison H, Cameron K, Basten A, (1988), Alpha-interferon (Wellferon) as an adjunct to standard surgical therapy in the management of recurrent respiratory papillomatosis. Ann Otol Rhinol Laryngol, 97:376–380.

Bennett S, Bishop S, Lumpkin S, (1987), Phonatory characteristics associated with bilateral diffuse polypoid degeneration. Laryngoscope, 97:446–450.

Bernstein L, Bernstein RS, (1985), Interviewing, A Guide for Health Professionals (4th ed.), Norwalk, CT: Appleton-Century-Crofts.

Bless DM, Miller J, (1972), Influence of mechanical and linguistic factors on lung volume effects during speech. Paper presented at convention of American Speech Language Hearing Association, San Francisco.

Bless DM, Hunker C, Weismer G, (1981), Comparison of noninvasive methods to obtain chestwall displacement and aerodynamic measures during speech. In: Transcripts of the Tenth Symposium: Care of the Professional Voice, Lawrence V (ed.), New York: The Voice Foundation, pp. 43–51.

Bless DM, Hirano M, (1982), Verbal instructions: A critical variable in obtaining optimal performance for maximum phonation time. Paper presented at convention of American Speech Language Hearing Association, Toronto.

Bless DM, Abbs JH, (eds.), (1983), Vocal Fold Physiology: Contemporary Research and Clinical Issues. San Diego: College Hill Press.

Bless DM, Brandenburg JH, (1983), Stroboscopic evaluation of ''functional'' voice disorders. Paper presented at the Middle section of the Triologic Society, Madison, WI.

Bless DM, Hirano M, Feder RJ, (1987), Videostroboscopic evaluation of the larynx. Ear Nose Throat J, 66:289–296.

Blitzer A, Lovelace RE, Brin MF, Fahn S, Fink ME, (1985), Electromyographic findings in focal laryngeal dystonia (spastic dysphonia). Ann Otol Rhinol Laryngol, 94:591–594.

Blitzer A, Brin MF, Fahn S, Lovelace RE, (1988), Localized injections of botulinum toxin for the treatment of focal laryngeal dystonia (spastic dysphonia). Laryngoscope, 98:193–197.

Bloch P, (1965), Neuro-psychiatric aspects of spastic dysphonia. Folia Phoniatr, 17:301–364.

Blum RH, (1960), The Management of the Doctor-Patient Relationship, New York: McGraw-Hill.

Boone DR, (1977), The Voice and Voice Therapy (2nd ed.), Englewood Cliffs, NJ: Prentice-Hall.

Boone DR, (1983), The Voice and Voice Therapy (3rd ed.), Englewood Cliffs, NJ: Prentice-Hall.

Boone DR, (1987), Human Communication and Its Disorders, Englewood Cliffs, NJ: Prentice-Hall.

Boone DR, (1988), Respiratory training in voice therapy. J Voice, 2:20–25.

Botez MI, Barbeau A, (1971), Role of subcortical structures and particularly of the thalamus in the mechanisms of speech and language. Int J Neurol, 8:300–320.

Bouchayer M, Cornut G, Witzig E, Loire R, Roch J, Bastian R, (1985), Epidermoid cysts, sulci and mucosal bridges of the true vocal cord: A report of 157 cases. Laryngoscope, 95:1087–1094.

Brandt JF, Ruder KF, Shipp T, (1969), Vocal loudness and effort in continuous speech. J Acoust Soc Am, 46:1543–1548.

Brantigan CO, Brantigan TA, Joseph N, (1982), Effects of beta blockade and beta stimulation on stage fright. Am J Med, 72:88–94.

Brewer DW, Gould L, (1974), Pyriform sinus: Functional visualization. Ann Otol Rhinol Laryngol, 83:720–724.

Brewer DW, McCall GN, (1974), Visible laryngeal changes during voice therapy. Ann Otol Rhinol Laryngol, 83:423–427.

Brewer DW, Brodnitz F, Gould WJ, Lawrence VL, Monaghan J, Pratt D, Titze IR, Vaughan C, (1979), Medical care for professional voice: Panel discussion. In: Transcripts of the Seventh Symposium: Care of the Professional Voice, Lawrence V (ed.), New York: The Voice Foundation, pp. 8–38.

Briant TDR, Blair RL, Cole P, Singer L, (1983), Laboratory investigation of abnormal voice. J Otolaryngol, 12:285–290.

Broad DJ, (1973), Phonation. In: Normal Aspects of Speech, Hearing and Language, Minifie FD, Hixon TJ, Williams F (eds.), Englewood Cliffs, NJ: Prentice-Hall, pp. 127–167.

Brodie K, Colton RH, Swisher L, (1988), Reliability of inverse filtered and EGG measurements of vocal function. Unpublished manuscript.

Brodnitz F, (1976), Spastic dysphonia. Ann Otolaryngol, 85:210–214.

Brown JE, Simonson J, (1963), Organic voice tremor. Neurology, 13:520–525.

Brown JR, Darley FL, Aronson AE, (1970), Ataxic dysarthria. Int J Neurol, 7:302–318.

Browne, K, Freeling P, (1976), The Doctor-Patient Relationship (2nd ed.), New York: Churchill Livingstone.

Burch PR, (1981), Passive smoking and lung cancer. Br Med J, 282:1393.

Canter GJ, (1963), Speech characteristics of patients with Parkinson's disease I. Intensity, pitch and duration. J Speech Hear Disord, 28:221–229.

Canter GJ, (1965), Speech characteristics of patients with Parkinson's disease II: Physiological support for speech. J Speech Hear Disord, 30:44–49.

Carpenter R, McDonald T, Howard F, (1978), The otolaryngologic presentation of amyotrophic lateral sclerosis. Otolaryngology, 86:479–484.

Carrow E, Rivera V, Mauldin M, Shamblin L, (1974), Deviant speech characteristics in motor neuron disease. Arch Otolaryngol, 100:212–218.

Caruso A, Burton EK, (1987), Temporal acoustic measures of dysarthia associated with amyotrophic lateral sclerosis. J Speech Hear Res, 30:80–87.

Case, JL, (1984), Clinical Management of Voice Disorders, Rockville, MD: Aspen Publications.

Casper JK, Brewer DW, Conture EG, (1981), Speech therapy patient evaluation techniques with the fiberscope. In: Transcripts of the Tenth Symposium: Care of the Professional Voice (Part II), Lawrence V (ed.), New York: The Voice Foundation, pp. 136–140.

Casper JK, (1983), Frequency perturbation in normal speakers: A descriptive and methodological study. Ph.D. dissertation, Syracuse University, Syracuse, NY.

Casper JK, Colton RH, Brewer DW, (1985), Selected therapy techniques and laryngeal physiological changes in patients with vocal fold immobility. In: Transcripts of the Fourteenth Symposium: Care of the Professional Voice (Part II), Lawrence V (ed.), New York: The Voice Foundation, pp. 318–323.

Casper JK, Brewer DW, Colton RH, (1987a), Variations in normal human laryngeal anatomy and physiology as viewed fiberscopically. J Voice, 1:180–185.

Casper JK, Brewer DW, Colton RH, (1987b), Pitfalls and problems in flexible fiberoptic videolaryngoscopy. J Voice, 1:347–352.

Casper JK, Colton RH, Brewer DW, Woo P,

(1989), Investigation of selected voice therapy techniques. Paper presented at the Eighteenth Annual Symposium: Care of the Professional Voice, Philadelphia.

Chapey R, Salzberg A, (1981), The speech clinician's use of fiberoptics in indirect laryngoscopy. J Commun Dis, 14:87–90.

Charcot M, (1881), Lectures on the Diseases of the Nervous System, London: The New Sydenham Society.

Cherry J, Margulies S, (1968), Contact ulcers of the larynx. Laryngoscope, 73:1937–1940.

Chevrie-Muller C, Arabia-Guidet C, Pfauwadel M, (1987), Can one recover from spasmodic dysphonia? Br J Disord Comm, 22:117–128.

Chiari H, (1896), Ueber Veranderungen des Kleinhirns des Pons und der Medulla Oblongata in Folge von congenitaler Hydrocephalie des Grosshirns. Denkschr Akad Wiss Wien, 63:71–116.

Childers DG, Naik J, Larar J, Krishnamurthy A, Moore GP, (1983), Electroglottography, speech and ultra high speed cinematography. In: Vocal Fold Physiology: Biomechanics, Acoustics and Phonatory Control, Titze I, Scherer R (eds.), Denver: Denver Center for the Performing Arts, pp. 202–220.

Childers DG, Smith AM, Moore GP, (1984), Relationships between electroglottograph, speech, and vocal cord contact. Folia Phoniatr, 36:105–118.

Childers DG, Krishnamurthy AK, (1985), A critical review of electroglottography. CRC Crit Reviews Bioengineering, 12:131–161.

Chipman SF, Carey S, (1975), Anatomy of a stimulus domain: The relation between multidimensional and unidimensional scaling of noise bands. Perception Psychophysics, 17:417–424.

Chisnall B, (1977), Increase in house fires. Fire Protection, 4:119–121.

Chodosh PL, (1977), Gastro-esophageal-pharyngeal reflux. Laryngoscope, 87:1418–1427.

Christopher KL, Wood RP II, Eckert RC, Blager FB, Raney RA, Souhrada JF, (1983), Vocal cord dysfunction presenting as asthma. N Engl J Med, 308:1566–1570.

Cisler J, (1927), Sur les troubles du language articulé et de la phonation au cours de l'encephalite épidémique. Arch Inter Laryngol, 33:1054–1057.

Close LG, Catlin FI, Cohn AM, (1980), Acute and chronic effects of ammonia burns on the respiratory tract. Arch Otol, 106:151–158.

Cohen SR, Geller KA, Birns JW, Thompson JW, (1982), Laryngeal paralysis in children: A long term retrospective study. Ann Otol Rhinol Laryngol, 91:417–424.

Coleman RF, Wendahl R, (1967), Vocal roughness and stimulus duration. Speech Monogr, 34:85–92.

Coleman RF, Mabis JH, Hinson JK, (1977), Fundamental frequency-sound pressure level profiles of adult male and female voices. J Speech Hear Res, 20:197–204.

Coleman RO, (1971), Male and female voice quality and its relationship to vowel formant frequencies. J Speech Hear Res, 14:565–577.

Coleman RO, (1973), Speaker identification in the absence of inter-subject differences in glottal source characteristics. J Acoust Soc Am, 53:1741–1743.

Coleman RO, (1976), A comparison of the contributions of two voice quality characteristics to the perception of maleness and femaleness in the voice. J Speech Hear Res, 19:168–180.

Colton RH, (1972), Phonational range in the modal and falsetto registers. J Speech Hear Res, 15:708–713.

Colton RH, (1973), Vocal intensity in the modal and falsetto registers. J Speech Hear Res, 25:62–70.

Colton RH, Brown WS, (1973), Some relationships between vocal effort and intraoral air pressure. J Acoust Soc Am, 53:296.

Colton RH, Sagerman R, Chung C, Young Y, Reed G, (1978), Voice change after radiotherapy. Radiology, 127:821–824.

Colton RH, Estill J, (1981), Elements of voice quality: Perceptual, acoustic and physiologic aspects. In: Speech and Language: Advances in Basic Research and Practice (Vol. 5), Lass N (ed.), New York: Academic Press, pp. 311–403.

Colton RH, Estill JE, Gertsman L, (1981), Identification of four selected voice qualities by spectral analysis. Paper presented at Vocal Fold Physiology Conference, Madison, WI.

Colton RH, (1982), Acoustic characteristics of older speakers. Unpublished manuscript.

Colton RH, Reed G, Sagerman R, Chung C, (1982), An investigation of voice change after radiotherapy. Final report, Grant # CA17962, National Cancer Institute, National Institutes of Health, Bethesda, MD.

Colton RH, Brewer D, Rothenberg M, (1983), Evaluating vocal function. J Otolaryngol, 12:291–294.

Colton RH, Brewer DW, (1985), Fiberoptic/vibratory relationships in patients with voice disorders. In: Transcripts of the Fourteenth Symposium: Care of the Professional Voice (Part I), Lawrence V (ed.), New York: The Voice Foundation, pp. 271–275.

Colton RH, Brewer DW, Rothenberg M, (1985), Vibratory characteristics of patients with voice disorders. Unpublished manuscript.

Colton RH, (1987), The role of pitch in the discrimination of voice quality. J Voice, 1:240–245.

Colton RH, (1988), Physiological mechanisms of

vocal frequency control: The role of tension. J Voice, 2:208–220.

Conrad WC, (1984), The importance of applying supraglottal resistance for producing controlled phonation. In: Transcripts of the Thirteenth Symposium Care of the Professional Voice (Part I), Lawrence V (ed.), New York: The Voice Foundation, pp. 19–24.

Conture EG, Cudahy E, Caruso A, Schwartz H, Brewer D, Casper J, (1981), Computer assisted measures of video taped data: A description and case study. In: Transcripts of the Tenth Symposium: Care of the Professional Voice (Part II), Lawrence V (ed.), New York: The Voice Foundation, pp. 129–135.

Conture EG, Schwartz H, Brewer D, (1985), Laryngeal behavior during stuttering: A further study. J Speech Hear Res, 28:233–240.

Cooper D, Titze, I,(1983), Generation and transfer of heat in the vocal folds. In: Vocal Fold Physiology Biomechanics, Acoustics and Phonatory Control, Titze I, Shearer R (eds.), Denver: The Denver Center for the Performing Arts, pp. 318–327.

Cooper M, (1973), Modern Techniques of Vocal Rehabilitation, Springfield, IL: Charles C Thomas.

Cooper M, Cooper MH, (eds.), (1977), Approaches to Vocal Rehabilitation, Springfield, IL: Charles C Thomas.

Cooper M, (1984), Change Your Voice, Change Your Life, New York: Macmillan.

Cotton RT, Richardson MA, (1981), Congenital laryngeal anomalies. Otolaryngol Clin North Am, 14:203–218.

Crapo RO, (1981), Smoke inhalation injuries. JAMA, 246:1694–1696.

Critichley M, (1949), Observations on essential (heredofamilial) tremor. Brain, 72:9–139.

Crumley RL, (1983), Phrenic nerve graft for bilateral vocal cord paralysis. Laryngoscope, 93:425–428.

Cudmore RE, Vivori E, (1981), Inhalation injury to the respiratory tract of children. Prog Ped Surg, 14:173–188.

Cummings CW, (1986), Bilateral vocal cord paralysis/ankylosis. In: Otolaryngology—Head Neck Surgery (Vol. 3), Cummings C, Fredrickson J, Harker L, Krause C, Schuller D (eds.), St. Louis: CV Mosby Company, pp. 2181–2189.

Damste PH, (1964), Virilization of the voice due to anabolic steroids. Folia Phoniatr, 16:10–18.

Damste PH, (1967), Voice change in adult women caused by virilizing agents. J Speech Hear Disord, 32:126–132.

Damste PH, (1970), Phonogram: A new method for evaluating voice characteristics. Otologia (Fukuoka), 18:428–440.

Daniloff R, Schuckers G, Feth L, (1980), The Physiology of Speech and Hearing: An Introduction, Englewood Cliffs, NJ: Prentice-Hall.

Darley F, Aronson A, Brown J, (1968), Motor speech signs in neurologic disease. Med Clin North Am, 52:835–844.

Darley FL, Aronson AE, Brown JR, (1969a), Clusters of deviant speech dimensions in the dysarthrias. J Speech Hear Res, 12:462–496.

Darley FL, Aronson AE, Brown JR, (1969b), Differential diagnostic patterns of dysarthria. J Speech Hear Res, 12:246–269.

Darley FL, Brown JR, Goldstein NH, (1972), Dysarthria in multiple sclerosis. J Speech Hear Res, 15:229–245.

Darley FL, Aronson AE, Brown JR,(1975), Motor Speech Disorders. Philadelphia: WB Saunders.

Darley FL, Spriestersbach DC, (1978), Diagnostic Methods in Speech Pathology (2nd ed.), New York: Harper & Row.

Davis PJ, Boone DR, Carroll RL, Darvenzia P, Harrison GA, (1988), Adductor spastic dysphonia: Heterogeneity of physiologic and phonatory characteristics. Ann Otol Rhinol Laryngol, 97:179–185.

Davis SB, (1981), Acoustic characteristics of normal and pathological voices. In: Proceedings of the Conference on the Assessment of Vocal Pathology, Ludlow CL, Hart MO (eds.), Rockville, MD: American Speech Language Hearing Association, pp. 97–115.

Dedo HH, (1976), Recurrent nerve section for spastic dysphonia. Ann Otol Rhinol Laryngol, 85:451–459.

Dedo HH, Izdebski K, Townsend JJ, (1977), Recurrent laryngeal nerve histopathology in spastic dysphonia. Ann Otol Rhinol Laryngol, 86:806–812.

Dedo HH, Townsend J, Izdebski K, (1978), Current evidence for the organic etiology of spastic dysphonia. Otolaryngology, 86:875–880.

Dedo HH, Izdebski K, (1981), Surgical treatment of spastic dysphonia. Contemp Surg, 18:75–90.

Dedo HH, Izdebski K, (1983), Problems with surgical (RLN section) treatment of spastic dysphonia. Laryngoscope, 93:268–271.

Dejonckere PH, Lebacq J, (1985), Electroglottography and vocal nodules: An attempt to quantify the shape of the signal. Folia Phoniatr, 37:195–200.

Delahunty JE, Cherry J, (1968), Experimentally produced vocal cord granulomas. Laryngoscope, 78:1941–1947.

Delahunty JE, (1972), Acid laryngitis. J Laryng Otol, 86:335–342.

DeWeese DD, Saunders WH, (1982), Textbook of Otolaryngology (6th ed.), St. Louis: CV Mosby.

Dickson DR, Maue-Dickson WM, (1982), Anatomical and Physiological Bases of Speech, Boston: Little, Brown & Co.

Diehl CF, (1960), Voice and Personality, In: Psychological and Psychiatric Aspects of Speech and Hearing, Barbara DA (ed.), Springfield, IL: Charles C Thomas, pp. 171–203.

Dordain M, Dordain G,(1972), L'epreuve du A tenu au cours des tremblements de la voix (tremblement idiopathique et dyskinesie volitionnelle. Leurs rapports avec la dysphonie spasmodique). Rev Laryngol Otol Rhinol (Bord), 93:167–182.

Dyer RF, Esch VH, (1976), Polyvinyl chloride toxicity in fires. JAMA, 235:393–397.

Eccles JC, (1977), The Understanding of the Brain, New York: McGraw-Hill, pp. 121–145.

Eckel F, Boone DR, (1981), The s/z ratio as an indicator of laryngeal pathology. J Speech Hear Disord, 46:147–149.

Emanuel F, Sansone F, (1969), Some spectral features of normal and simulated "rough" vowels. Folia Phoniatr, 21:401–415.

Faaborg-Andersen K, (1957), Electromyographic investigation of intrinsic laryngeal muscles in humans: An investigation of subjects with normally movable vocal cords and patients with vocal cord paresis. Acta Physiol (Scand), 41(Suppl 140):1–148.

Fairbanks GF, Herbert EL, Hammond JM, (1949), An acoustical study of vocal pitch in seven-and eight-year old girls. Child Develop, 20:71–78.

Fairbanks GF, Wiley JH, Lassman FM,(1949), An acoustical study of vocal pitch in 7 and 8 year old boys. Child Develop, 20:63–69.

Fairbanks GF, (1960), Voice and Articulation Drillbook (2nd ed.), New York: Harper & Row.

Fant G, (1960), Acoustic Theory of Speech Production, The Hague: Mouton.

Farmakides MN, Boone DR, (1960), Speech problems of patients with multiple sclerosis. J Speech Hear Disord, 25:385–390.

Feder R, (1986), On standardizing the laryngeal examination. Arch Otolaryngol Head Neck Surg, 112:145.

Feder RJ, Michell MJ, (1984), Hyperfunctional, hyperacidic and intubation granulomas. Arch Otolaryngol, 110:582–584.

Fendler M, Shearer W, (1988), Reliability of the s/z ratio in normal children's voices. Lang Speech Hear Ser Sch, 19:2–4.

Fex S, (1970), Judging the movements of vocal cords in laryngeal paralysis. Acta Otolaryngol, 263(suppl):82–83.

Finitzo T, Pool KD, Freeman FJ, Cannito MP, Schaefer SD, (1987), Spasmodic dysphonia subsequent to head trauma. Arch Otolaryngol Head Neck Surg, 113:1107–1110.

Finitzo-Hieber T, Freeman FJ, Gerling IJ, Dobson L, Schaefer S,(1982), Auditory brainstem response abnormalities in adductor spasmodic dysphonia. Am J Otolaryngol, 3:26–30.

Finnegan DE, (1984), Maximum phonation time for children with normal voices. J Commun Disord, 17:309–317.

Finnegan DE, (1985), Maximum phonation time for children with normal voices. Folia Phoniatr, 37:209–215.

Fitch JL, Holbrook A, (1970), Modal vocal fundamental frequency of young adults. Arch Otolaryngol, 92:379–382.

Fitz-Hugh GS, Smith DE, Chiong AT, (1958), Pathology of three hundred clinically benign lesions of the vocal cords. Laryngoscope, 68:855–875.

Flynn PT, (1983), Speech-language pathologists and primary prevention: From ideas to action. Lang Speech Hear Ser Sch, 14:99–104.

Freeman F, (1988), Voice therapy techniques: Fact and fallacy. Paper presented at convention of the American Speech Language Hearing Association, Boston.

Freud ED, (1962), Functions and dysfunctions of the ventricular folds. J Speech Hear Disord, 27:334–340.

Friedmann I, (1973), Granulomas of the larynx. In: Otolaryngology (Vol. 3), Paparella MM, Shumrick DA (eds.), Philadelphia: WB Saunders, pp. 616–630.

Fritzell B, Hammerberg B, Wedin L, (1977), Clinical application of acoustic voice analysis I: Background and perceptual factors. Quarterly Progress and Status Report, Stockholm Speech Transmission Laboratory, Royal Institute of Technology, Stockholm, Sweden, 2–3:31–38.

Fritzell B, Feuer E, Haglund S, Knutsson E, Schiratzki H, (1982), Experiences with recurrent laryngeal nerve section for spastic dysphonia. Folia Phoniatr, 34:160–167.

Fritzell B, Fant G, (eds.), (1986), Voice Acoustics and Dysphonia. J Phonetics, 14(Suppl).

Froeschels E, (1952), Chewing method as therapy. Arch Otol, 56:427–434.

Fujimura O, (1981), Body-cover theory of the vocal fold and its phonetic implications. In: Vocal Fold Physiology, Stevens K, Hirano M (eds.), Tokyo: University of Tokyo Press, pp. 271–288.

Fulton J, Dow R, (1937), The cerebellum: A summary of functional localization. Yale J Biol Med, 10:89–119.

Furukawa M, (1967), Studies on the mechanism of phonation in excised larynges. Pract Otol (Kyoto) 60:145–181.

Garcia M, (1855), Observations of the human voice. Philosophical Mag J Science, 10:511–513.

Gardner E, (1963), Fundamentals of Neurology, Philadelphia: WB Saunders.

Garfinkle T, Kimmelman C, (1982), Neurologic disorders: Amyotrophic lateral sclerosis, myasthenia gravis, multiple sclerosis and poliomyelitis. Am J Otolaryngol, 3:204–212.

Gates GA, Saegert J, Wilson N, Johnson L, Sheppard A, Hearne EA, (1985), The effect of beta blockade on singing performance. Ann Otol Rhinol Laryngol, 94:570–574.

Gates GA, Montalbo PJ, (1987), The effect of low-dose beta blockade on performance anxiety in singers. J Voice, 1:105–108.

Giger HL, (1984), The value of phonetogram studies in clinical work. In: Transcripts of the Thirteenth Symposium: Care of the Professional Voice (Part II), Lawrence V (ed.), New York: The Voice Foundation, pp. 367–370.

Glacer HS, Siegel MJ, (1986), Radiology of the larynx. In: Otolaryngology—Head Neck Surgery, Cummings C, Fredrickson J, Harker L, Krause C, Schuller D (eds.), St. Louis: CV Mosby, pp. 1847–1865.

Golden GS, (1977), Tourette syndrome: The pediatric perspective. Am J Disord Childhood, 131:531–534.

Gould WJ, (1987), Surgery in professional singers. ENT J, 66:327–332.

Gramming P, Gauffin J, Sundberg J, (1986), An attempt to improve the clinical usefulness of phonetograms. J Phonetics, 14:421–428.

Gramming P, Sundberg J, (1987), Spectrum factors relevant to phonetogram measurement. Quarterly Progress and Status Report, Royal Institute of Technology, Stockholm, Sweden, 2–3:39–61.

Gramming P, (1988), The phonetogram: An experimental and clinical study. Ph.D. dissertation, Lund University, Malmo, Sweden.

Grob W, (1953), Course and management of myasthenia gravis. JAMA, 153:529–532.

Grob W, (1961), Myasthenia gravis. Arch Int Med, 108:615–638.

Guidi AM, Bannister R, Gibson WPR, Payne JK, (1981), Laryngeal electromyography in multiple system atrophy with autonomic failure. J Neurol Neurosurg Psychiatr, 44:49–53.

Hallewell J, Cole TB, (1970), Isolated head and neck symptoms due to hiatus hernia. Arch Otolaryngol, 92:499–501.

Hamlet SL, (1972), Vocal fold articulatory activity during whispered speech. Arch Otol, 95:211–312.

Hamlet SL, (1981), Ultra-sound assessment of phonatory function. Proceedings of the Conference on Vocal Pathology, ASHA Reports 11:128–140.

Hammarberg B, Fritzell B, Gauffin J, Sundberg J, Wedin L, (1980), Perceptual and acoustic correlates of abnormal voice qualities. Acta Otolaryngol, 90:441–451.

Hammarberg B, Fritzell B, Schiratzki H, (1984), Teflon injection in 16 patients with paralytic dysphonia, perceptual and acoustic evaluation. J Speech Hear Disord, 49:72–82.

Hammarberg B, Fritzell B, Gauffin J, Sundberg J, (1986), Acoustic and perceptual analysis of vocal dysfunction. J Phonetics, 14:533–548.

Hammond EC, (1966), Smoking in relation to the death rate of 1 million men and women. National Cancer Institute Monogr, 19:127–204.

Hanson DG, Gerratt BR, Ward PH, (1983), Glottographic measurement of vocal dysfunction: A preliminary report. Ann Otol Rhinol Laryngol, 92:413–420.

Hanson DG, Gerratt BR, Ward PH, (1984), Cineradiographic observations of laryngeal function in Parkinson's disease. Laryngoscope, 94:348–353.

Hanson DG, Ludlow C, Bassich C, (1984), Vocal fold paresis in Shy-Drager syndrome. Ann Otol Rhinol Laryngol, 92:85–90.

Hanson DG, Ward PH, Gerratt BR, Berci G, Berke GS, (1989), Diagnosis of neuromuscular impairment. In: Geriatric Otorhinolaryngology, Goldstein JC, Kashima HK, Koopman CF (eds.), Toronto: BC Decker, pp. 71–78.

Hanson WR, Metter EJ, (1980), DAF as instrumental treatment for dysarthria in progressive supranuclear palsy: A case report. J Speech Hear Disord, 45:268–276.

Harden RJ, (1975), Comparison of glottal area changes of measures from ultra high-speed photographs and photoelectric glottographs. J Speech Hear Res, 18:728–738.

Hartman DE, Aronson AE, (1981), Clinical investigations of intermittent breathy dysphonia. J Speech Hear Disord, 46:428–432.

Hartman DE, Vishwanat B, (1984), Spastic dysphonia and essential (voice) tremor treated with primidone. Arch Otolaryngol, 110:394–397.

Hartman DE, Abbs JH, Vishwanat B, (1988), Clinical investigations of adductor spastic dysphonia. Ann Otol Rhinol Laryngol, 97:247–252.

Hatcinski VC, Thomsen IV, Buch NH, (1975), The nature of primary vocal tremor. Can J Neurol Sci, 2:195–197.

Heaver L, (1959), Spastic dysphonia II: Psychiatric considerations. Logos, 2:15–24.

Hecker MH, Kreul EJ, (1971), Descriptions of the speech of patients with cancer of the vocal folds I: Measures of fundamental frequency. J Acoust Soc Am, 49:1275–1282.

Henschen TL, Burton NG, (1978), Treatment of spastic dysphonia by EMG biofeedback. Biofeedback & Self-Regulation, 3:91–96.

Hersen M, Turner SM, (1985), Diagnostic Interviewing, New York: Plenum Press.

Hibi SR, Bless DM, Hirano M, Yoshida T, (1988), Distortions of videofiberoscopy imaging: Reconstruction and correction. J Voice, 2:168–175.

Hill A, (1938), The heat of shortening and the dynamic constants of muscle. Proc Royal Soc, 126:136–195.

Hillman RE, Weinberg B, (1981), A new procedure for venting a reflectionless tube. J Acoust Soc Am, 69:1449–1451.

Hirano M, Koike Y, von Leden H, (1968), Maximum phonation time and air usage during phonation. Folia Phoniatr, 20:185–201.

Hirano M, (1974), Morphological structure of the vocal cord as a vibrator and its variations. Folia Phoniatr, 26:89–94.

Hirano M, Yoshida Y, Matsushita H, Nakajima T, (1974), An apparatus for high speed cinematography of the vocal cords. Ann Otol, 83:12–18.

Hirano M, (1975), Phonosurgery: Basic and clinical investigations. Otologia (Fukuoka), 21:239–242.

Hirano M, Kakita Y, Kawasaki H, Matsushita H, (1977), Vocal cord vibration: Behavior of the layer-structured vibrator in normal and pathological conditions, (16 mm film, also available on videotape), New York: The Voice Foundation.

Hirano M, Kurita S, Matsuo K, Nagata K, (1980), Laryngeal tissue reaction to stress. In: Transcripts of the Seventh Symposium: Care of the Professional Voice (Part II), Lawrence V (ed.), New York: The Voice Foundation, pp. 10–20.

Hirano M, (1981a), Clinical Examination of Voice, Vienna, Austria: Springer-Verlag.

Hirano M, (1981b), Structure of the vocal fold in normal and disease states: Anatomical and physical studies. In: Proceedings of the Conference on the Assessment of Vocal Pathology, Ludlow C, Hart M (eds.), Rockville, MD: American Speech Language Association, pp. 11–30.

Hirano M, Kurita S, Matsuo K, Nagata K, (1981), Vocal fold polyp and polypoid vocal fold (Reinke's edema). J Research in Singing, 4:33–44.

Hirano M, (1983), Epithelial hyperplasia of the larynx. In: Illustrated Handbook of Clinical Otolaryngology (Vol. 4), Hirano M (ed.), Tokyo: Medical View, pp. 100–101.

Hirano M, Feder R, Bless DM, (1983), Clinical evaluation of patients with voice disorders: Stroboscopic evaluation. Paper presented at the convention of the American Speech Language Hearing Association, Cincinnati.

Hirano M, Kurita S, Nakashima T, (1983), Growth, development and aging of human vocal fold. In: Vocal Fold Physiology, Bless DM, Abbs JW (eds.), San Diego: College Hill Press, pp. 22–43.

Hirano M, Matsuo K, Kahita Y, Kawasaki H, Kurita S, (1983), Vibratory behavior versus structure of the vocal fold. In: Vocal Fold Phys-

iology, Titze I, Scherer R (eds.), Denver: Denver Center for the Performing Arts, pp. 26–40.

Hirano M, Kurita S, Kyokawa K, Sato K, (1986), Posterior glottis: Morphological study in excised human larynges. Ann Otol Rhinol Laryngol, 95:576–581.

Hirano M, (1988), Endolaryngeal microsurgery. In: Otolaryngology (Vol. 3), English GM, (ed.), Philadelphia: JB Lippincott, Chapter 43, pp. 1–22.

Hirano M, (1989), Surgical alteration of voice quality. In: Otolaryngology—Head and Neck Surgery (Update I), Cummings CW, Frederickson JM, Harker LA, Krause CJ, Schuller DE (eds.), St Louis: CV Mosby, pp. 239–264.

Hiroto I, Hirano M, Tomita H, (1968), Electromyographic investigation of human vocal cord paralysis. Ann Otol, 77:296–304.

Hiroto I, (1976), Surgical voice improvement for unilateral recurrent laryngeal nerve paralysis. Otologia (Fukuoka), 22:473–474.

Hixon T, (1987), Respiratory Function in Speech and Song, Boston: Little, Brown & Co.

Holbrook A, Rolnick MI, Bailey CW, (1974), Treatment of vocal abuse disorders using a vocal intensity controller. J Speech Hear Disord, 39:298–303.

Holinger LD, (1987), Congenital anomalies of the larynx. In: Otolaryngology (Vol. 3), English GM (ed.), Philadelphia: JB Lippincott, Chapter 15, pp. 1–15.

Holinger P, Brown WT, (1967), Congenital webs cysts, laryngoceles, and other anomalies of the larynx. Ann Otol Rhinol Laryngol, 76:744–752.

Hollien H, (1962), The relationship of vocal fold thickness to absolute fundamental frequency of phonation. In: Proceedings Fourth International Congress of Phonetic Sciences, The Hague: Mouton, pp. 173–177.

Hollien H, Colton RH, (1969), Four laminagraphic studies of vocal fold thickness. Folia Phoniatr, 21:179–198.

Hollien H, Dew D, Philips P, (1971), Phonational frequency ranges of adults. J Speech Hear Res, 14:755–760.

Hollien H, Shipp T, (1972), Speaking fundamental frequency and chronologic age in males. J Speech Hear Res, 15:155–159.

Hollien H, Jackson B, (1973), Normative data on the speaking fundamental frequency characteristics of young adult males. J Phonetics, 19:117–120.

Hollien H, Michel J, Doherty ET, (1973), A method of analyzing vocal jitter in sustained phonation. J Phonetics, 1:85–91.

Hollien H, (1974), On vocal registers. J Phonetics, 2:25–43.

Holmberg ES, Hillman RE, Perkell JS, (1988), Glottal airflow and transglottal air pressure measurements for male and female speakers in soft, normal and loud voice. J Acoust Soc Am, 84:511–529.

Horii Y, Cooke PA, (1978), Some airflow, volume and duration characteristics of oral reading. J Speech Hear Res, 21:470–481.

Horii Y, (1979), Fundamental frequency perturbation observed in sustained phonation. J Speech Hear Res, 22:5–19.

Horii Y, (1980), Vocal shimmer in sustained phonation. J Speech Hear Res, 23:202–209.

Horii Y, (1982), Jitter and shimmer differences among sustained vowels. J Speech Hear Res, 25:12–14.

Horii Y, (1983), Some acoustic characteristics of oral reading by ten- to twelve-year-old children. J Commun Disord, 16:257–267.

House AS, (1959), Note on optimal vocal frequency. J Speech Hear Res, 2:55–60.

House EL, Pansky B, (1967), A Functional Approach to Neuroanatomy, New York: McGraw-Hill.

Hufnagle J, Hufnagle K, (1982), Whisper: Is it harmful to the vocal mechanism? Paper presented at the convention of the American Speech Language Hearing Association, Toronto.

Hufnagle J, Hufnagle K, (1988), S/Z ratio in dysphonic children with and without vocal nodules. Lang Speech Hear Ser Sch, 19:418–422.

Hunt JL, Agee RN, Pruitt BA, (1975), Fiberoptic bronchoscopy in acute inhalation injury. J Trauma, 15:641–648.

Irwin RJ, Mills AW, (1965), Matching loudness and vocal level: An experiment requiring no apparatus. Br J Psychol, 56:143–146.

Isshiki N, (1964), Regulatory mechanism of voice intensity regulation. J Speech Hear Res, 7:17–29.

Isshiki N, von Leden H, (1964), Hoarseness: Aerodynamic studies. Arch Otolaryngol, 80:206–213.

Isshiki N, (1965), Vocal intensity and air flow rate. Folia Phoniatr, 17:92–104.

Isshiki N, (1977), Functional Surgery of the Larynx: With Special Reference to Percutaneous Approach, Kyoto: Maeda Press.

Isshiki N, Tanabe M, Ishizaka K, Board C, (1977), Clinical significance of asymmetrical tension of the vocal cords. Ann Otol Rhinol Laryngol, 86:1–9.

Ivers RR, Goldstein NP, (1963), Multiple sclerosis: A current appraisal of symptoms and signs. Proc Staff Meetings Mayo Clin, 38:457–466.

Iwata S, von Leden H, Williams D, (1972), Air flow measurement during phonation. J Commun Disord, 5:67–79.

Iwata S, Esaki T, Iwami K, Mimura Y, (1976), Air flow studies in patients with laryngeal diseases during phonation. J Nagoya Cy Univ Med Assoc, 26:398–406.

Iwata S, Esaki T, Iwami K, Takasu T, (1976), Laryngeal function in patients with laryngeal polyps after laryngomicrosurgery. Pract Otol (Kyoto), 69:499–506.

Izdebski K, Dedo HH, (1979), Characteristics of vocal tremor in spastic dysphonia: A preliminary study. In: Transcripts of the Eighth Symposium: Care of the Professional Voice (Part III), Lawrence V (ed.), New York: The Voice Foundation, pp. 17–23.

Izdebski K, (1981), Magnetic sound recording in laryngology. Am J Otolaryngol, 2:48–53.

Izdebski K, Dedo HH, Shipp T, (1981), Postoperative and follow-up studies of spastic dysphonia patients treated by recurrent nerve section. Otolaryngol Head Neck Surg, 89:96–101.

Izdebski K, (1983), Practical techniques of office voice recording. Otolaryngol Head Neck Surg, 91:638–642.

Izdebski K, (1984), Overpressure and breathiness in spastic dysphonia. Acta Otolaryngol (Stockh), 97:373–378.

Jackson CL, (1941), Vocal nodules. Transactions Am Laryngol Assoc, 63:185–193.

Jacobsen E, (1938), Progressive Relaxation (2nd ed.), Chicago: University of Chicago Press.

Jako GJ, (1972), Laser surgery of the vocal cords. An experimental study with carbon dioxide lasers on dogs. Laryngoscope, 82:2204–2216.

James IM, Pearson RM, Griffith DNM, Newburg P, (1977), Effect of osprenolol on stage-fright in musicians. Lancet, 2:952–954.

Janzen VD, Rae RE, Hudson AJ, (1988), Otolaryngologic manifestations of amyotrophic lateral sclerosis. J Otolaryngol, 17:41–42.

Jarema AD, Kennedy JL, Shoulson I, (1985), Acoustic and aerodynamic measurements of hyperkinetic dysarthria in Huntington's disease. Paper presented at the convention of the American Speech Language Hearing Association, Washington, DC.

Jensen JR, (1960), A study of certain motor-speech aspects of the speech of multiple sclerotic patients. Ph.D. dissertation, University of Wisconsin, Madison, WI.

Johns ME, Rood SR, (1987), Vocal Cord Paralysis: Diagnosis and Management, Washington, DC: American Academy of Otolaryngology—Head & Neck Surg Foundation, Inc.

Johnson TS, (1983), Treatment of vocal abuse in children. In: Current Therapy of Communication Disorders Voice Disorders, Perkins WH (ed.), New York: Thieme-Stratton, pp. 3–11.

Johnson TS, (1985), Voice disorders: The measurement of clinical progress. In: Speech Disorders in Adults: Recent Advances, Costello J, (ed), San Diego: College Hill Press, pp. 127–154.

Kahane J, (1981), Anatomic and physiologic changes in the aging peripheral speech mechanism. In: Aging Communication Processes and Disorders, Beasley D, Davis G (eds.), New York: Grune & Stratton, pp. 22–45.

Kahane J, (1982), Anatomy and physiology of the organs of the peripheral speech mechanism. In: Speech, Language and Hearing (Vol. 1), Lass NJ, McReynolds LV, Northern JL, Yoder DE (eds.), Philadelphia: WB Saunders, pp. 109–155.

Kahane J, Mayo R, (1989), The need for aggressive pursuit of healthy childhood voices. Lang Speech Hear Ser Sch, 20:102–107.

Kahn HA, (1966), The Dorn study of smoking and mortality amoung US veterans: A report on eight 1/2 years of observation. National Cancer Institute Monogr, 19:1–125.

Kakita Y, Hirano H, Okmaru K, (1981), Physical properities of the vocal fold tissue: Measurements on excised larynges. In: Vocal Fold Physiology, Stevens KN, Hirano M (eds.), Tokyo: University of Tokyo Press, pp. 377–397.

Kallen IA, (1932), Laryngostroboscopy. Arch Otolaryngol, 16:791–807.

Kammermeier MA, (1969), A comparison of phonatory phenomena among groups of neurologically impaired speakers. Ph.D. dissertation, University of Minnesota, Minneapolis, MN.

Keaton AL, (1983), The physiology of imagery. In: Transcripts of the Twelfth Symposium: Care of the Professional Voice (Part II), Lawrence V (ed.), New York: The Voice Foundation, pp. 281–283.

Kellman RM, Leopold DA, (1982), Paradoxical vocal cord motion: An important cause of stridor. Laryngoscope, 92:58–60.

Kempster GB, Kistler D, (1983), Selected acoustic characteristics of pathological and normal speakers: A reanalysis. J Speech Hear Res, 26:159–160.

Kempster GB, (1984), A multidimensional analysis of vocal quality in two dysphonic groups. Ph.D. dissertation, Northwestern University, Evanston, IL.

Kempster GB, Larson CR, Kistler MK, (1988), Effects of electrical stimulation of cricothyroid and thyroarytenoid muscles on voice fundamental frequency. J Voice, 2:221–229.

Kent RD, Netsell R, (1975), A case study of an ataxic dysarthric: Cineradiographic and spectrographic observations. J Speech Hear Disord, 40:115–134.

Kent RD, Netsell R, Abbs JH, (1979), Acoustic characteristics of dysarthria associated with cerebellar disease. J Speech Hear Res, 22:627–648.

Kent RD, Kent J, Rosenbek J, (1987), Maximum performance tests of speech production. J Speech Hear Res, 52:367–387.

Kim KM, Kakita Y, Hirano M,(1982), Sound spectrographic analysis of the voice of patients with recurrent laryngeal nerve paralysis. Folia Phoniatr, 34:124–133.

Kitajima K, (1981), Quantitative evaluation of the noise level in the pathologic voice. Folia Phoniatr, 33:115–124.

Kitzing P, (1985), Stroboscopy—a pertinent laryngological examination. J Otolaryngol, 14:151–157.

Kleinsasser O, (1968), Microlaryngoscopy and Endolaryngeal Microsurgery, Philadelphia: WB Saunders.

Kleinsasser O, (1987), Surgery in unilateral vocal cord paralysis. Paper presented at the International Symposium on Phonosurgery, Cairo, Egypt.

Klingholz F, Martin F, (1985), Quantitative spectral evaluation of shimmer and jitter. J Speech Hear Res, 28:169–174.

Koike Y, (1967a), Applications of some acoustic measures for the evaluation of laryngeal dysfunction. J Acoust Soc Am, 42:1209.

Koike Y, (1967b), Experimental studies on vocal attack. Practica Otologica (Kyoto), 60:663–688.

Koike Y, Hirano M, von Leden H, (1967), Vocal initiation: Acoustic and aerodynamic investigations of normal subjects. Folia Phoniatr, 19:171–182.

Koike Y, Hirano M, (1968), Significance of the vocal velocity index. Folia Phoniatr, 20:285–296.

Koike Y, Takahashi H, Calcaterra T, (1977), Acoustic measures for detecting laryngeal pathology. Acta Otolaryngol, 84:105–117.

Kojima H, Gould WJ, Lambiase A, (1979), Computer analysis of hoarseness. J Acoust Soc Am, 65:67.

Kojima H, Gould WJ, Lambiase A, Isshiki N, (1980), Computer analysis of hoarseness. Acta Otolaryngol, 89:547–554.

Komiyama S, (1972), Phonogram: A new method of evaluating voice characteristics. Otologia (Fukuoka), 18:428–440.

Kooper R, Sullivan CA, (1986), Professional liability: Management and prevention. In: Prospering in Private Practice, Butler KG (ed.), Rockville, MD: Aspen Publications, pp. 59–80.

Kornhuber HH, (1977), A reconsideration of the cortical and subcortical mechanisms involved in speech and aphasia. In: Language Specialization in Man: Cerebral ERPs, Progress in Clinical Neurophysiology (Vol. 3), Desmedt JE (ed.), Basel: Karger, pp. 28–35.

Kotby MN, Haugen LK, (1970), The mechanics of laryngeal function. Acta Otolaryngol, 70:203–211.

Koufman JA, (1986), Laryngoplasty for vocal cord medialization: Alternative to Teflon. Laryngoscope, 96:726–731.

Koufman JA, Wiener GJ, Wu WC, Castell DO,

(1988), Reflux laryngitis and its sequelae: The diagnostic role of ambulatory 24 hour pH monitoring. J Voice, 2:78–79.

Kreindler A, Pruskauer-Apostol B, (1971), Neurologic and psychopathologic aspects of compulsive crying and laughter in pseudobulbar palsy patients. Revue Roumaine de Neurologie, 8:125–139.

Kurita S, (1980), Layer structure of the human vocal fold: Morphological investigation. Otologia (Fukuoka), 26:973–997.

Kuroki K, (1969), Subglottic pressure of normal and pathological larynges. Otologia (Fukuoka), 15:54–74.

Kurtzke JF, Beebe GW, Nagler B, Auth TL, Kurland LT, Nefzger MD, (1972), Studies on the natural history of multiple sclerosis. Acta Neurol (Scand), 48:19–46.

Kushner D, Michel JF, (1978), Maximum phonation time in 100 adults. Paper presented at the convention of the American Speech Language Hearing Association, San Francisco.

Ladefoged P, McKinney NP, (1963), Loudness, sound pressure and subglottal pressure in speech. J Acoust Soc Am, 35:454–460.

Lane HL, Catania AC, Stevens SS, (1961), Voice level: Autophonic scale, perceived loudness and effects of side tone. J Acoust Soc Am, 33:160–177.

Lang AE, Marsden CD, (1983), Spasmodic dysphonia in Gilles de la Tourette's disease. Arch Neurol, 40:51–52.

Langworthy OR, Hesser FH, (1940), Syndrome of pseudobulbar palsy: An anatomic and physiologic analysis. Arch Int Med, 65:106–121.

Larson CR, Sutton D, Lindeman RC, (1978), Cerebellar regulation of phonation in rhesus monkey (*Macaca mulatta*). Exp Brain Res, 33:1–18.

Larson CR, (1985), The midbrain periaqueductal gray: A brainstem structure involved in vocalization. J Speech Hear Res, 28:241–249.

Larson CR, Kistler MK, (1986), The relationship of periaqueductal gray neurons to vocalization and laryngeal EMG in the behaving monkey. Exp Brain Res, 63:596–606.

Larson CR, (1988), Brain mechanisms involved in the control of vocalization. J Voice, 2:301–311.

Larsson T, Sjogren T, (1960), Essential tremor: A clinical and genetic population study. Acta Psychiatr Neurol (Scand), 36 (Suppl 144): 1–176.

Launer P, (1971), Maximum phonation time in children. Master's thesis, State University of New York, Buffalo, NY.

Laver J, (1980), The Phonetic Description of Voice Quality, New York: Cambridge University Press.

Lawrence VL, (1987), Common medications with laryngeal effects. ENT J, 66:318–322.

Leanderson R, Meyerson BA, Persson A, (1972), Lip muscle function in Parkinsonian dysarthria. Acta Otolaryngol, 74:350 357.

Lechtenberg R, Gilman S, (1978), Speech disorders in cerebellar disease. Ann Neurol, 3:285–290.

Lee KJ, (1973), The Otolaryngology Boards, New York: Medical Exam Publishing Co.

Lehmann, QH, (1965), Reverse phonation: A new maneuver for examining the larynx. Radiology, 84:215–222.

LeJeune FE, Guice CE, Samuels PM, (1983), Early experiences with vocal ligament tightening. Ann Otol Rhinol Laryngol, 92:475–477.

Leonard RJ, Ringel RL, (1979), Vocal shadowing under conditions of normal and altered laryngeal sensation. J Speech Hear Res, 22:794–817.

Lester B, (1985), Introduction: There's more to crying than meets the ear. In: Infant Crying, Lester B, Boukydis CF (eds.), New York: Plenum Press, pp. 1–28.

Levine L, Hatlali JM, Zaggy M, (1985), Myasthenia gravis presenting as intermittent laryngeal paralysis. In: Transcripts of the Fourteeth Symposium: Care of the Professional Voice (Part II), Lawrence V (ed.), New York: The Voice Foundation, pp. 348–351.

Levinson D, (1987), A Guide to the Clinical Interview, Philadelphia: WB Saunders.

Lewis K, Casteel R, McMahon J, (1982), Duration of sustained /a/ related to the number of trials. Folia Phoniatr, 34:41–48.

Lewy RB, (1976), Experiments with vocal cord injection. Ann Otolaryngol, 85:440–450.

Liden S, Gottfries C, (1974), Beta-blocking agents in the treatment of catecholamine-induced symptoms in musicians. Lancet, 2:529.

Lieberman P, (1963), Some acoustic measures of the fundamental periodicity of normal and pathologic larynges. J Acoust Soc Am, 35:344–353.

Lieberman P, (1968), Vocal cord motion in man. Ann NY Acad Sci, 155:28–38.

Linebaugh C, (1979), The dysarthrias of Shy-Drager syndrome. J Speech Hear Disord, 44:55–60.

Linville SE, Fisher H, (1985), Acoustic characteristics of perceived versus actual aging: Controlled phonation by adult females. J Acoust Soc Am, 78:40–48.

Logemann JA, Fisher HB, Boches B, Blonsky ER, (1978), Frequency and cooccurrence of vocal tract dysfunctions in the speech of a large sample of Parkinson patients. J Speech Hear Res, 43:47–57.

Logemann JA, (1983), Evaluation and Treatment of Swallowing Disorders, San Diego: College Hill Press.

Longridge NS, (1987), Bilateral vocal cord paralysis in Shy-Drager syndrome. J Otolaryngol, 16:146–148.

Lowenthal G, (1958), The treatment of polypoid laryngitis. Laryngoscope, 68:1095–1104.

Luchsinger R, Arnold GE, (1965), Voice Speech Language Clinical Communicology: Its Physiology and Pathology, Belmont, CA: Wadsworth.

Ludlow C, Hart M, (1981), Research needs for the assessment of phonatory function. In: Proceedings of the Conference on Vocal Assessment of Vocal Pathology, Ludlow C, Hart M (eds.), ASHA Reports, 11:3–8.

Ludlow CL, Coulter D, Gentges F, (1983), Differential sensitivity of frequency perturbation to laryngeal neoplasms and neuropathologies. In: Vocal Fold Physiology: Contemporary Research and Clinical Issues, Bless D, Abbs J (eds.), San Diego: College Hill Press, pp. 381–392.

Ludlow CL, Connor NP, Coulter D, (1984), A preliminary investigation into the validity of an optimum frequency for phonatory functioning in patients with laryngeal pathology. Transcripts of the Twelfth Symposium: Care of the Professional Voice (Part II), Lawrence V (ed.), New York: The Voice Foundation, pp. 155–168.

Ludlow CL, Bassich CJ, Connor NP, Coulter DC, (1986), Phonatory characteristics of vocal fold tremor. J Phonetics, 14:509–516.

Ludlow, CL, Schulz, GM, Naunton, RF, (1988), The effects of diazepam on intrinsic laryngeal muscle activation during respiration and speech. J Voice, 2:70–77.

Mahshie J, Conture E, (1983), Deaf speakers' laryngeal behavior. J Speech Hear Res, 26:550–559.

Maple FF, (1985), Dynamic Interviewing: An Introduction to Counseling, Beverly Hills, CA: Sage Publications.

Markel N, Meisels M, Houck J, (1964), Judging personality from voice quality. J Abn Soc Psychol, 69:458–463.

Markel N, Bein M, Philips J, (1973), The relationship between words and tone-of-voice. Language and Speech, 16:15–21.

Marge M, (1984), The prevention of communication disorders. ASHA, 26:29–37.

Martin FG, (1983), Drugs and the voice. In: Transcripts of the Twelfth Symposium: Care of the Professional Voice (Part I), Lawrence V (ed.), New York: The Voice Foundation, pp. 124–132.

Martin FG, (1984), The influence of drugs on voice (Part II). In: Transcripts of the Thirteenth Symposium: Care of the Professional Voice (Part II), Lawrence V (ed.), New York: The Voice Foundation, pp. 191–201.

Martin FG, (1988), Tutorial: Drugs and vocal function. J Voice, 2:338–344.

Maxwell S, Locke J, (1969), Voice in myasthenia gravis. Laryngoscope, 79:1902–1906.

McCall G, Colton RH, Rabuzzi D, (1972), Preliminary EMG investigation of certain intrinsic and extrinsic laryngeal muscles in patients with spasmodic dysphonia. J Acoust Soc Am, 53:345.

McClean MD, (1988), Neuromotor aspects of speech production and dysarthria. In: Clinical Management of Dysarthric Speakers, Yorkston KM, Beukelman DR, Bell KR (eds.), Boston: College Hill Press, pp. 19–58.

McFarlane SC, Fujiki M, Brinton B, (1984), Coping with Communicative Handicaps: Resources for the Practicing Clinician, San Diego: College Hill Press.

McGlone RE, Hollien H, (1963), Vocal pitch characteristics of aged women. J Speech Hear Res, 6:164–170.

Merritt HH, (1979), A Textbook of Neurology (6th ed.), Philadelphia: Lea & Febiger.

Merson RM, Ginsberg AP, (1979), Spasmodic dysphonia: Abductor type. A clinical report of acoustic, aerodynamic & perceptual characteristics. Laryngoscope, 89:129–139.

Metz DE, Whitehead RL, Peterson DH, (1980), An optical illumination system for high speed laryngeal cinematography. J Acoust Soc Am, 67:719–720.

Meurman Y, (1952), Operative mediofixation of the vocal cord in complete unilateral paralysis. Arch Otolaryngol, 55:544.

Miehlke VA, Arnold R, (1982), Chirurgie des Nervus recurrense-ein Ausblick. In: Hals-Nasen-Ohren-Heilkunde in Praxis and Klinik (Band 4 Teil 1), Berendes J, Link R, Zollner F (eds.), Stuttgart: Georg Thieme Verlag, pp. 6.1–6.24

Millar JHD, (1971), Multiple Sclerosis: A Disease Acquired in Childhood, Springfield, IL: Charles C Thomas.

Miller JE, Mathews MV, (1963), Investigation of the glottal waveshape by automatic inverse filtering. J Acoust Soc Am, 35:1876.

Miller RL, (1959), Nature of the vocal cord wave. J Acoust Soc Am, 31:667–677.

Miller RP, Gray SD, Cotton RT, Myer CM, (1988), Airway reconstruction following laryngotracheal thermal trauma. Laryngoscope, 98:826–829.

Miller SQ, Madison CL, (1984), Public school voice clinics, II: Diagnosis and recommendations—a 10 year review. Lang Speech Hear Ser Sch, 15:58–64.

Minifie FD, Hixon TJ, Williams F, (1983), Normal Aspects of Speech, Hearing and Language, Englewood Cliffs, NJ: Prentice-Hall.

Minifie FD, (1984), Against the clinical use of optimal pitch. In: Transcripts of the Twelfth Symposium: Care of the Professional Voice (Part II), Lawrence V (ed.), New York: The Voice Foundation, pp. 148–154.

Moll KL, Peterson GE, (1969), Speaker and listener judgments of vowel levels. Phonetica, 19:104–117.

Monday LA, Cornut G, Bouchayer M, Roch JB, (1983), Epidermoid cysts of the vocal cords. Ann Otol Rhinol Laryngol, 92:124–127.

Monoson P, Zemlin WR, (1984), Quantitative study of whisper. Folia Phoniatr, 36:53–65.

Moore GP, (1937), A short history of laryngeal investigation. Quart J Speech, 23:531–564.

Moore GP, von Leden H, (1958), Dynamic variations of the vibratory pattern in the normal larynx. Folia Phoniatr, 10:205–238.

Moore GP, (1977), Have the major issues in voice disorders been answered by research in speech science? A 50-year retrospective, J Speech Hear Disord, 42:152–160.

Moore GP, Cannon KA, Wilson LI, (1979), Vocal fold vibration in the presence of vocal nodules. In: Transcripts of the Eighth Symposium: Care of the Professional Voice (Part III), Lawrence V (ed.), New York: The Voice Foundation, pp. 24–31.

Moore GP, Hicks DM, Abbott TB, (1985), Defects of speech and language. In: Diseases of the Nose, Throat, Ear, Head and Neck (13th ed.), Ballenger JJ (ed.), Philadelphia: Lea & Febiger, pp. 692–731.

Moore GP, (1986), Voice disorders. In: Human Communication Disorders: An Introduction (2nd ed.), Shames GA, Wiig EH (eds.), Columbus, OH: Merrill, pp. 183–241.

Morrison MD, Rammage LA, Belisle GM, Pullan CB, Nichol H, (1983), Muscular tension dysphonia. J Otolaryngol, 12:302–306.

Murry T, (1978), Speaking fundamental frequency characteristics associated with voice pathologies. J Speech Hear Disord, 43:374–379.

Murry T, Doherty ET, (1980), Selected acoustic characteristics of pathological and normal speakers. J Speech Hear Res, 23:361–369.

Murry T, (1982), Phonation: Remediation. In: Speech, Language and Hearing (Vol. 2), Lass N, McReynolds LV, Northern J, Yoder DE (eds.), New York: WB Saunders, pp. 489–498.

Mysak ED, (1959), Pitch and duration characteristics of older males. J Speech Hear Res, 2:46–54.

Nagler W, (1987), Dr. Nagler's Body Maintenance and Repair Book, New York: Simon & Schuster.

Neiman GS, Edeson B, (1981), Procedural aspects of eliciting maximum phonation time. Folia Phoniatr, 33:285–293.

Nielsen VM, Hojslet PE, Karlsmose M, (1986), Surgical treatment of Reinke's oedema (long-term results). J Laryngol Otol, 100:187–190.

Nilson H, Schneiderman CR, (1983), Classroom program for the prevention of vocal abuse in elementary school children. Lang Speech Hear Ser Sch, 14:172–178.

Noffsinger D, Olsen WO, Carhart R, Hart CW, Sahgal V, (1972), Auditory and vestibular aberrations in multiple sclerosis. Acta Otolaryngol, (Suppl 303):1–63.

Ortega JD, DeRosier E, Park S, Larson C, (1988), Brainstem mechanisms of laryngeal control as revealed by microstimulation studies. In: Vocal Fold Physiology: Voice Production, Mechanisms and Function, Fujimura O (ed.), New York: Raven Press, pp. 19–28.

Osserman KE, (1958), Myasthenia Gravis, New York: Grune & Stratton.

Pahn J, (1966), Zur entwicklung und behandlung funktioneller singstimmerkrankugen. Folia Phoniatr, 18:117–130.

Painter C, (1986), The laryngeal vestibule and voice quality. Arch Otorhinolaryngol, 243:329–337.

Painter C, (1988), Electroglottogram waveform types. Arch Otorhinolaryngol, 245:116–121.

Papp P, (1983), The Process of Change, New York: Guilford Press.

Parnes SM, Lavarato AB, Myers EN, (1978), Study of spastic dysphonia using videofiberoptic laryngoscopy. Ann Otol Rhinol Laryngol, 87:322–326.

Peacher G, (1947), Contact ulcer of the larynx I: History. J Speech Hear Disord, 12:67–76.

Penfield W, Roberts L, (1959), Speech and Brain Mechanisms, Princeton: Princeton University Press.

Perkins W, (1971), Speech Pathology: An Applied Behavioral Science, St. Louis: CV Mosby.

Perkins WH, (1983), Quantification of vocal behavior: A foundation for clinical management of voice. In: Vocal Fold Physiology: Contemporary Research and Clinical Issues, Bless DM , Abbs J (eds.), San Diego: College Hill Press, pp. 425–431.

Perkins WH, (1985), Assessment and treatment of voice disorders: State of the art. In: Speech Disorders in Adults, Costello J (ed.), San Diego: College Hill Press, pp. 79–112.

Perlman AL, Titze IR, Cooper DS, (1984), Elasticity of canine vocal fold tissue. J Speech Hear Res, 27:212–219.

Perlman AL, Titze IR, (1988), Development of an in vitro technique for measuring elastic properties of vocal fold tissue. J Speech Hear Res, 31:288–298.

Plomp R, (1976), Aspects of Tone Sensation, New York: Academic Press.

Prater RJ, Swift RW, (1984), Manual of Voice Therapy, Boston: Little, Brown & Co.

Pressman JJ, (1942), Physiology of vocal cords in phonation and respiration. Arch Otol, 35:355–398.

Pressman JJ, Kelemen G, (1955), Physiology of the larynx. Physiol Rev, 35:506–554.

Prosek R, Montgomery A, Walden B, Schwartz

D, (1978), EMG biofeedback in the treatment of hyperfunctional voice disorders. J Speech Hear Disord, 43:282–294.

Ptacek PH, Sander EK, (1963), Maximum duration of phonation. J Speech Hear Disord, 28:171–182.

Ptacek PH, Sander EK, Maloney WH, Jackson CCR, (1966), Phonatory and related changes with advanced age. J Speech Hear Disord, 9:353–360.

Punt N, (1983), Laryngology applied to singers and actors. J Laryngol Otol, (Suppl 6).

Ramig L, Ringel R, (1983), Effects of physiological aging on selected acoustic characteristics of voice. J Speech Hear Res, 26:22–30.

Ramig L, (1986), Acoustic analysis of phonation in patients with Huntington's disease. Ann Otol Rhinol Laryngol, 95:288–293.

Rastatter MP, Hyman M, (1982), Maximum phoneme duration of /s/ and /z/ by children with vocal nodules. Lang Speech Hear Serv Sch, 13:197–199.

Ravits J, (1988), Myasthenia gravis. A well-understood neuromuscular disorder. Postgrad Med, 83:219–223.

Reed C, (1980), Voice therapy: A need for research. J Speech Hear Disord, 45:157–169.

Reich A, Lerman J, (1978), Teflon laryngoplasty: An acoustical and perceptual case study. J Speech Hear Res, 43:496–505.

Reich AR, (1982), Evaluating and preventing dysphonia in the artist/athlete. Short course at the annual meeting of the American Speech Language Hearing Association, Toronto.

Reich AR, Mason JA, Polen SB, (1986) Task administration variables affecting phonation time measures in 3rd grade girls with normal voice quality. Lang Speech Hear Serv Sch, 17:262–269.

Reik T, (1948), Listening with the Third Ear, New York: Farrar, Strauss & Giroux.

Reiser DE, Schroder AK, (1980), Patient Interviewing, The Human Dimension, Baltimore: Williams & Wilkins.

Riklan M, Levita E, (1969), Subcortical Correlates of Human Behavior, Baltimore: Williams & Wilkins.

Robe E, Brumlik J, Moore GP, (1960), A study of spastic dysphonia. Laryngoscope, 70:219–245.

Rogers JH, Stell PM, (1978), Paradoxical movement of the vocal cords as a cause of stridor. J Laryngol Otol, 92:157–158.

Rontal M, Rontal E, Leuchter W, Rolnick M, (1978), Voice spectrography in the evaluation of myasthenia gravis of the larynx. Arch Otolaryngol, 87:722–728.

Rosenfield D, (1987), Neurolaryngology. ENT J, 66:323–326.

Rosenthal RS, (1978), Malpractice: Cause and its prevention. Laryngoscope, 88:1–11.

Rothenberg M, (1968), The breath stream dynamics of simple-released plosive production. Bibliotheca Phonetica, 6:(whole volume).

Rothenberg M, (1973), A new inverse filtering technique for deriving the glottal airflow during voicing. J Acoust Soc Am, 53:1632–1645.

Rothenberg M, (1977), Measurement of air flow during speech. J Speech Hear Res, 2:155–176.

Rothenberg M, (1981), Some relations between glottal air flow and vocal fold contact area. In: Proceedings of the Conference on the Assessment of Vocal Pathology, Ludlow CL, Hart M (eds.), Rockville, MD: American Speech Language Hearing Association, pp. 88–96.

Rothenberg M, (1982), Interpolating subglottal pressure from oral pressure. J Speech Hear Disord, 47:218–224.

Rothenberg M, Mahshie JJ, (1988), Monitoring vocal fold abduction through vocal fold contact area. J Speech Hear Res, 31:338–351.

Rubin HJ, (1964), Role of the laryngologist in management of dysfunctions of the singing voice. Eye, Ear, Nose and Throat Monthly, 43:45–55.

Rullan A, (1955), Vocal cord paralysis of intrathoracic origin. Bul Assoc Med Puerto Rico, 47:39–44.

Rullan A, (1956), Associated laryngeal paralysis: Presentation of a case of bilateral abductor paralysis in a patient with the Arnold-Chiari deformity. Arch Otolaryngol, 64:207–212.

Sackner MA, (1980), Monitoring of ventilation without physical connection to the airway. In: Diagnostic Techniques in Pulmonary Disease, Sackner MA (ed.), New York: Marcel Dekker, pp. 503–537.

Saito S, Ogino M, Ishikura M, Niino Y, Fukuda H, (1966), Endolaryngeal microsurgery. J Jpn Bronchoesophagol Soc, 17:253–266.

Saito S, (1977), Phonosurgery; Basic study of the mechanism of phonation and endolaryngeal microsurgery. Otologia (Fukuoka), 23:171–384.

Salamy JN, Sessions RB, (1980), Spastic dysphonia. J Fluency Disord, 5:281–290.

Sander EK, (1989), Arguments against the aggressive pursuit of voice treatment for children. Lang Speech Hear Serv Sch, 20:94–101.

Sasaki CT, Carlson RD, (1986), Malignant neoplasms of the larynx. In: Otolaryngology—Head and Neck Surgery (Vol. 3), Cummings, C, Frederickson L, Harker L, Krause C, Schuller D (eds.), St. Louis: CV Mosby, pp. 1987–2017.

Sataloff RT, (1987a), Clinical evaluation of the professional singer. ENT J, 66:267–277.

Sataloff RT, (1987b), Common diagnoses and treatments in professional singers. ENT J, 66:278–288.

Sataloff RT, (1987c), The professional voice III:

Common diagnoses and treatments. J Voice, 1:283–292.

Sawashima M, Sato M, Funasaka S, Totsuk G, (1958), Electromyographic study of the human larynx and its clinical application. J Otolaryngology (Japan), 61:1357–1364.

Sawashima M, (1966), Measurements of phonation time. Japanese J Logopedics Phoniatr, 7:23–29.

Sawashima M, Totsuka G, Kobayashi T, Hirose M, (1968), Reconstructive surgery for hoarseness due to unilateral vocal cord paralysis. Arch Otolaryngol, 87:289.

Sawashima M, Abramson A, Cooper FS, Lisker L, (1970), Observing laryngeal adjustments during running speech by use of a fiberoptics system. Phonetica, 22:193–201.

Sawashima M, Hirose H, (1981), Abduction-adduction of the glottis in speech and voice production. In: Vocal Fold Physiology, Stevens KN, Hirano M (eds.), Tokyo: University of Tokyo Press, pp. 329–346.

Saxman J, Burk KW, (1967), Speaking fundamental frequency characteristics of middle aged women. Folia Phoniatr, 19:167–172.

Schaefer SD, (1983), Neuropathology of spasmodic dysphonia. Laryngoscope, 93:1183–1202.

Schaefer SD, Freeman F, Finitzo T, Close L, Cannito M, Ross E, Reisch H, Maravilla K, (1985), Magnetic resonance imaging findings and correlations in spasmodic dysphonia patients. Ann Otol Rhinol Laryngol, 94:595–601.

Schaefer SD, Freeman FJ, (1987), Spasmodic dysphonia. Otolaryngol Clin North Am, 20:161–178.

Schiffman SS, Reynolds ML, Young FW, (1981), Introduction to Multidimensional Scaling: Theory, Methods, Applications, New York: Academic Press.

Schilling R, (1925), Experimentell-phonetische Untersuchunger bei Erkrankunger des extrapyramidalen Systems. Arch Psychiatr Nevenkr, 75:419–471.

Schmidt, P, Klingholz, F, Martin, F, (1988), Influence of pitch, voice sound pressure and vowel quality on maximum phonation time. J Voice, 1:245–249.

Schutte H, Seidner W, (1983), Recommendation by the Union of European Phoniatricians (UEP): Standardizing voice area measurement/phonetography. Folia Phoniatr, 35:286–288.

Senturia DH, Wilson FB, (1968), Otorhinolaryngologic findings in children with voice deviations. Ann Otol Rhinol Laryngol, 77:1–15.

Shapiro SL, (1973), On the management of professional voice disorders. Eye, Ear, Nose and Throat Monthly, 52:328–331.

Sharbrough FW, Stockard JJ, Aronson AE, (1975), Brainstem auditory evoked responses in spastic dysphonia. Trans Am Neurol Assoc, 103:198–201.

Shearer WH, (1972), Diagnosis and treatment of voice disorders in school children. J Speech Hear Disord, 37:215–228.

Shearer WH, (1983), S/z ratio for detection of vocal nodules. Folia Phoniatr, 35:172.

Shigemori Y, (1977), Some tests related to the air usage during phonation: Clinical investigations. Otologia (Fukuoka), 23:138–166.

Shipp T, Huntington D, (1965), Some acoustic and perceptual factors in acute laryngitic hoarseness. J Speech Hear Disord, 30:350–359.

Shipp T, Hollien H, (1969), Perception of the aging male voice. J Speech Hear Res, 12:703–710.

Shipp T, McGlone R, (1971), Laryngeal dynamics associated with voice frequency change. J Speech Hear Res, 14:761–768.

Shipp T, (1975), Vertical laryngeal position during continuous and discrete vocal frequency change. J Speech Hear Res, 18:707–718.

Shipp T, Izdebski K, (1975), Vocal frequency and vertical larynx positioning in singers and non-singers. J Acoust Soc Am, 58:1104–1106.

Shipp T, Mueller P, Zwitman D, (1980), Intermittent abductory dysphonia. J Speech Hear Disord, 45:283.

Shipp T, (1987), Vertical laryngeal position: Research findings and application for singers. J Voice, 1:217–219.

Shipp T, Guinn L, Sundberg J, Titze IR, (1987), Discussion: Vertical laryngeal position—research findings and their relationship to singing. J Voice, 1:220–222.

Shipp T, Izdebski K, Schutte HK, Morrissey P, (1988), Subglottal air pressure in spastic dysphonia speech. Folia Phoniatr, 40:105–110.

Shy GM, Drager G, (1960), A neurological syndrome associated with orthostatic hypotension. AMA Arch Neurol, 2:511–527.

Simkin B, (1964), Corticosteroids in clinical practice. Eye, Ear, Nose and Throat Monthly, 43:47–54.

Siribodhi C, Sundmaker W, Atkins JP, Bonner FL, (1963), Electromyographic studies of laryngeal paralysis and regeneration of laryngeal motor nerve in dogs. Laryngoscope, 73:148–164.

Smitheran J, Hixon T, (1981), A clinical method for estimating airway resistance during vowel production. J Speech Hear Disord, 46:138–146.

Snidecor JC, (1943), A comparative study of the pitch and duration characteristics of impromptu speaking and oral reading. Speech Monogr, 10:50–57.

Snow J, Marano M, Balogh K, (1966), Post-intubation granuloma of the larynx. Anes Analg Current Researches, 45:426–429.

Solomon NP, McCall GN, Trosset MW, Gray WC, (1989), Laryngeal configuration and constriction during two types of whispering. J Speech Hear Res, 32:161–174.

Sondi MM, (1975), Measurement of the glottal waveform. J Acoust Soc Am, 57:228–232.

Sonnesson B, (1959), A method for studying the vibratory movements of the vocal cords. J Laryngol Otology, 73:732–737.

Sonnesson B, (1960), On the anatomy and vibratory pattern of the human vocal folds. Acta Otolaryngol, (Suppl 156):1–80.

Spector GJ, Ogura JH, (1985), Tumors of the larynx and laryngopharynx. In: Diseases of the Nose, Throat, Ear, Head, and Neck (13th ed.), Ballenger JJ (ed.), Philadelphia: Lea & Febiger, pp. 549–602.

Stemple J, Weiler E, Whitehead W, Komray R, (1980), EMG biofeedback training with patients exhibiting a hyperfunctional voice disorder. Laryngoscope, 90:471–476.

Stevens KN, House A, (1961), An acoustical theory of vowel production and some of its implications. J Speech Hear Res, 4:303–320.

Stoicheff M, (1981), Speaking fundamental frequency characteristics of nonsmoking female adults. J Speech Hear Res, 24:437–441.

Stoicheff M, Giampi A, Passi J, Fredrickson J, (1983), The irradiated larynx and voice: A perceptual study. J Speech Hear Res, 26:482–485.

Stone, RE, (1983), Issues in clinical assessment of laryngeal function: Contraindications for subscribing to maximum phonation time and optimum fundamental frequency. In: Vocal Fold Physiology: Contemporary Research and Clinical Issues, Bless DM, Abbs J (eds.), San Diego: College Hill Press, pp. 410–424.

Stradling J, Chadwick G, Quirk C, Phillips T, (1985), Respiratory inductive plethysmography: Calibration techniques, their validation and the effects of posture. Bull European de Physiopathologie Respiratoire, 21:317–324.

Strong MS, Jako GJ, (1972) Laser surgery in the larynx: Early clinical experience with continous CO_2 laser. Ann Otol Rhinol Laryngol 81:791–798.

Stuart WD, (1965), The otolaryngologic aspects of myasthenia gravis. Laryngoscope, 75:112–121.

Sundberg J, (1974), Articulatory interpretation of the ''singing formant.'' J Acoust Soc Am, 55:838–844.

Sundberg J, Askenfelt A, (1983), Larynx height and voice source: A relationship. In: Vocal Fold Physiology: Contemporary Research and Clinical Issues, Bless DM, Abbs J (eds.), San Diego: College Hill Press, pp. 307–316.

Tait NA, Michel JF, Carpenter MA, (1980), Maximum duration of sustained /s/ and /z/ in children. J Speech Hear Disord, 45:239–246.

Takahashi H, Koike Y, (1975), Some perceptual dimensions and acoustical correlates of pathologic voices. Acta Otolaryngol, 338:1–24.

Tanaka S, Gould W, (1985), Vocal efficiency and aerodynamic aspects in voice disorders. Ann Otol Laryngol, 94:29–33.

Teter, DL, (1976), Voice disorders. In: Otolaryngology: A Textbook, English GM (ed.), Hagerstown, NY: Harper & Row, pp. 584–599.

Thomas JE, Schirger A, (1970), Idiopathic orthostatic hypotension: A study of its natural history in 57 neurologically affected patients. Arch Neurol, 22:289–293.

Thurman WL, (1958), Frequency intensity relationships and optimum pitch level. J Speech Hear Res, 1:117–123.

Timcke R, von Leden H, Moore GP, (1958), Laryngeal vibrations: Measurements of the glottic wave I: The normal vibratory cycle. Arch Otolaryngol, 68:1–19.

Titze I, (1981), Heat generation in the vocal folds and its possible effect on vocal endurance. In: Transcripts of the Tenth Symposium: Care of the Professional Voice (Part I), Lawrence V (ed.), New York: The Voice Foundation, pp. 52–59.

Toogood JH, Jennings BA, Greenway RW, Chuang L, (1980), Candidiasis and dysphonia complicating beclomethasone treatment of asthma. J Allergy Clin Immun, 65:145–153.

Toohill RJ, (1975), The psychosomatic aspects of children with vocal nodules. Arch Otolaryngol, 101:591–595.

Tucker HM, (1978), Human laryngeal reinnervation: Long term experience with the nerve-muscle pedicle technique. Laryngoscope, 88:598–604.

Tucker HM, (1980), Vocal cord paralysis-etiology and management—1979. Laryngoscope, 90:585–590.

Tucker HM, Rusnov M, (1981), Laryngeal reinnervation for unilateral vocal cord paralysis: Long term results. Ann Otol Rhinol Laryngol, 90:457–459.

Tucker H, (1985), Anterior commissure laryngoplasty for adjustment of vocal fold tension. Ann Otol Rhinol Laryngol, 94:547–549.

Ungerleider S, (1986), Athletes in motion: Training for the Olympic games with mind and body: Two case studies. Paper presented at International Conference on Mental Health and Technology, British Columbia.

US Department of Health and Human Services, (1982), The health consequences of smoking: Cancer, a report of the Surgeon General, (Public Health Service), Washington, DC: Government Printing Office, pp. vi-viii, 63–78.

US Department of Health and Human Services, (1986), The health consequences of involuntary smoking, a report of the surgeon general, (Public Health Service), Washington, DC: Government Printing Office, pp. vii-ix, 5-8, 227–252.

Vallancien B, Gautheron B, Pasternak L, Guisez D, Paley B, (1971), Comparaison des signaux microphoniques, diaphanographiques et glottographiques avec application au laryngographe. Folia Phoniatr, 23:371–380.

van den Berg J, (1956), Direct and indirect determination of the mean subglottic pressure. Folia Phoniatr, 8:1–24.

van den Berg JW, (1958), Myoelastic-aerodynamic theory of voice production. J Speech Hear Res, 1:227–244.

van den Berg JW, Tan TS, (1959), Results of experiments with human larynges. Pract Otorhinolaryngol, 21:425–450.

Vaughan CW, (1982), Diagnosis and treatment of organic voice disorders. N Engl J Med, 307:863–866.

von Leden H, Moore GP, (1960), Contact ulcer of the larynx. Arch Otolaryngol, 72:746–752.

von Leden H, Moore GP, Timcke R, (1960), Laryngeal vibrations: Measurements of the glottic wave III: The pathologic larynx. Arch Otolaryngol, 71:16–35.

von Leden H, Moore GP, (1961a), The mechanics of the cricoarytenoid joint. Arch Otolaryngol, 73:541–550.

von Leden H, Moore, GP, (1961b), Vibratory pattern of the vocal cords in unilateral laryngeal paralysis. Acta Otolaryngol, 53:493–506.

von Leden H, Isshiki N, (1965), An analysis of cough at the level of the larynx. Arch Otolaryngol, 81:616–625.

von Leden H, LeCover M, Ringel RL, Isshiki N, (1966), Improvement in laryngeal cinematography. Arch Otolaryngol, 83:482–487.

von Leden H, Yanagihara N, Werner-Kukuk E, (1967), Teflon in unilateral vocal cord paralysis. Arch Otolaryngol, 85:110–118.

von Leden H, Poyle PJ, Goff WF, Miller AH, (1969), Symposium on surgery for the improvement of voice. Transactions of the Pacific Coast Oto-Ophthalmological Soc, 50:351–362.

Ward PH, Cannon D, Lindsay JR, (1965), The vestibular system in multiple sclerosis. Laryngoscope, 75:1031–1046.

Ward PH, Sanders JW, Goldman R, Moore GP, (1969), Diplophonia. Ann Otol Rhinol Laryngol, 78:771–777.

Ward PH, Zwitman D, Hanson D, Berci G, (1980), Contact ulcers and granulomas of the larynx: New insights into their etiology as a basis for more rational treatment. Otolaryngol Head-Neck Surg, 88:262–269.

Ward PH, Hanson D, Berci G, (1981), Observations on central neurologic etiology for laryngeal dysfunction. Ann Otolaryngol, 90:430–441.

Ward PH, Berci G, (1982), Observations on the pathogenesis of chronic nonspecific pharyngitis and laryngitis. Laryngosope, 92:1377–1382.

Warren RM, (1962), Are autophonic judgments based on loudness? Am J Psychol, 75:452–456.

Warren WR, Gutmann L, Cody RC, (1977), Stapedius reflex decay in myasthenia gravis. Arch Neurol, 34:496–497.

Warr-Leeper GA, McShea RS, Leeper H, (1979), The incidence of voice and speech deviations in a middle school population. Lang Speech Hear Serv Sch, 10:14–20.

Watkin K, Ewanowski S, (1979), Effects of triamcinolone acetonide on the voice. J Speech Hear Res, 22:446–455.

Watson H, (1979), The technology of respiratory inductive plethysmography. 3rd International Symposium on Ambulatory Monitoring, Middlesex, United Kingdom, pp. 1–24.

Watson PJ, Hixon TJ, Maher MZ, (1987), To breathe or not to breathe—that is the question: An investigation of speech breathing kinematics in world class Shakespearean actors. J Voice, 1:269–272.

Watterson T, Hensen-Magorian HJ, McFarlane SC, (1988), A demographic description of laryngeal contact ulcers. Paper given at convention of American Speech Language Hearing Association, Boston.

Wechsler E, (1976), A Laryngographic study of voice disorders. Br J Commun Disord, 12:9–22.

Weiler G, (1984), Histomorphology findings in the inner laryngeal muscles in sudden infant death (SIDS). Beitr Gerichtl Med, 42:65–70.

Wendahl RW, (1963), Laryngeal analog synthesis of harsh voice quality. Folia Phoniatr, 15:241–250.

Wendahl RW, (1966), Some parameters of auditory roughness. Folia Phoniatr, 18:26–32.

Wendahl RW, Coleman RF, (1967), Vocal cord spectra derived from glottal-area waveforms and subglottal photocell monitoring. J Acoust Soc Am, 41:1113.

Weymuller EA, (1988), Laryngeal injury from prolonged endotracheal intubation. Laryngoscope, 98(Supp 45).

Williams AJ, Hanson D, Calne D, (1979), Vocal cord paralysis in the Shy-Drager syndrome. J Neurosurg Psychiatr, 42:151–153.

Williams AJ, Baghat MS, DeStableforth CRM, Shenoi PM, Skinner C, (1983), Dysphonia caused by inhaled steroids: Recognition of a characteristic laryngeal abnormality. Thorax, 38:813–821.

Williams RT, Farquharson IM, Anthony J, (1975), Fiberoptic laryngoscopy in the assessment of laryngeal disorder. J Laryngol, 89:299–306.

Wilner LK, Sataloff RT, (1987), Speech-language pathology and the professional voice. ENT J, 66:313–317.

Wilson DK, (1979), Voice Problems of Children (2nd ed.), Baltimore: Williams & Wilkins.

Wilson DK, (1987), Voice Problems of Children (3rd ed.), Baltimore: Williams & Wilkins.

Wilson FB, Lamb MM, (1973), Comparison of personality characteristics of children with and without vocal nodules on Rorschach protocol interpretation. Paper presented at the convention of the American Speech Language Hearing Association, Atlanta.

Wilson FB, Rice MA, (1977), A Programmed Approach to Voice Therapy, Austin, TX: Learning Concepts.

Wilson FB, Oldring DJ, Mueller K, (1980), Recurrent laryngeal nerve dissection: A case report involving return of spastic dysphonia after initial surgery. J Speech Hear Disord, 45:112–118.

Wilson FB, Wellen CJ, Kimbarow ML, (1983), Perception of the fundamental frequencies of children's voices by trained and untrained listeners. J Otolaryngol, 12:341–344.

Wolfe V, Bacon M, (1976), Spectrographic comparison of two types of spastic dysphonia. J Speech Hear Disord, 41:325–332.

Wolfe V, Steinfatt T, (1987), Prediction of vocal severity within and across voice types. J Speech Hear Res, 30:230–240.

Wolfe V, Ratusnik DL, (1988), Acoustic and perceptual measurements of roughness influencing judgments of pitch. J Speech Hear Disord, 53:15–22.

Wolski W, (1967), Hypernasality as the presenting symptom of myasthenia gravis. J Speech Hear Res, 32:36–38.

Woo P, Colton R, Shangold L, (1987) Phonatory airflow analysis in patients with laryngeal disease. Ann Otol Rhinol Laryngol, 96:549–555.

Workinger MS, (1986), Acoustic analysis of the dysarthria in children with athetoid and spastic cerebral palsy. Ph.D. dissertation, University of Wisconsin, Madison, WI.

Wright HN, Colton RH, (1972a), Some parameters of autophonic level. Paper presented at the convention of the American Speech Language Hearing Association, San Francisco.

Wright HN, Colton RH, (1972b), Some parameters of vocal effort. J Acoust Soc Am, 51:141.

Wyke B, (1967), Recent advances in the neurology of phonation: Phonatory reflex mechanisms in the larynx. Br J Disord Commun, 2:2–14.

Wyke B, (1969), Deus ex machina vocis. An analysis of the laryngeal reflex mechanisms of speech. Br J Disord Commun, 4:3–20.

Wynder EL, Covey LS, Mabuchi K, Mushinski M, (1976), Environmental factors in cancer of the larynx: A second look. Cancer, 38:1591–1601.

Wynder EL, Stellman SD, (1977), Comparative epidemiology of tobacco-related cancers. Cancer Res, 37:4608–4622.

Yanagihara N, (1967), Significance of harmonic changes and noise components in hoarseness. J Speech Hear Res, 10:531–541.

Yanagihara N, Koike Y, (1967), The regulation of sustained phonation. Folia Phoniatr, 19:1–18.

Yanagihara N, von Leden H, (1967), Respiration and phonation. Folia Phoniatr, 19:153–166.

Yoshida Y, Mitsumasu T, Hirano M, Morimoto M, Kanaseki T, (1987), Afferent connections to the nucleus ambiguus in the brainstem of the cat—an HRP study. In: Laryngeal Function in Phonation and Respiration, Baer T, Sasaki C, Harris K (eds.), San Diego: College Hill Press, pp. 45–61.

Young MA, Bless DM, McNeil MR, Braun SR, (1983), Relation of physical condition to age-related voice changes. Folia Phoniatr, 35:185.

Yumoto E, Gould WJ, Baer T, (1982), Harmonics-to-noise ratio as an index of the degree of hoarseness. J Acoust Soc Am, 71:1544–1550.

Yumoto E, Sasaki Y, Okamura H, (1984), Harmonics-to-noise ratio and psychological measurement of the degree of hoarseness. J Speech Hear Res, 27:2–6.

Zemlin W, (1962), A comparison of the periodic function of vocal fold vibration in a multiple sclerosis and a normal population. Ph.D. dissertation, University of Minnesota, Minneapolis, MN.

Zemlin WR, (1988), Speech and Hearing Science: Anatomy and Physiology (3rd ed.), Englewood Cliffs, NJ: Prentice-Hall.

Zwitman DH, (1979), Bilateral cord dysfunctions: Abductor type spastic dysphonia. J Speech Hear Disord, 44:373–378.

INDEX

Page numbers in *italics* denote figures; those followed by "t" denote tables.

Abuse of voice, 81–85, *105*
　chronic laryngitis, 84
　education for prevention of, 268–269
　excessive, prolonged loudness, 82
　excessive coughing/throat clearing, 83–84
　excessive use with swelling/inflammation/
　　tissue changes, 82–83
　medical management of, 233–234
　reduction/elimination of, 259
　screaming/noise making, 84
　sports/exercise enthusiast, 84–85
　voice therapy for, 242–243
Acanthosis, 59
Acoustic spectrum, 23–24
　analysis of, 189–191, *190*
　in spastic dysphonia, 130–131, *131–132*
Air pressure, 26
　measurement of, 315t, 316
Airflow, 26
　average rates of, 314–315, 314t–315t
　drug effects on, 87
　vibratory, 316
Allergies, 231–232
Aminoglycosides, 89
Amplitude, 22–23
　dynamic range, 22–23, *23*
　overall sound pressure level, 22, *22*
　variability of, 22
Amplitude perturbation, 23, 188
　normative data on, 312, 312t
Amyotrophic lateral sclerosis, 120–122
Anatomical malformations, 30
Anatomy, laryngeal, 271–283, *283*
　cartilages, 51, 273–277
　cavities, 282
　folds, 282
　laryngographic/fiberoptic anatomy, 282–283,
　　283
　muscles, 51–52, *52*
　　extrinsic, 272–273, *273*, 274t
　　intrinsic, 278–280, 279t
　vocal folds, 280–282, *281*

Androgens, 89
Anesthetics, 87
Anterior commissure advancement, 228, *228*
Anterior commissure tendon, 56
Anterior glottal web
　endolaryngeal surgery for, 231, *232*
　thyrotomy for, 231, *233*
Antidepressants, 88
Antihistamines, 88
Antihypertensive agents, 88–89
Antipsychotics, 88
Antispasmodic agents, 88
Antitussive agents, 88
Aphonia, 14, 18
　differential diagnosis of, 41–43
　of psychological origin, 80–81
　signs of, 43t
Apraxia, phonatory, 31
Aqueduct of Sylvius, 298
Arnold-Chiari malformation, 110–111, 127
Aryepiglottic muscle, 52
Arytenoid cartilage, 51, 275, *276*
　rotation of, *225*, 225–226
Arytenoidectomy, 226, *227*
Arytenoideus muscle, 278, 279t
Aspirate initiation technique, 249–250
Aspirin, 90
Ataxic dysphonia, 125–127
Avellis's syndrome, 137t
Axonotmesis, 67–68

Babinski-Nageotte syndrome, 137t
Bernoulli effect, 286–287
Beta blockers, 90
Birth control pills, 246
Bonnier's syndrome, 137t
Brainstem, *300*, 300–301
Breathiness, 14, 17
　differential diagnosis of, 38–40
　signs of, 39t–40t
Breathing
　clavicular, 263

Breathing—*continued*
    therapy, 255–256, *258*
Breathy phonation, 249
Broca's area, 297

Cancer
    carcinoma, 66, *67, 161*, 161–163, *163*
        classification of, 162, 162t
        etiology of, 161–162
        signs of, 162
        surgery for, 217–218, *220*
        treatment for, 162–163
    other tumors, 163–164
Cartilages, laryngeal, 51, 273–277, *276–277*
    arytenoid, 51, 275–276
    corniculate, 277
    cricoid, 51, 275
    cuneiform, 277
    epiglottis, 51, 52, 276–277
    thyroid, 51, 275
Cavities, laryngeal, 282
Cerebellum, 301–304, *303*
    disorders of
        Arnold-Chiari malformation, 127
        ataxic dysphonia, 125–127
Cestan-Chenais syndrome, 137t
Chant-talk technique, 251
Chemical tracheobronchitis, 158. *See also*
        Inhalation injuries
Chemotherepeutic agents, 89
Chewing technique, 250–251
Clavicular breathing, 263
Collet-Sicard syndrome, 138t
Colliculi, 298
Confidential voice, 249
Congenital anomalies, 30
Contact ulcer, 102–104
    voice therapy for, 241
Corniculate cartilage, 277
Corticosteroids, 87–88
Coughing
    excessive, 83–84
        voice therapy for, 241
    therapeutic, 254–255
Cricoarytenoid joint
    ankylosis of, 157–158
    movements by, 275, *277*
Cricoid cartilage, 51, 275, *276–277*
Cricothyroid approximation technique, 227, *227*
Cricothyroid muscle, 51, 278–280, 279t
Crying, 3
CSpeech, 184, 187, 188
Cuneiform cartilage, 277
Cysts
    epidermoid, 62, *64*
        surgery for, 214–215, *216*
    intracordal, 96–97

Decongestants, 87–88
Depressant drugs, 86–87
Diagnostic procedures, 165–210. *See also*
        specific procedures
    examination, 175–183
    history taking, 165–175
    imaging, 208–209

    laboratory testing
        acoustic studies, 184–191
        physiological studies, 191–193
        respiratory studies, 193–195
    neurological testing, 208
    noninstrumental testing, 195–205
    psychiatric testing, 206–208
    summary of, 209–210
    voice sample recording, 205–206
Diazepam, 87
Diencephalon, 298
Differential diagnosis, 11–50
    case studies of, 32–47
        aphonia, 41–43
        breathiness, 38–40
        hoarseness, 32–36
        pitch breaks or falsetto, 43–44
        reduced phonational range, 40–41
        strain/struggle voice, 45–46
        tremor, 47
        vocal fatigue, 36–38
    definition of, 12
    etiology, 12
    process of, 11
    signs of voice problems, 49t–50t. *See also*
            Signs of voice problems
        acoustic, 18–25
        definition of, 13
        interrelationships of, 31
        laryngoscopic, 29–31
        perceptual, 15–18
        physiological, 26–27
        stroboscopic, 27–29
    symptoms of voice problems, 13–14, 14t
        definition of, 12–13
        vs. signs, 13
Digastric muscle, 272, *273*, 274t
Digital manipulation technique, 252–253
Diplophonia, 18
Diuretics, 87–88
    ototoxic, 89
Drug effects, 85–90
    on airflow, 87
    of aspirin, 90
    of beta blockers, 90
    on coordination and proprioception, 86–87
        anesthetics, 87
        depressants, 86–87
        diazepam, 87
        stimulants, 86
    on fluid balance, 87–88
        corticosteroids, 87–88
        decongestants, 87–88
        diuretics, 87–88
        steroid inhalants, 88
    on hearing, 89
        aminoglycosides, 89
        chemotherapeutic agents, 89
        diuretics, 89
    of herbal teas, 89–90
    principles of, 86
    of tobacco and marijuana, 90
    on upper respiratory tract secretions, 88–89
        antidepressants, 88
        antihistamines, 88
        antihypertensives, 88–89

antipsychotics, 88
antispasmodic agents, 88
antitussive agents, 88
wetting agents, 89
on vocal fold structure, 89
androgens, 89
Dynamic range, 22–23, *23*
Dysphonia. *See also* specific types
ataxic, 125–127
of psychological origin, 42, 80–81, 206–208
spastic, 127–133

Edema, 82–83, 97–99
Reinke's 62, *63*, 97–98, *98*
surgery for, 214, *215*
Elderly persons
drug responses of, 86
vocal fold structure in, 59, *60*
voice changes in, 5
Electroglottography, 191
Electromyography, 27, 193, *194*
Epidermoid cyst, 62, *64*
surgery for, 214–215, *216*
Epiglottis, 51, 52, 276–277
Epiglottitis, 101
Epithelial hyperplasia/dysplasia, 59, *61*
surgery for, 216–217, *218*
Examination procedures, 175–183
direct laryngoscopy, 177
flexible fiberoptic laryngoscopy, 177–180, *178–179*
indirect laryngoscopy, 176–177
recording of, 321–322
stroboscopy, 180–182, *181*
ultra-high-speed photography, 182–183, *183*
ultrasound, 183
videofluoroscopy, 182
Extrapyramidal disorders
amyotrophic lateral sclerosis, 120–122
Huntington's chorea, 122–125
parkinsonism, 115–117
Shy-Drager syndrome, 117–119

Fall time, 24
Falsetto. *See* Pitch breaks
Forms
examination record, 321–322
fiberoptic assessment protocol, 326
referral form, 319
stroboscopic assessment chart, 327
telephone contact sheet, 318
voice history, 320, 323–325
Fundamental frequency, 19
breaks in, 25
definition of, 184
mean, 19–20, *20*, 184
measurement of, 184–185, *185*
perturbation, 19, 21–22
measurement of, 188
normative data on, 311t, 311–312
phonational range, 14, 21, 184
measurement of, 185, *186*
normative data on, 311t, 312
standard deviation of, 184
variability of, 20
normative data on, 309–310, 310t

vocal fold length and, 287–288, *289*
vocal fold mass and, 288, *289*
vocal fold tension and, 288–290, *290*

Gag reflex, 2
Gard-Gignoux syndrome, 138t
Gargling, 254–255
Gastroesophageal reflux, 233
Geniohyoid muscle, 272, *273*, 274t
Gilles de la Tourette syndrome, 136
Glottal coup, 75
Glottal fry, 78–79
Glottis
closure of, 28
posterior wall of, 53, *54*
Granulomas, 62–64, *65*, 153–154
surgery for, 215–216, *217*
voice therapy for, 241

Hard glottal attack, 75
Harmonics-to-noise ratio, 23
measurement of, 189
Herbal teas, 89–90
Histology, laryngeal, 51–59
cartilage, 51
epiglottis, 52, *53*
mucosa, 52
muscle, 51–52, *52*
posterior wall of glottis, 53, *54*
subglottic region, 54, *54*
ventricular fold, 52, *53*
vocal fold
in adults, 55–57, *55–57*
in elderly, 59, *60*
in newborns, 57–59, *58*
Histopathology, 59–69, 70t–72t
of carcinomas, 66, *67*
of epidermoid cyst, 62, *64*
of epithelial hyperplasia and dysplasia, 59, *61*
of neuromuscular diseases, 66–68
of nonspecific granuloma, 62–64, *65*
of papilloma, 66, *67*
of Reinke's edema, 62, *63*
of sulcus vocalis, 64–65, *66*
of vocal fold nodules, 59–60, *62*
of vocal fold polyps, 60–62, *63*
of vocal fold scar, 65
vocal physiology implications of, 68–69
History taking, 165–175
case history, 165–175
associated symptoms/sensations, 172
developmental history of problem, 169
duration of problem, 171
effect of problem, 169
onset of problem, 170–171
problem identification, 168–169
variability vs. consistency of problem, 171–172
form for, 320
interview process, 165–168
listening skills for, 167–168, 195–197
what patient brings to, 166
what professional brings to, 167
patient history, 172–175
health status, 173–174
psychological history, 175

History taking, patient history—*continued*
  recreational history, 175
  social history, 175
  substance use, 174
  surgical history, 174
  vocation, 174
  voice use, 172–173
  patient questionnaires, 168
Hoarseness, 14, 17
  differential diagnosis of, 32–36
  signs of, 34t–35t
Hughlings-Jackson syndrome, 137t
Humming technique, 251–252
Huntington's chorea, 122–125
Hyperkeratosis. *See* Keratosis
Hypothyroidism, 245
Hypotonia, 127

Imagery technique, 253–254
Imaging modalities, 208–209
Infections, 231
Inhalation injuries, 158–161
  case study of, 160–161
  laryngeal/supraglottal edema due to, 159
  long-term effects of, 160
  symptoms of, 159
  timing of voice therapy in, 159–160
Interarytenoid muscle, 51
Interviewing, 165–175. *See also* History taking
Intracordal cysts, 96–97
Intubation injuries
  in burn/inhalation injury patients, 159–160
  granulomas, 153–154, *154*
Inverse filtering procedure, 192–193, *193*
Isometric therapy, 254

Jitter. *See* Perturbation

Kay Series of Sona-graphs, 189
Keratosis, 59, 151–153
Klinkert syndrome, 138t

Laboratory testing
  acoustic studies, 184–191
    acoustic spectrum, 189–191, *190*
    fundamental frequency, 184–185, *185*
    perturbation, 188
    phonational range, 185, *186*
    spectrograms, 188–189, *189*
    vocal intensity, 185–188, *187*
  physiological studies, 191–193
    electroglottography, 191
    electromyography, 193, *194*
    inverse filtering, 192–193, *193*
    photoglottography, 191–192
  respiratory studies, 193–195
    air volumes and capacities, 193–195
    respiratory movements, 195, *195*
Lamina propria, 54–56, 280, *281*
Laryngeal web, 30
Laryngitis, 5, 99–101
  chronic, 84, *100*
  complications of, 101
  other forms of, 101
  voice misuse and, 81
Laryngograph, 191

Laryngomalacia, 30
Laryngoscopy
  direct, 177
  flexible fiberoptic, 177–180, *178–179*
    protocol for, 326
  indirect, 176–177
Larynx
  anatomy of, 271–283, *283*
  anteroposterior dimensions of, 30
  anteroposterior squeezing of, 76
  biological importance of, 1–2
  cancer of, *161*, 161–163, *163*
  cavities of, 282
  examination of, 175–183
  folds of, 282
  high position of, 75–76
  histology of, 51–59
  histopathology of, 59–69, 70t–72t
  involuntary activity of, 31
  laryngographic/fiberoptic anatomy of, 282–283, *283*
  muscle function in, 27
  normal-appearing, 31
  spasms of, 246–247
  vertical position of, 30
  voice and, 2–3
Lateral cricoarytenoid muscle, 51, 278, 279t
Laughing, 254–255
Leukoplakia, 59
Listening skills, 167–168, 195–197
Loudness, 16–17
  alteration of, 199
  excessive, prolonged, 82
  mechanisms of change of, 290–292, *292*
  monoloudness, 16
  reduction of, 259
  variations of, 4, 16–17

Mackenzie syndrome, 137t
Macula flava
  anterior, 56
  posterior, 57
Magnetometry, 195
Magnitude estimation method, 203–204
Malpractice, 269–270
Marijuana, 90
Massage technique, 252–253
Medical procedures, 231–234
Menstruation, 246
Mesencephalon, 298
Micro Speech Lab, 184, *185*, 187
Microphones, 206
Misuse of voice, 73–81, 74t
  antecedents of, 81
  anteroposterior laryngeal squeezing, 76
  aphonia/dysphonia of psychological origin, 80–81
  education for prevention of, 268–269
  evolution of, 81
  excessive talking, 79
  hard glottal attack/glottal coup, 75
  high laryngeal position, 75–76
  inappropriate pitch level, 76–79
    lack of pitch variability, 79
    persistent glottal fry, 78–79
    puberphonia, 77–78

increased tension/strain, 74
ventricular phonation, 80
voice therapy for, 242–243
Mucosal wave, 28
Multiple sclerosis, 136–140
Muscles, laryngeal, 51–52, *52*
  extrinsic, 272–273, *273*, 274t
    infrahyoid, 272–273
    innervation of, 304
    suprahyoid, 272
  function of, 27
  intrinsic, 278–280, 279t
Myasthenia gravis, 140–142
Mylohyoid muscle, 272, *273*, 274t

Nervous system. *See also* specific disorders
  afferent vs. efferent components of, 108
  brainstem and medulla disorders
    essential tremor, 134–136
    other syndromes, 136, 137t–138t
    spastic dysphonia, 127–133
  central vs. peripheral, 107
  cerebellar disorders, 125–127
    Arnold-Chiari malformation, 127
    ataxic dysphonia, 125–127
  dysfunction of, 108
  extrapyramidal disorders, 115–125
    amyotrophic lateral sclerosis, 120–122
    Huntington's chorea, 122–125
    parkinsonism, 115–117
    Shy-Drager syndrome, 117–119
  generalized/unknown location disorders, 136–140
    Gilles de la Tourette syndrome, 136
    multiple sclerosis, 136–140
  management for disorders of, 234
  muscle and myoneural junction disorders, 140–142
    myasthenia gravis, 140–142
  peripheral nerve lesions, 143–148
  pseudobulbar palsy, 112–115
  role of, 107–108
    in phonation and speech, 109–110
  voice pathology and organization of, 110–112, *111*
Neuroanatomy, 110–112, *111*, 297–307
  brainstem, *300*, 300–301
  cerebellum, 301–304, *303*
  cortical mechanisms, 297–298, *299*
  midbrain mechanisms, 298, *300*
  subcortical mechanisms, 298, *300–302*
  vagus nerve, 304–306, *305*, 306t
Neuroapraxia, 66–67
Neurolaryngology, 7
Neurological testing, 208
Nodules, *91*, 91–94
  histopathology of, 59–60, *62*
  voice therapy for, 240
  vs. polyps, 91–92
Noise
  definition of, 23
  generation of, 23–24
Noninstrumental testing, 195–205
  critical listening and description, 195–197
  critical observations and descriptions, 197–198
  diagnostic therapy tasks, 198–199

altering pitch, 198–199
altering vocal loudness, 199
phonation with effortful glottal closure, 199
"placing the voice," 199
production of reflexive sounds, 198
of maximum phonation time, 199–200
of s/z ratio, 200–201
scaling, 201–202
  of pitch, 202–203
  of vocal effort, 203–205, *204*

Omohyoid muscle, 272, *273*, 274t
Organic conditions, 151–164
  ankylosis of cricoarytenoid joint, 157–158
  carcinoma, 161–163
  granulomas, 153–154
  keratosis, 151–153
  pachydermia laryngis, 155
  papilloma, 155–157
  trauma, 158–161
  tumors, 163–164
Otolaryngology, 7
Ototoxic drugs, 89

Pachydermia laryngis, 59, 155
Papilloma, 66, *67*, 155–157
  surgery for, 217, *219*
Parkinsonism, 110, 115–117
Perturbation
  amplitude, 23, 188, 312, 312t
  frequency, 19, 21–22
  measurement of, 188
  normative data on, 311t, 311–312
Phonation
  breathy, 249
  easy initiation of, 249–250
  on inhalation, 257
  neurologic diseases affecting, 107–149
  organic diseases affecting, 151–164
  ventricular, 8, 264
Phonation time, 24–25
  measurement of, 199–200
  normative data on, 313–314, 314t
Phonational range, 21
  measurement of, 185, *186*
  normative data on, 311t, 312
  reduced, 14
    differential diagnosis of, 40–41
    signs of, 41t
Phonatory apraxia, 31
Phonatory physiology, 5–6, 285–295
  glottal tone initiation, 285–287, *286*
    Bernoulli effect, 286–287
    collapsible tube analogy, 287
    conditions required for, 285–286
  mechanisms of loudness change, 290–292, *292*
  mechanisms of quality variation, 292–293, *293–294*
  mechanisms of vocal frequency change, 287–290
    vocal fold length and, 287–288, *289*
    vocal fold mass and, 288, *289*
    vocal fold tension and, 288–290, *290*
Phonosurgery, 212–231. *See also* Surgical procedures
Photoglottography, 191–192

Phrenic nerve damage, 42
Pitch, 15–16
    alteration of, 198–199
    easy production of falsetto, 253
    inappropriate, 14, 15–16, 76–79
        lack of pitch variability, 79
        persistent glottal fry, 78–79
        puberphonia, 77–78
    measurement of, 77
    monopitch, 15
    optimum, 76–77, 265–267
        definition of, 265
        methods for determination of, 265–266
        studies of, 266
    scaling of, 202–203
    subjective perceptions of, 266–267
Pitch breaks, 14, 16
    differential diagnosis of, 43–44
    signs of, 44t
"Placing the voice," 199
Plethysmography, 195, *195*
PM Pitch Analyzer, 184, 187, 188
Polyps, 94–96, *95*
    histopathology of, 60–62, *63*
    surgery for, 213, *213–214*
    voice therapy for, 241
    vs. nodules, 91–92
Posterior cricoarytenoid muscle, 51, 278, 279t
Pregnancy, 246
Pressure technique, 252–253
Preventive techniques, 268–269
    primary vs. secondary, 268–269
    smoking cessation, 268
    training to avoid abusive behaviors, 268–269
    voice training for singers, 269
Propranolol, 90
Pseudobulbar palsy, 112–115
Psychiatric testing, 206–208
Psychogenic voice disorder, 42, 80–81, 206–208
Psychotherapy, 7
Puberphonia, 44, 77–78
Pulling technique, 254
Pulse register, 78–79
Pushing technique, 254
Pyriform sinuses, 30

Quality, 17–18
    breathiness, 14, 17
    descriptions of, 196–197, 292
    determinants of, 292–293
    diplophonia, 18
    hoarseness/roughness, 14, 17
    mechanisms of variation of, 292–293, *293–294*
    strain/struggle behavior, 14, 17–18
    sudden interruption of voicing, 18
    tension, 17
    tremor, 14, 17
    variations of, 4

Radiology, 7
Recurrent laryngeal nerve, 304, 306t
    anesthesia of, 45–46
    section of, 229–230
Referral form, 319
Reinke's edema, 62, *63*, 97–98, *98*
    surgery for, 214, *215*

Reinke's space, 55
Relaxation techniques, 256–257
Respiration
    analysis of, 193–195
        air volumes and capacities, 193–195
        respiratory movements, 195, *195*
    breathing therapy, 255–256, *258*
    normative data on, 314–316
        air pressure, 315t, 316
        average flow rates, 314–315, 314t–315t
        vibratory airflow, 315t, 316
    observation of, 198
Rise time, 24
Rolandic area, 297

s/z ratio, 24–25
    in adults, 200
    in children, 200–201
    measurement of, 200–201
    normative data on, 313, 313t
Scaling, 201–202
    interval scale, 202
    multidimensional, 202
    ordinal scale, 201–202
    of pitch, 202–203
    ratio scale, 202
    visual analog scale, 202
    of vocal effort, 203–205, *204*, 261
Schmidt's syndrome, 137t
"Screamer's nodes," 84
Screaming, 84
Shimmer. *See* Amplitude perturbation
Shy-Drager syndrome, 110, 117–119
Sigh, 249–250
Signs of voice problems, 49t–50t
    acoustic, 18–25, 19t
        amplitude, 22–23
        frequency breaks, 25
        fundamental frequency, 19–22
        normal acoustics, 25
        phonation time, 24–25
        spectral noise, 23–24
        tremor, 24
        vocal rise or fall time, 24
        voice stoppages, 25
    interrelationships of, 31
    laryngoscopic, 29t, 29–31
        anteroposterior laryngeal dimensions, 30
        involuntary laryngeal activity, 31
        malformations/anomalies, 30
        normal-appearing larynx, 31
        phonatory apraxia, 31
        pyriform changes, 30
        tissue changes, 29
        ventricular folds, 30
        vertical laryngeal position, 30
        vocal fold approximation, 29
        vocal fold lengthening, 30
        vocal fold movement, 29
    perceptual, 15–18, 16t
        loudness, 16–17
        nonphonatory perceptions, 18
        pitch, 15–16
        quality, 17–18
    physiological, 26t, 26–27
        aerodynamics, 26

muscle activity, 27
vibratory characteristics, 27
stroboscopic, 27–29, 28t
amplitude of vocal fold movement, 28
glottic closure, 28
mucosal wave, 28
periodicity of vocal folds, 29
phase closure of vocal folds, 28
phase symmetry of vocal folds, 29
vertical level of vocal folds, 28
vibratory behavior, 28
Singing, 2
coaches for, 7
training for, 269
vertical laryngeal height in, 75
vocal demands of, 173
Smoking, 90, 232, 268
Sound pressure level, 22, *22*. *See also* Vocal
intensity
Spastic dysphonia, 45, 127–133
acoustic signs of, 129–131
fundamental frequency, 129–130
spectrum, 130–131, *131–132*
vocal intensity, 130
adductor vs. abductor types of, 129
description of, 127–129
etiology of, 128–129
laryngoscopic signs of, 132–133
nomenclature of, 129
other neurological signs in, 133
pathophysiology of, 133
perceptual signs and symptoms of, 129, *130*
physiological signs of, 131–132
primary voice symptom of, 127
recurrent laryngeal nerve section for, 229–230
stroboscopic signs of, 133
voice therapy for, 244
Spectrograms, 188–189, *189*
Speech
evolution of, 1–2
role of nervous system in, 109–110
Spirometry, 194
Sternohyoid muscle, 272, *273*, 274t
Sternothyroid muscle, 272, *273*, 274t
Steroid inhalants, 88
Stimulant drugs, 86
Strain/struggle voice, 14, 17–18
differential diagnosis of, 45–46
signs of, 46t
Stridor, 18, 197
Stroboscopic evaluation, 27–29, 28t, 180–182,
181
form for, 327
Stylohyoid muscle, 272, *273*, 274t
Subglottal cavity, 282
Subglottal stenosis, 30
Sulcus vocalis, *101*, 101–102
histopathology of, 64–65, *66*
intrafold injection for, 222
Superior laryngeal nerve, 304, 306t
Suprabulbar palsy, 112–115. *See also*
Pseudobulbar palsy
Supraglottal cavity, 282
Suprasegmentals, 197
Surgical procedures, 212–231
anterior commissure advancement, 228, *228*

for anterior glottal web, 231
for benign neoplasms, 217, *219*
concept of phonosurgery, 212–213
cricothyroid approximation, 227, *227*
for epidermoid cyst, 214–215, *216*
for epithelial hyperplasia and dysplasia, 216–
217, *218*
for glottal carcinoma, 217–218, *220*
laryngeal reconstruction, 230–231
neuromuscular surgery for vocal fold
paralysis, 228–229
for nonspecific granuloma, 215–216, *217*
recurrent laryngeal nerve section for
spasmodic dysphonia, 229–230
for Reinke's edema, 214, *215*
vocal fold lateralization, 226
vocal fold medialization, 218–226
for vocal fold polyp, 213, *213–214*
for vocal fold slackening, 228
for vocal fold tensing, 227–228
Sydenham's chorea, 122. *See also* Huntington's
chorea
Symptoms of voice problems, 13–14, 14t
definition of, 12–13
vs. signs, 13
SynchroVoice, 191

Talbot's law, 180
Talking
from diaphragm, 263–264
excessive, 79
reducing amount of, 259
Tape recorders, 205–206
Tapia's syndrome, 138t
Telephone contact form, 318
Tension, 17, 74
fundamental frequency and, 288–290, *290*
Thalamus, 298, *301–302*
Thermal injuries, 158–161
Throat clearing
excessive, 18, 83–84
voice therapy for, 241
therapeutic, 254–255
Thyroarytenoid muscle, 51, 279t, 280
Thyroepiglottic muscle, 52
Thyrohyoid muscle, 272, *273*, 274t
Thyroid cartilage, 51, 275, *276–277*
medial shift of, 223–225, *224–225*
Tobacco exposure, 90, 232, 268
Transsexual voice, 245
Trauma, 158–161, *159*
blunt or penetrating, 158
inhalation and thermal, 158–161
Tremor, 14, 17, 24, *25*
differential diagnosis of, 47
essential, 134–136
signs of, 48t

Ultra-high-speed photography, 182–183, *183*
Ultrasound, 183
"Um-hum" technique, 255

Vagus nerve, 304–306, *305*, 306t
Ventricles of Morgagni, 282
Ventricular folds, 30, 282, *283*
histology of, 52, *53*

Ventricular phonation, 80, 264
Vernet's syndrome, 138t
Vibration, 27
Videofluoroscopy, 182
Villarets syndrome, 138t
Virilization, 246
Visi-Pitch, 184, 187, 188
Vocal effort scaling, 203–205, *204*, 261
Vocal fatigue, 14
　differential diagnosis of, 36–38
　signs of, 37t
Vocal fold lateralization, 226
　arytenoidectomy, 226, *227*
　laterofixation of vocal fold, 226, *226*
Vocal fold medialization, 218–226
　intrafold injection, 219–222, *220–222*
　　indications for, 219
　　injection materials for, 219
　　for sulcus vocalis, 222
　　transcutaneous, 221, *222*
　　transoral under direct laryngoscope, 220–221, *221*
　　transoral using laryngeal mirror, 219, *220*
　　for unilateral vocal fold paralysis, 221–222, *222*
　surgical techniques, 223–226
　　medial shift of thyroid cartilage, 223–225
　　rotation of arytenoid cartilage, *225*, 225–226
　　surgical augmentation, 223, *223–224*
Vocal fold paralysis, 30, 66–68, *68*, 143–148
　neuromuscular surgery for, 228–229, *229–230*
　unilateral
　　crossing of midline, 264–265
　　intrafold injection for, 219–222
　　voice therapy for, 243–244
Vocal folds
　amplitude of, 28
　anatomy of, 280–282, *281*
　approximation of, 29
　edema/inflammation of, 62, *63*, 82–83, 97–99, *98*
　　medical management of, 231–234
　false. *See* Ventricular folds
　lengthening of, 30
　movement of, 29
　mucosal wave of, 28
　nodules of, 59–60, *62*, *91*, 91–94
　paradoxical motion of, 246–247
　periodicity of, 29
　phase closure of, 28
　phase symmetry of, 29
　polyps of, 60–62, *63*, *94–95*, 94–96
　scars of, 65
　structure of
　　in adults, 55–57, *55–57*
　　development of, 58–59
　　effect of androgens on, 89
　　in elderly, 59, *60*
　　in newborns, 57–59, *58*
　tissue changes in, 29
　vertical level of, 28
　vibratory behavior of, 28
Vocal hygiene, 257–260, *259*
　manipulating environment, 260
　reducing amount of talking, 259
　reducing loudness, 259
　reducing vocal abuse, 259–260

Vocal intensity
　amplitude perturbation, 23, 188
　　normative data on, 312, 312t
　intensity range, measurement of, 186
　maximum intensity level, normative data on, 312, 313t
　maximum phonation duration, 24–25
　　measurement of, 199–200
　　normative data on, 313–314, 314t
　mean intensity level, measurement of, 186
　measurement of, 185–188, *187*
　normative data on, 312–314, 312–314t
Vocal ligament, 55
Vocal process, 57
Vocal rehabilitation, 235–270
　anatomical/physiological bases of, 236–237
　for changes in laryngeal tissue/structure, 240–242
　　combined treatment, 241
　　goals of, 241–242
　　nature of intervention, 242
　　as only therapy, 240–241
　for children, 240–241
　criteria for termination of, 261–263
　documentation of therapy, 270
　efficacy of, 248
　guidelines for, 237–239
　　feedback, 237–238
　　modeling therapy tasks, 238
　　patient education, 237
　　patient practice, 238
　　patient selection, 239
　　patient verbalization, 237
　　prognostic statement, 238–239
　　stepwise therapy, 238
　　tape recording therapy sessions, 238
　individualization of, 247
　malpractice and, 269–270
　for misuse/abuse problems, 242–243
　　goals of, 242–243
　　nature of intervention, 243
　　as only therapy, 242
　for neurological problems, 243–245
　　goals of, 244
　　nature of intervention, 244–245
　prognosis of, 239
　for special problems, 245–247
　　hypothyroidism, 245
　　menstruation/pregnancy/birth control pill use, 246
　　paradoxical vocal fold motion/laryngeal spasm, 246–247
　　transsexual voice, 245
　　virilization, 246
　techniques of, 247–261
　　breathing, 255–256, *258*
　　breathy phonation, 249
　　chant-talk, 251
　chewing, 250–251
　digital manipulation/pressure/massage, 252–253
　easy production of high-pitched sounds, 253
　energizing the voice, 260–261
　hum and nasal consonants, 251–252
　imagery, 253–254
　laughing/coughing/throat clearing/gargling/reflexive acts, 254–255

nonspecificity of, 248
phonating on inhalation, 257
pushing/pulling/isometrics, 254
relaxation, 256–257
sigh/aspirate initiation/easy initiation of
    phonation, 249–250
"um-hum," 255
vocal effort, 261
vocal hygiene, 257–260, *259*
whispering, 255
yawn/sigh, 250
Vocal tics, 197
Vocalis muscle, 55, *281*, 282
Voice
    abuse of, 81–85. *See also* Abuse of voice
    disciplines involved with, 6–8
        team approach, *9*
        traditional approach, *8*
    effect of drugs on, 85–90. *See also* Drug
        effects
    emotionality of, 2–3
    energizing of, 260–261
    larynx and, 2–3
    life changes in, 3–5

adult, 4
elderly, 5
infant and child, 3–4
misuse of, 73–81. *See also* Misuse of voice
normal, 235–236
production of, 5–6
"weak," 260
Voice box. *See* Larynx
Voice Identification instruments, 189
Voice sample recording, 205–206
    environment for, 206
    microphones for, 206
    tape recorders for, 205–206
    tasks for, 206
Voice stoppages, 25
Voiscope, 191

Wallenberg's syndrome, 137t
Whispering
    harmfulness of, 267–268
    therapeutic technique of, 255

Yawn/sigh technique, 250